MODERN EPIDEMIOLOGY

MODERN EPIDEMIOLOGY

KENNETH J. ROTHMAN

Professor, Department of Family and Community Medicine,
University of Massachusetts Medical School,
Worcester, Massachusetts

LITTLE, BROWN AND COMPANY
Boston/Toronto

Library of Congress Catalog Card No. 85-82480

ISBN 0-316-75776-4

Printed in the United States of America

DON

CONTENTS

PREFACE

The tenets of epidemiology, like those of every other science, have become established piecemeal. Some are more useful than others, and some exist in mutual conflict. In this book my aim has been to weave the diverse threads of epidemiologic concepts and research methods into a single fabric. I have tried to reconcile conflicting ideas and unify the conceptual foundation, omitting needless partitions. In particular, I have labored to tie the statistical topics of epidemiologic analysis—which have a way of generating their own special goals, momentum, and lingo—to the basic goals of epidemiologic research. I have also ventured to reconcile epidemiologic principles with the broader goals and methods of scientific inquiry, as I understand them. In sewing the final cloth, I have been mindful that I cannot succeed fully, but rather must fail in my attempts to varying degrees. Intent readers will surely find holes in the fabric and an incorrect stitch here and there. Some of these irregularities undoubtedly reflect inadequate understanding or communication on my part. Some mark conceptual areas, such as confounding and interaction between causes, where development is progressing rapidly. I hope that such problems are few, and small enough not to impair the overall usefulness of the work.

Throughout this book I have strived to make the material accessible to a novice to the field. Whenever possible the descriptions are verbal rather than mathematical, despite the quantitative objectives of research. The first eight chapters deal with fundamental issues of epidemiologic conceptualization, measurement, and study design, and should be comprehensible even to those who lack previous training in epidemiology or statistics; the second eight chapters address the somewhat more technical issues of epidemiologic data analysis, but even these topics are presented with step by step explanations and simplicity as a central objective.

Chapters 1 through 5 form an introductory unit on basic epidemiologic concepts and tools. Chapter 1 places epidemiology in its historical perspective. Chapter 2 ventures into the philosophic foundation for epidemiology, providing a model for causal action that serves as a platform for understanding etiology and its quantitative description. Chapters 3 through 5 continue with the fundamental measures of epidemiology (incidence, prevalence, and risk) and the measures derived from them to quantify causal actions.

Chapters 6 through 8 form a second unit that deals with epidemiologic studies. The basic types of studies are presented in Chapter 6, where I have pursued steadfastly the objective of a unified approach, stressing the theoretical connections among study types. Chapters 7 and 8 explore the issues of study design without resorting to mathematical notation. They emphasize the sources of error in effect estimates as well as the quantitative nature of most aspects of study design.

Chapters 9 through 16 deal with data analysis. In this section some reliance on mathematical formulations has been unavoidable, and I have assumed a basic knowledge of the relevant statistical distributions. Nevertheless, the fundamental statistical principles are introduced and explained in Chapters 9 and 10 using as little notation as possible. Chapter 11 introduces the basic analytic formulations for crude data, which are extended in Chapters 12 and 13 for stratified and matched data. Chapters 11 through 13 cover the routine analytic tasks that an epidemiologist faces; consequently, these are the most technical chapters in the book. Various approaches are described in detail, so that these chapters can be used as a reference for researchers, as well as an instructional guide to the fundamental analytic methods.

The final three chapters turn to more advanced analytic topics, but the emphasis is not so much on formulas as on analytic strategies. Thus, Chapter 14 on multivariate analysis is probably the least technical description of multivariate analysis in any textbook; it provides practical guidance on choosing, constructing, and interpreting multivariate models. Chapters 15 and 16 deal with the advanced topics of interaction and "dose-response" evaluation, but the emphasis once again is on the principles and pitfalls of such analyses, rather than on the technical aspects of the requisite calculations. I could not avoid formulas entirely and still provide an adequate discussion of these topics, but the formulas presented illustrate approaches of conceptual simplicity amenable to a pencil-and-paper solution.

In my efforts to tie together epidemiologic concepts for all these topics, I have encountered some fossilized divisions that I consider no longer useful. For example, a rift has separated the traditional area of infectious disease epidemiology from the more recent and growing area of "chronic" disease epidemiology. I have never been persuaded of any rationale for this distinction. The terms "infectious" and "chronic" are neither mutually exclusive nor collectively exhaustive alternatives. Many diseases are both infectious and chronic; some, such as fatal traumatic injury, are neither. "Chronic" has sometimes been taken to mean a long induction period, rather than a long period of manifestation, but this redefinition still fails to make a meaningful distinction between two conceptually different types of epidemiology. Although some specialized methods have been developed solely to study the spread of infectious illness, whatever distinctions exist between traditional and modern areas of epidemiology are certainly less important than the broad base of concepts that are shared. This book does not deal with models for epidemic spread, but focuses on the general epidemiologic concepts that apply to all diseases, infectious or not, chronic or not, and to causes that have short or long induction periods.

Another distinction that has been used to categorize epidemiologic work is its classification into descriptive and analytic epidemiology. My view is that this demarcation is also best forgotten. It has been used in reference both to specific study variables (so-called "descriptive" variables being distinguished from putative causes) and to entire studies, but in neither context does it hold as a sensible classification scheme. No qualitative distinction, other than a completely arbitrary one, distinguishes "descriptive" variables from more fundamental risk factors. Any disease determinant can be specified in terms of more proximal determinants or previously unsuspected confounding factors. The division of epidemiologic research into descriptive and analytic compartments has given rise to the illusion that there are different sets of research principles that apply to descriptive and analytic studies. This notion devolves from a mechanical view of scientific research, and diverges from prevailing doctrines of scientific philosophy. For example, the view that "descriptive data" from "exploratory studies" generate hypotheses, whereas the data from "analytic studies" are used to test hypotheses, does not cohere with a broader understanding of science. Hypotheses are not generated by data; they are proposed by scientists. The process by which scientists use their imagination to create hypotheses has no formal methodology and is certainly not prescriptive. Any study, whether considered exploratory or not, can serve to refute a hypothesis. It is not useful to regard some studies merely as "hypothesis generating" and others as "hypothesis testing," because the inexorable advance of scientific knowlege cannot be constrained by such rigidities.

I believe that epidemiology is much more coherent than these traditional divisions would suggest. Even the stark contrast between follow-up studies and case-control studies has been softened as understanding of the basic principles of epidemiology has progressed. In writing this book, my greatest hope is to convey to the reader the conviction that epidemiologic principles can be understood as an integrated substrate of logical ideas, rather than as a jumble of isolated and sometimes conflicting postulates.

K. J. R.

ACKNOWLEDGMENTS

Interchange of ideas is essential in scientific discourse, and the preparation of this book has been no exception. I have benefited from illuminating discussions over many years with colleagues, students, and teachers, beginning long before this project took shape.

My intent to write a book solidified in 1980. Since the inception of the New England Epidemiology Institute Summer Program in 1981, I have used successive drafts of this book for my course handout each summer. Every cohort of participants in the program has been a dedicated and enthusiastic body of critics, offering me numerous suggestions, criticisms, and corrections. I am appreciative of their unflagging encouragement and their honesty.

I showed early drafts of the book to Anders Ahlbom, who was especially helpful in finding the right perspective and level of detail. Anders continued to provide constructive suggestions and motivation during years of writing and revising; his suggestions have invariably proved to be on target. Peter Boyle also offered useful comments on the first drafts, propelling me to continue. Cristina Cann, my co-worker for nearly a decade, has tirelessly corrected draft after draft; many times I felt sure that I taxed her endless patience too heavily, especially as I gradually became preoccupied with the writing, but she never complained. Her empathy was truly a gift.

Three colleagues have been my mainstay for conceptual accuracy and clarity. Sander Greenland has brought his penetrating insight into epidemiology to bear on the final two drafts of the book, eagerly sending me mountains of constructive criticism. Sander's encyclopedic knowledge of the literature and his renowned mastery of the thorny statistical aspects of epidemiologic analysis are without equal. Stephan Lanes and Charles Poole of Epidemiology Resources Inc. have been my closest colleagues during the past two years; their comments have prompted the most sweeping revisions. Steve has elucidated the philosophic underpinnings of epidemiology for me, and educated me about the nature of causal inference in science. Charles has shown me that the conceptual basis for the study of causal interactions is a straightforward extension of the same concepts applied to single component causes, a crucial unifying concept. Both Steve and Charles have been highly influential to me in each of these areas, as well as for many other topics, including the rapidly evolving subjects of confounding and case-control studies. I was extremely fortunate to be able to prevail upon such willing and trenchant critics, whose concern for ideas and language and whose understanding of epidemiology have been invaluable.

Many other colleagues have offered important suggestions. I received feedback on an early draft from Janet Lang, and on a later draft from Elizabeth Delzell, Tricia Hartge, D'Arcy Holman, and Noel Weiss. Alec Walker contributed extensive comments and helped me to smooth several rough edges. I gleaned useful insights from reading some doctoral dissertations, especially those of Oswald Siu and Walt Willett of Harvard. I often discussed puzzling points with colleagues; in addition to those mentioned above, I am grateful to Suresh Moolgavkar and James Robins for their helpful advice.

Curtis Vouwie, Senior Medical Editor of Little, Brown and Company, has been a guiding light since I first contacted him with a rough draft of the first third of the book. His editorial encouragement through the several years' gestation of the finished work indicates that, should he ever tire of being an editor, he has a career waiting as an obstetrician.

I am also grateful to the New England Journal of Medicine for permission to use parts of my 1978 editorial, "A show of confidence," volume 299, pages 1362–1363, and to the W. B. Saunders Company for permission to use part of my chapter, "Causation and Causal Inference," from the book *Cancer Epidemiology and Prevention,* edited by Schottenfeld and Fraumeni.

MODERN EPIDEMIOLOGY

1. THE EMERGENCE OF EPIDEMIOLOGY

Among the sciences, epidemiology is an embryo. Although some excellent epidemiologic studies were conducted before the twentieth century, a systematized body of epidemiologic principles by which to design and judge such studies has begun to form only in the last two decades. These principles have evolved in tandem with an explosion of epidemiologic activity covering a wide range of health problems.

After the Second World War, the United States initiated many large-scale epidemiologic studies. A number of these studies have had far-reaching influence on the health of today's citizens. For example, the community intervention trials of fluoride supplementation in water that were started during the 1940s have led to widespread primary prevention of dental caries [Ast, 1965]. The Framingham Heart Study, initiated in 1949 to study risk factors for cardiovascular disease, is the most notable of several long-term follow-up studies of cardiovascular disease that have contributed importantly to understanding the etiology of this staggering public-health problem [Dawber et al., 1957; Kannel et al., 1961; Kannel et al., 1970; McKee et al., 1971]. This remarkable study is continuing to produce valuable findings 35 years after it was begun [Kannel et al., 1984] and has undoubtedly contributed essential knowledge that has stemmed the United States epidemic of cardiovascular mortality, which peaked in the mid 1960s [Stallones, 1980]. The largest formal human experiment ever conducted was the Salk vaccine field trial in 1954, with nearly a million school children as subjects [Francis et al., 1957]. This study provided the practical basis for the prevention of paralytic poliomyelitis.

The same era saw the first epidemiologic studies linking smoking and health, eventually leading to the landmark report *Smoking and Health,* issued by the Surgeon General in 1964 [U.S. Dept. of Health, Education and Welfare, 1964]. Since that time epidemiologic research has steadily attracted public attention. Along with a rising tide of social concern about environmental issues and health in general, epidemiologic studies on many subjects have been vaulted to prominence by the news media. Some of these studies were controversial, although the media may have been partly responsible in many cases for fueling the controversy. A few of the biggest attention-getters were studies related to

the efficacy of oral antidiabetic medication
the effect of diethylstilbestrol (DES) on offspring
clustering and infectious transmission of Hodgkin's disease
reserpine and breast cancer
Legionnaire's disease
low-level ionizing radiation and leukemia
saccharin and bladder cancer
swine flu vaccination and Guillain-Barré syndrome
hormonal drugs in pregnancy and birth defects
tampons and toxic-shock syndrome

Bendectin and birth defects
hazardous waste disposal sites
replacement estrogens and endometrial cancer
coffee drinking and pancreatic cancer
passive smoking
Agent Orange
Acquired Immune Deficiency Syndrome (AIDS)

Despite the surge of epidemiologic activity in recent years, there is still abundant evidence that, as a science, epidemiology remains in an early stage of development. In established sciences, one does not find wide disagreement and confusion about the most basic concepts or measures. Whereas physicists agree on the definition of mass or energy, epidemiologists often disagree on definitions of incidence (not to mention the definition of epidemiology itself). In 1975, a paper appeared in the *American Journal of Epidemiology* entitled "Definition of rates: some remarks on their use and misuse" [Elandt-Johnson, 1975]. No revolutionary concepts or definitions were proposed, but the paper was useful because so many readers did not know the definitions of the basic measures used in epidemiology. It is notable that all but one of the introductory texts published in the decade since Elandt-Johnson's paper appeared continue to corrupt the definitions of the basic measures that she discussed. Clear concepts of causation and related ideas such as induction period, like the definitions of basic measures, are fundamental to an understanding of epidemiologic research. Nevertheless, even these underpinnings have not yet been integrated into the conceptual bedrock of the discipline. Disagreement about basic conceptual and methodologic points has led, in some instances, to profound differences in the interpretation of data. In 1978, a controversy erupted about whether exogenous estrogens are carcinogenic to the endometrium: Several case-control studies had reported an extremely strong association, with up to a 15-fold increase in risk, but one group argued that a selection bias accounted for nearly the entire effect [Smith et al., 1975; Ziel and Finkle, 1975; Mack et al., 1976; Horwitz and Feinstein, 1978; Hutchison and Rothman, 1978; Jick et al., 1979; Greenland and Neutra, 1981]. Disagreement and confusion about basic ideas in epidemiology does not necessarily attest to the thick-headedness of epidemiologists; a more charitable interpretation would be that the basic ideas fundamental to the new science have not yet displaced the complacent languor of traditional thinking.

Why has epidemiology been so slow to blossom? The answer lies partially in the difficulty of conducting epidemiologic research. Measures of disease incidence are the basic building blocks of epidemiologic inferences. These measures involve the observation of disease occurrence in relation to the people and time spans in which they occur. This is not a simple process. Typically, disease occurs rarely in the person-time experience (see Chap. 3), so that considerable time and effort are needed to make the basic measurements. Epidemiologists also face the problem of obtaining cooperation from other people to make their observations. The investigator has no control over the "experimental" setting and usually must reckon with limitations imposed by budget and concerns for the privacy of subjects. The end product of such an excruciating and often frustrating exercise is just the first step in accumulating epidemiologic knowledge.

Such difficulties have long discouraged epidemiologic research and will continue to do so. Economies of scale resulting from these observational problems have favored epidemiologic research in settings where medical records and vital statistics are carefully collected and available for use, or where the wealth of society can support the expensive efforts needed to gather the necessary information. The logistic problems encountered in measuring disease incidence have also led to the ascendance of the case-control study as a central tool of modern epidemiology. Case-control research is in many ways emblematic of the modern synthesis of epidemiologic concepts. The methodology of case-control studies has a sound theoretical basis, and as a means of increasing measurement efficiency in epidemiology, it is an attractive option. Unfortunately, the case-control approach has often been misunderstood to be a second-rate substitute for follow-up studies. Only through a firm conceptual grounding in epidemiologic principles can the student of epidemiology see that there is no basis for this derogation of case-control research. Since this type of understanding, covering a wide range, is critical to the successful conduct and interpretation of epidemiologic research of all types, a focus on epidemiologic concepts and methods is crucial to anyone who aspires to understand modern epidemiology.

The past two decades have also seen rapid growth in the understanding and synthesis of epidemiologic concepts. The main stimulus for the growth of theory seems to have been practice: The explosion of epidemiologic activity accentuated the need to improve understanding of the theoretical underpinnings. For example, the signal studies on smoking and lung cancer in the early 1950s were scientifically noteworthy not only for their substantive findings but also because they demonstrated the efficacy and great efficiency of the case-control study [Wynder and Graham, 1950; Doll and Hill, 1952]. Likewise, analysis of data from the Framingham Heart Study stimulated the development of the most popular multivariate methodology used today, multiple logistic regression analysis [Cornfield, 1962; Truett et al., 1967].

The fundamental concepts of epidemiology depend little on other scientific disciplines, nor do they depend on empirical results. Thus, the capacity to formulate a theory of epidemiologic concepts has been possible for centuries; that it is a twentieth century phenomenon is independent of any recent scientific and technical breakthroughs. Rather, the economic development of the prosperous nations in the twentieth century afforded the luxury of conducting epidemiologic research, which in turn motivated the conceptual development that is the scientific "emergence" of epidemiology.

Until recently, virtually all epidemiologists were physicians. Their interest in epidemiology was typically focused on the occurrence patterns of a particular disease. Perhaps because these researchers subordinated an interest in epidemiologic principles to their substantive goals in understanding disease etiology, there was no movement to pursue the development of a theory of epidemiologic investigation. Many epidemiologic investigations, now best forgotten, were designed and conducted poorly for want of such a theory.

Historically, physicians have collaborated fruitfully with statisticians, who contributed expertise in making observations on large populations as well as in data analysis. Much of the theoretical development of modern epidemiology was contributed by statisticians—Cornfield, Mantel, Cox, Breslow, and Prentice are a few of the outstanding contributors. The influence of statistical thinking in epidemiology has not been wholly positive, however. It was natural for statisticians, bringing their skills to bear on epidemiologic problems, to borrow methods with which they were familiar in other areas of application. These methods often became incorporated into epidemiologic practice, not always with a sound basis in theory.

One example of the negative influence of statistical thinking in epidemiologic practice is the dominance of statistical hypothesis testing in epidemiologic data analysis. The motivation for the development of statistical hypothesis testing was to provide a basis for decision making in agricultural and quality-control experiments. These experiments were designed to answer questions that called for specific actions, so that the results had to be classified, if possible, into qualitatively discrete categories. Thus arose the practice of declaring associations in data as "statistically significant" or "nonsignificant," using arbitrary criteria that became conventional. The notion of statistical significance has come to pervade epidemiologic thinking as well as that of other disciplines. Unfortunately, statistical hypothesis testing is a mode of analysis that offers less insight into epidemiologic data than alternative methods that emphasize estimation of interpretable measures.

Another example of the misapplication of statistics in epidemiology has been in the area of multivariate analysis. Statistical methodology in multivariate modeling has often been transferred wholesale to epidemiology without giving sufficient thought to the underlying epidemiologic concepts. Many practices common in multivariate analysis are often inappropriate in an epidemiologic context: The use of continuous independent variates, product terms to evaluate interactions, stepwise algorithms to determine the model, and variance reduction to evaluate the model are all potentially problematic. Multivariate analysis is an important analytic tool for the epidemiologist, but it cannot be used appropriately without first considering the epidemiologic principles that govern its use. Today, notwithstanding the important contributions to the field by many who consider themselves first as statisticians or physicians, epidemiologists have achieved a separate identity. Being either a physician or a statistician or even both simultaneously is not sufficient qualification for being an epidemiologist. What is sufficient is a theoretical understanding of the principles of epidemiologic research and the experience to apply them.

Epidemiology has established a toehold as a scientific discipline. Whereas epidemiologic results were once greeted mainly with skepticism, they are now generally accorded some degree of respect. At midcentury, epidemiologists had trouble persuading the scientific community of a relation between smoking and lung cancer. By 1984, the situation had changed so much that a weak epidemiologic association observed between beta-carotene and cancer occurrence was the stimulus for a biochemical hypothesis on anti-oxidants, which was published in *Science*. The paper begins with the observation that

[E]pidemiological studies indicate that the incidence of cancer may be slightly lower among individuals with an above-average intake of beta-carotene and other carotenoids [Burton and Ingold, 1984].

The respectability evinced by this integration of epidemiology into the fold of the biologic sciences stems in large part from the emergence of a clearer understanding of the epidemiologic concepts that have become the basis of modern epidemiology.

REFERENCES

Ast, D. B. Dental public health. In P. E. Sartwell (ed.), *Preventive Medicine and Public Health* (9th ed.). New York: Meredith, 1965.

Burton, G. W., and Ingold, K. U. Beta-carotene: An unusual type of lipid antioxidant. *Science* 1984; 224:569–573.

Cornfield, J. Joint dependence of the risk of coronary heart disease on serum cholesterol and systolic blood pressure: A discriminant function analysis. *Fed. Proc.* 1962; 21:58–61.

Dawber, T. R., Moore, F. E., and Mann, G. V. II. Coronary heart disease in the Framingham study. *Am. J. Public Health* 1957; 47:4–24.

Doll, R., and Hill, A. B. A study of the aetiology of carcinoma of the lung. *Br. Med. J.* 1952; 2:1271–1286.

Elandt-Johnson, R. C. Definition of rates: some remarks on their use and misuse. *Am. J. Epidemiol.* 1975; 102:267–271.

Francis, T., Napier, J. A., Voight, B. S., et al. Evaluation of the 1954 Field Trial of Poliomyelitis Vaccine. Final Report. Ann Arbor: Poliomyelitis Vaccine Evaluation Center, University of Michigan, 1957.

Greenland, S., and Neutra, R. An analysis of detection bias and proposed corrections in the study of estrogens and endometrial cancer. *J. Chron. Dis.* 1981; 34:433–438.

Horwitz, R. I., and Feinstein, A. R. Alternative analytic methods for case-control studies of estrogens and endometrial cancer. *N. Engl. J. Med.* 1978; 299:1089–1094.

Hutchison, G. B., and Rothman, K. J. Correcting a bias? *N. Engl. J. Med.* 1978; 299:1129–1130.

Jick, H., Watkins, R. N., Hunter, J. R., et al. Replacement estrogens and endometrial cancer. *N. Engl. J. Med.* 1979; 300:218–222.

Kannel, W. B., Dawber, T. R., Kagan, A., et al. Factors of risk in the development of coronary heart disease—six year follow-up experience: The Framingham study. *Ann. Intern. Med.* 1961; 55:33–50.

Kannel, W. B., Wolf, P. A., Verter, J., et al. Epidemiologic assessment of the role of blood pressure in stroke: The Framingham study. *J.A.M.A.* 1970; 214:301–310.

Kannel, W. B., and Abbott, R. D. Incidence and prognosis of unrecognized myocardial infarction. An update on the Framingham study. *N. Engl. J. Med.* 1984; 311:1144–1147.

Mack, T. M., Pike, M. C., Henderson, B. E., et al. Estrogens and endometrial cancer in a retirement community. *N. Engl. J. Med.* 1976; 294:1262–1267.

McKee, P. A., Castelli, W. P., McNamara, P. M., et al. The natural history of congestive heart failure: The Framingham study. *N. Engl. J. Med.* 1971; 285:1441–1446.

Smith, D. C., Prentice, R., Thompson, D. J., et al. Association of exogenous estrogen and endometrial carcinoma. *N. Engl. J. Med.* 1975; 293:1164–1167.

Stallones, R. A. The rise and fall of ischemic heart disease. *Sci. American* 1980; 243:(5)53–59.

Truett, J., Cornfield, J., and Kannel, W. A multivariate analysis of the risk of coronary heart disease in Framingham. *J. Chron. Dis.* 1967; 20:511–524.

U.S. Department of Health, Education and Welfare. Smoking and Health: Report of the Advisory Committee to the Surgeon General of the Public Health Service. Public Health Service Publication No. 1103. Washington, D.C. Government Printing Office, 1964.

Wynder, E. L., and Graham, E. A. Tobacco smoking as a possible etiologic factor in bronchogenic carcinoma. A study of six hundred and eighty-four proved cases. *J.A.M.A.* 1950; 143:329–336.

Ziel, H. K., and Finkle, W. D. Increased risk of endometrial carcinoma among users of conjugated estrogens. *N. Engl. J. Med.* 1975; 293:1167–1170.

2. CAUSAL INFERENCE IN EPIDEMIOLOGY

In *The Magic Years,* Selma Fraiberg [1959] characterizes every toddler as a scientist, busily fulfilling an earnest mission to develop a logical structure for the strange objects and events that make up the world that he or she inhabits. None of us is born with any concept of causal connections. As a youngster, each person develops an inventory of causal explanations that brings meaning to the events that are perceived and ultimately leads to increasing power to control those events. Parents can attest to the delight that children take in forming causal hypotheses and then meticulously testing them, often through exasperating repetitions that are motivated mainly by the joy of scientific confirmation. At a certain age, a child will, upon entering a new room, search for a wall switch to operate the electric lighting, and upon finding one that does, repeatedly switch it on and off merely to confirm the discovery beyond any reasonable doubt. Experiments such as those designed to test the effect of gravity on free-falling liquids are usually conducted with careful attention, varying the initial conditions in subtle ways and reducing extraneous influences whenever possible by conducting the experiments safely removed from parental interference. The fruit of these scientific labors is the essential system of causal beliefs that enables each of us to navigate our complex world.

Although the method of proposing and testing causal theories is mastered intuitively by every youngster, the inferential process involved has been the subject of philosophic debate throughout the history of scientific philosophy. It is worthwhile to consider briefly the history of ideas describing the inductive process that characterizes causal inference, to understand better the modern view and its implications for epidemiology.

PHILOSOPHY OF SCIENTIFIC INFERENCE

The dominant scientific philosophy from the birth of historic scientific inquiry until the beginning of the scientific revolution was the doctrine of *rationalism.* According to this doctrine, scientific knowledge accumulated through reason and intuition rather than by empirical observation. In ancient Greece, the only prominent empirical science was astronomy. Nevertheless, even the observation of the heavens was belittled by Plato, who considered celestial observations an unreliable source of knowledge compared with reason [Reichenbach, 1951]. The highest form of knowledge was considered to be mathematics, a system of knowledge built upon a framework of axioms by deductive logic. The geometry of Euclid exemplifies the rationalist ideal.

Skeptics of rationalism who believed that perceptions of natural phenomena are the source and ultimate judge of knowledge developed a competing doctrine known as *empiricism.* The great pioneers of modern empiricism were Francis Bacon, John Locke, and David Hume. Bacon saw that earlier empiricists, though they exalted empirical science, overemphasized observation to the extent that logic played little role in the accumulation of knowledge. Bacon likened the rationalists to spiders, spinning cobwebs out of their own substance, and the older empiricists to ants, collecting material without being able to find an order in it. He envisioned a new empiricist that he likened to a bee, collecting material, digesting it, and adding to it from its own substance, thus creating a product of higher quality. According to Bacon, reason introduces abstract relations of order to observational knowledge. Bacon is famous for saying "knowledge is power," by which he meant that abstract relations imply prediction. Thus, "fire is hot" is not merely descriptive of fire but also predictive of the nature of fires not yet observed. Prediction is obtainable by a process known as *inductive inference* or *inductive logic*. Unlike deductive logic, inductive logic is not self-contained and therefore is open to error. On the other hand, deductive logic, being self-contained, cannot alone establish a theory of prediction, since it has no connection to the natural world.

Bacon formalized the process of inductive inference, demonstrating how deductive logic could never be predictive without the fruits of inductive inference. John Locke popularized the inductive methods that Bacon formalized and helped establish empiricism as the prevailing doctrine of scientific philosophy. Hume was the critic: He pointed out that inductive inference does not carry a "logical necessity," by which he meant that induction did not carry the logical force of a deductive argument. He also demonstrated that it is a circular argument to claim that inductive logic is a valid process even without a logical necessity simply because it seems to work well: No amount of experience with inductive logic could be used to justify logically its validity. Hume thus made it clear that inductive logic cannot establish a fundamental connection between cause and effect. No number of repetitions of a particular sequence of events, such as turning a light on by pushing a switch, can establish a causal connection between the action of the switch and the turning on of the light. No matter how many times the light comes on after the switch has been pressed, the possibility of coincidental occurrence cannot be ruled out. This incompleteness in inductive logic became known as "Hume's problem."

Various philosophers have tried to provide answers to Hume's problem. The school of logical positivism that emerged from the Vienna Circle of philosophers incorporated the symbolic logic of Russell and Whitehead's *Principia Mathematica* into its analysis of the verification of scientific propositions. The tenet of this philosophy was that the meaningfulness of a proposition hinged on the empirical verifiability of the proposition according to logical principles. This view was inadequate as a philosophy of science, however, because, as Hume had indicated, no amount of empirical evidence can verify conclusively the type of universal proposition that is a scientific law [Popper, 1965]. Hume's problem remained unanswered by this approach.

Confronting the hopelessness of conclusive verification, some philosophers of science adopted a graduated system of verifiability, embodied by the logic of probabilities proposed by Rudolph Carnap. Under this philosophy, scientific propositions are evaluated on a probability scale. Upon empirical testing, hypotheses become more or less probable depending on the outcome of the test. The description by Heisenberg of the "uncertainty principle" and the acceptance of quantum mechanics by physicists early in the twentieth century fostered this probabilistic view of scientific confirmation. Philosophers, influenced strongly by contemporary physicists, abandoned the search for causality:

The picture of scientific method drafted by modern philosophy is very different from traditional conceptions. Gone is the ideal of the scientist who knows the absolute truth. The happenings of nature are like rolling dice rather than like revolving stars; they are controlled by probability laws, not by causality, and the scientist resembles a gambler more than a prophet [Reichenbach, 1951].

The notion of verifiability by probabilistic logic did not take root. The inadequacy of this philosophy was revealed by Karl Popper, who demonstrated that statements of probabilistic confirmation, being neither axioms nor observations, are themselves scientific statements requiring probability judgments [Popper, 1965]. The resulting "infinite regress" did not resolve Hume's criticism of the inductive process.

Popper proposed a more persuasive solution to Hume's problem. Popper accepted Hume's point that induction based on confirmation of a cause-effect relation, or confirmation of a hypothesis, never occurs. Furthermore, he asserted that knowledge accumulates only by falsification. According to this view, hypotheses about the empirical world are never proved by inductive logic (in fact, empirical hypotheses can never be "proved" at all in the sense that something is proved in deductive logic or in mathematics), but they can be disproved, that is, falsified. The testing of hypotheses occurs by attempting to falsify them. The strategy involves forming the hypothesis by intuition and conjecture, using deductive logic to infer predictions from the hypothesis, and comparing observations with the deduced predictions. Hypotheses that have been tested and not falsified are confirmed only in the sense that they remain reasonably good explanations of natural phenomena until they are falsified and replaced by other hypotheses that better explain the observations. The empirical content of a hypothesis, according to Popper, is measured by how falsifiable the hypothesis is. The hypothesis "God is one" has no empirical content because it cannot be falsified by any observations. Hypotheses that make many prohibitions about what can happen are more falsifiable and therefore have more empirical content, whereas hypotheses that make few prohibitions have little empirical content. Lack of empirical content, however, is not equivalent to lack of validity: A statement without empirical content relates to a realm outside of empirical science.

Popper also rejected the abandonment of causality. He argued forcefully that an indeterminist philosophy of science could have only negative consequences for the growth of knowledge, and that Heisenberg's "uncertainty principle" did not place strict limits on scientific discovery. For Popper, belief in causality was compatible with uncertainty, since scientific propositions are not proved: They are only tentative explanations, to be replaced eventually by better ones when observations falsify them. It is worth noting that at least one prominent physicist, like Popper, did not relinquish a belief in causality:

> . . . I should not want to be forced into abandoning strict causality without defending it more strongly than I have so far. I find the idea quite intolerable that an electron exposed to radiation should choose *of its own free will,* not only its moment to jump off, but also its direction. In that case, I would rather be a cobbler, or even an employee in a gaming house, than a physicist [Einstein, 1924].

Recent developments in theoretical physics seem to promise vindication of Einstein's faith in causality [Waldrop, 1985].

Popper's philosophy of science has many adherents, but recent scientific philosophers temper the strict falsificationism that he proposed. Brown [1977] cites three fundamental objections to the Popperian view: (1) refutation is not a certain process, since it depends on observations, which can be erroneous; (2) deduction may provide predictions from hypotheses, but no logical structure exists by which to compare predictions with observations; and (3) the infrastructure of the scientific laws in which new hypotheses are imbedded is itself falsifiable, so that the process of refutation amounts only to a *choice* between refuting the hypothesis or refuting the infrastructure from which the predictions emerge. The last point is the essential view of the post-Popperian philosophers, who argue that the acceptance or rejection of a scientific hypothesis comes through consensus of the scientific community [Brown, 1977] and that the prevailing scientific viewpoint, which Kuhn [1962] has referred to as "normal science," occasionally undergoes major shifts that amount to scientific revolutions. These revolutions signal a decision of the scientific community to discard the infrastructure rather than to falsify a new hypothesis that cannot be easily grafted onto it.

A GENERAL MODEL OF CAUSATION

Philosophers of science have clarified the understanding of the process of causal inference, but there remains the need, at least in epidemiology, to formulate a general and coherent model of causation to facilitate the conceptualization of epidemiologic problems. Without such a model, epidemiologic concepts such as causal interactions, induction time, and the proportion of disease attributable to specific causes would have no ontologic foundation.

We can define a cause of a disease as an event, condition, or character-istic that plays an essential role in producing an occurrence of the disease. Causality is a relative concept that can be understood only in relation to conceivable alternatives. Smoking one pack of cigarettes daily for 10 years may be thought of as a cause of lung cancer, since that amount of smoking may play an essential role in the occurrence of some cases of lung cancer. But this construction postulates some lesser degree of smoking, such as nonsmoking, as the alternative. Smoking only one pack of cigarettes daily for 10 years is a preventive of lung cancer if the alternative is to smoke 2 packs daily for the same period, because some cases of lung cancer that would have occurred from smoking 2 packs daily will not occur. Analo-gously, we cannot consider that taking oral contraceptives is a cause of death (by causing fatal cardiovascular disease) unless we know what the alternative is; if the alternative is childbirth, a life-threatening event, taking oral contraceptives may prevent death. Thus, causation and prevention are relative terms that should be viewed as two sides of the same coin.

Concept of Sufficient Cause and Component Causes

Concepts of cause and effect are established early in life. The child who repeatedly drops a toy and watches it fall or tips a glass and observes the milk spilling is applying his own method of reasoning to causal proposi-tions and in so doing is working out his own concept of causation. A char-acteristic of such early concepts is the assumption of a one-to-one corre-spondence between the observed cause and effect in the sense that each such cause is seen as necessary and sufficient in itself to produce the effect. Thus, the flick of a light switch makes the lights go on. The unseen causes that also operate to produce the effect are unappreciated: the need for an unspent bulb in the light fixture, wiring from the switch to the bulb, and voltage to produce a current when the circuit is closed. To achieve the effect of turning on the light, each of these is equally as important as mov-ing the switch because absence of any of these components of the causal constellation will prevent the effect. For many people, the roots of early causal thinking persist and become manifest in attempts to find single causes as explanations for observed phenomena. But experience and re-flection should easily persuade us that the cause of any effect must consist of a constellation of components that act in concert [Mill, 1862]. A "suffi-cient cause" may be defined as a set of minimal conditions and events that inevitably produce disease; "minimal" implies that none of the conditions or events is superfluous. In disease etiology, the completion of a sufficient cause may be considered equivalent to the onset of disease. For biologic effects, most and sometimes all of the components of a sufficient cause are unknown [Rothman, 1976].

For example, smoking is a cause of lung cancer, but by itself it is not a sufficient cause. First, the term *smoking* is too imprecise to be used in a causal description. One must specify the type of smoke, whether it is filtered or unfiltered, the manner and frequency of inhalation, and the duration of smoking. More important, smoking, even defined explicitly, will not cause cancer in everyone. So who are those who are "susceptible" to the effects of smoking, or, to put it in other terms, what are the other components of the causal constellation that act with smoking to produce lung cancer? When causal components remain unknown, there is an inclination to assign an equal risk to all individuals whose causal status for some components is known and identical. Thus, heavy cigarette smokers are said to have approximately a 10 percent lifetime risk of developing lung cancer. There is a tendency to think that all of us are subject to a 10 percent probability of lung cancer if we were to become heavy smokers, as if the outcome, aside from smoking, were purely a matter of chance. It is more constructive, however, to view the assignment of equal risks as reflecting nothing more than our ignorance about the determinants of lung cancer that interact with cigarette smoke. It is likely that some of us could engage in chain smoking for many decades without the slightest possibility of developing lung cancer. Others are or will become "primed" by presently unknown circumstances and need only to add cigarette smoke to the nearly sufficient constellation of causes to initiate lung cancer. In our ignorance of these hidden causal components, the best we can do in assessing risk is to assign the average value to everyone exposed to a given pattern of known causal risk indicators. As knowledge expands, the risk estimates assigned to people will approach one of the extreme values, zero or unity.

Each constellation of component causes represented in Figure 2-1 is minimally sufficient (i.e., there are no redundant or extraneous component causes) to produce the disease. Component causes may play a role in one, two or all three causal mechanisms.

Strength of Causes

Figure 2-1 does not depict aspects of the causal process such as sequence of action, dose, and other complexities. These aspects of the causal process can be accommodated by the model by an appropriate definition of each causal component. The model and diagram do facilitate an understanding of some important epidemiologic concepts. Imagine, for example, that in Sufficient Cause I, A, B, C, and D all are factors commonly present or experienced by people. Suppose E were rare. Although all factors are causes, E would appear to be a stronger determinant of disease because those with E differ greatly in risk from those without E. The other, more common component causes result in smaller differences in risk between those with and those without the causes because the rarity of E keeps the risks from all the other factors low. Thus, the apparent strength of a cause is determined by the relative prevalence of component causes. A rare factor becomes a strong cause if its complementary causes are common. It should

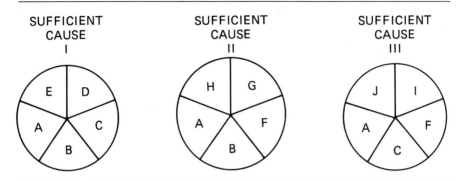

Fig. 2-1. Conceptual schematization of three sufficient causes for a disease [Rothman, 1976].

be apparent that, although it may have tremendous public health significance, the strength of a cause has little biologic significance in that the same causal mechanism is compatible with *any* of the component causes being strong or weak. The identity of the constituent components of the cause is the biology of causation, whereas the strength of a cause is a relative phenomenon that depends on the time- and place-specific distribution of component causes in a population.

Interaction Among Causes

Two component causes in a single sufficient cause are considered to have a mutual biologic interaction. The degree of observable interaction depends on the actual mechanisms responsible for disease. For example, in Figure 2-1, if G were a hypothetical substance that had not been created, no disease would occur from Sufficient Cause II; as a consequence, factors B and F are biologically independent. Now suppose that the prevalence of C is reduced because it is replaced by G or something that produced G. In this case the disease that occurs comes from Sufficient Cause II rather than from I or III, and as a consequence, B and F interact biologically. Thus, the extent of biologic interaction between two factors is in principle dependent on the relative prevalence of other factors.

Proportion of Disease Due to Specific Causes

In Figure 2-1, assuming that the three sufficient causes are the only ones operating, what proportion of disease is caused by A? The answer is all of it; without A, there is no disease. A is considered a "necessary cause." What proportion is due to B? B causes disease through two mechanisms, I and II, and all disease arising through either of these two mechanisms is due to B. This is not to say, of course, that all disease is due to A alone, or that a proportion of disease is due to B alone; no component cause acts alone.

It is understood that these factors interact with others in producing disease.

Recently it was proposed that as much as 40 percent of cancer is caused by occupational exposures. Many scientists argued against this claim [Higginson, 1980; Ephron, 1984]. One of the arguments used in rebuttal was as follows: x percent of cancer is caused by smoking, y percent by diet, z percent by alcohol, and so on; when all these percentages are added up, only a few percent are left for occupational causes. This argument is based on a naive view of cause and effect, which neglects interactions. There is, in fact, no upper limit to the sum that was being constructed; the total of the proportion of disease attributable to various causes is not 100 percent but infinity. Similarly, much publicity attended the pronouncement that 90 percent of cancer is environmentally caused [Higginson, 1960]; by extension of the previous argument, however, it is easy to show that 100 percent of any disease is environmentally caused, and 100 percent is inherited as well. Any other view is based on a naive understanding of causation.

Induction Period

The diagram of causes also gives us a model for conceptualizing the *induction period*, which may be defined as the period of time from causal action until disease initiation. If, in Sufficient Cause I, the sequence of action of the causes is A, B, C, D, and E, and we are studying the effect of B, which, let us assume, acts at a point in time, we do not observe the occurrence of disease immediately after B acts. Disease occurs only after the sequence is completed, so there will be a delay while C, D, and finally E act. When E acts, disease occurs. The interval between the action of B and the disease occurrence is the induction time for the effect of B. A clear example of a lengthy induction time is the cause-effect relation between exposure of a female fetus to diethylstilbestrol (DES) and the subsequent development of clear cell carcinoma of the vagina. The cancer occurs generally between the ages of 15 and 30. Since exposure occurs before birth, there is an induction time of 15 to 30 years. During this time, other causes presumably are operating; some evidence suggests that hormonal action during adolescence may be part of the mechanism [Rothman, 1981].

It is incorrect to characterize a disease as having a lengthy or brief induction time. The induction time can be conceptualized only in relation to a specific component cause. For each component cause, the induction time differs, and for the component cause that acts last, the induction time equals zero. If a component cause during adolescence that leads to clear cell carcinoma of the vagina among young women exposed to DES were identified, it would have a much shorter induction time for its carcinogenic action than DES. Thus, induction time characterizes a cause-effect pair rather than just the effect.

In carcinogenesis, the terms *initiator* and *promotor* have been used to refer to early-acting and late-acting component causes. Cancer has often been characterized as a disease process with a long induction time, but this is a misconception because any late-acting component in the causal process, such as a promotor, will have a short induction time, and the induction time must always be zero for at least one component cause, the last to act. (Disease, once initiated, will not necessarily be apparent. The time interval between disease occurrence and detection has been termed the *latent* period [Rothman, 1981], although others have used this term interchangeably with induction period. The latent period can be reduced by improved methods of disease detection.)

Empirical Content of the Model

According to Popper, the empirical content of a hypothesis or theory derives from the prohibitions that it makes on what can be observed. The model of causation proposed here makes numerous prohibitions about causal processes. It prohibits causes from occurring after effects. It states that unicausal effects are impossible if the setting of the effect of a specific component cause is interpreted to be part of the causal constellation. It prohibits a constant induction time for a disease in relation to its various component causes. The main utility of a model such as this lies in its ability to provide a conceptual framework for causal problems. The attempt to determine the proportion of disease attributable to various component causes is an example of a fallacy that is exposed by the model. As we shall see in Chapter 15, the evaluation of interactions is greatly clarified with the help of the model.

How does the model accommodate varying doses of a component cause? Since the model appears to deal qualitatively with the action of component causes, it might seem that dose variability cannot be taken into account. But this view is overly pessimistic. To account for dose variability, one need only to postulate a set of sufficient causes, each of which contains as a component a different dose of the agent in question. Small doses might require a larger set of complementary causes to complete a sufficient cause than large doses [Rothman, 1976]. It is not necessary to postulate an infinite set of sufficient causes to accommodate a spectrum of doses but only enough to accommodate the number of different mechanisms by which the different dose levels might bring about the disease. In this way the model could account for the phenomenon of a shorter induction period accompanying larger doses of exposure because there would be a smaller set of complementary components needed to complete the sufficient cause.

Stochastic thinkers might object to the intricacy of this deterministic model. A stochastic model could be invoked to describe a dose-response relation, for example, without a multitude of different mechanisms. A stochastic model would also accommodate the role of chance, which is apparently omitted from the causal model described above. Nevertheless, the deterministic model presented here does accommodate "chance," but it does so by reinterpreting chance in terms of deterministic action beyond the current limits of knowledge or observability. Thus, the outcome of a flip of a coin is usually considered a chance event, but theoretically the outcome can be determined completely by the application of physical laws and a sufficient description of the starting conditions. At first, it might seem that a deterministic model is more constricting than a stochastic one, since the deterministic model excludes random processes from causal mechanisms. One might argue, however, that just the reverse is true: Stochastic models accept the role of random events, and in doing so limit the scientific explanations that can be applied, since there will be no attempt to explain the random event. As noted above, Popper [1965] argued forcefully against accepting any indeterminist metaphysics for this reason, asserting that even Heisenberg's uncertainty principle and quantum theory should not and did not offer barriers to determinist explanations. Indeed, it now appears that even quantum theory may have a deterministic explanation [Waldrop, 1985]. Popper advised that ". . . we should abstain from issuing prohibitions that draw limits to the possibilities of research." Accepting random events as components of causal mechanisms does precisely that, whereas a determinist model can accommodate chance as ignorance of unidentified components—ignorance that is susceptible to elucidation as knowledge expands.

CAUSAL INFERENCE IN EPIDEMIOLOGY

Let us consider epidemiologic hypotheses in light of Popper's criterion for empirical content, which is equated with the prohibitions placed on what might occur. On this score, many epidemiologic propositions might seem to have little empirical content. For example, consider the proposition that cigarette smoking causes cardiovascular disease. What prohibitions does this statement make to give it content? It is clear that not all cigarette smokers will get cardiovascular disease and equally clear that some nonsmokers will develop cardiovascular disease. Therefore, the proposition cannot prohibit cardiovascular disease among nonsmokers or its absence among smokers. The proposition could be taken to mean that cigarette smokers, on the average, will develop more cardiovascular disease than nonsmokers. Does this statement prohibit finding the same rate of cardiovascular disease among smokers and nonsmokers, presuming that biases such as confounding and misclassification are inoperant? Not quite, since the effect of cigarette smoke could depend on a component cause that might be absent from the compared groups. One might suppose that at least the prohibition of a smaller rate of cardiovascular disease among smokers would be implied by the proposition. If one accepts, however, that a given factor could be both a cause and a preventive in different circumstances, even this prohibition cannot be attached to the statement.

With no prohibitions at all, the proposition would be devoid of meaning. The meaning must be derived from assumptions or observations about the complementary component causes as well as a more elaborate description of the causal agent, smoking, and the outcome, cardiovascular disease. This elaboration is, in part, the equivalent of a more detailed description of the characteristics of individuals susceptible to the cardiovascular effects of cigarette smoke.

Biologic knowledge about epidemiologic hypotheses is often scant, making the hypotheses themselves at times little more than vague statements of association between exposure and disease. These have few deducible consequences that can be falsified, apart from a simple iteration of the observation. How does one test the hypothesis that DES exposure of female fetuses in utero causes adenocarcinoma of the vagina, or that cigarette smoking causes cardiovascular disease? Not all epidemiologic hypotheses, of course, are simplistic. For example, the hypothesis that tampons cause toxic shock syndrome by acting as a culture medium for staphylococci leads to testable deductions about the frequency of changing tampons as well as the size and absorbency of the tampon. Even vague statements of association can be transformed into hypotheses with considerable content by rephrasing them as *null hypotheses*. For example, the statement "smoking is not a cause of lung cancer" is a highly specific, universally applicable statement that prohibits the existence of sufficient causes containing smoking in any form as a component. Any evidence indicating the existence of such sufficient causes would falsify the hypothesis. Popper's criterion for empirical content thus lends a scientific basis to the concept of the null hypothesis, which has often been viewed merely as a statistical crutch.

Despite philosophic injunctions concerning inductive inference, criteria have commonly been used to make such inferences. The justification offered has been that the exigencies of public health problems demand action and that despite imperfect knowledge causal inferences must be made. A commonly used set of standards has been advanced by Hill [1965]. The popularity of these standards as criteria for causal inference makes it worthwhile to examine them in detail.

Hill suggested that the following aspects of an association be considered in attempting to distinguish causal from noncausal associations: (1) strength, (2) consistency, (3) specificity, (4) temporality, (5) biologic gradient, (6) plausibility, (7) coherence, (8) experimental evidence, and (9) analogy.

1. Strength. By "strength of association," Hill means the magnitude of the ratio of incidence rates. Hill's argument is essentially that strong associations are more likely to be causal than weak associations because if they were due to confounding or some other bias, the biasing association would have to be even stronger and would therefore presumably be evident. Weak associations, on the other hand, are more likely to be explained

by undetected biases. Nevertheless, the fact that an association is weak does not rule out a causal connection. It has already been pointed out that the strength of an association is not a biologically consistent feature but rather a characteristic that depends on the relative prevalence of other causes.

2. Consistency. Consistency refers to the repeated observation of an association in different populations under different circumstances. Lack of consistency, however, does not rule out a causal association because some effects are produced by their causes only under unusual circumstances. More precisely, the effect of a causal agent cannot occur unless the complementary component causes act, or have already acted, to complete a sufficient cause. These conditions will not always be met. Furthermore, studies can be expected to differ in their results because they differ in their methodologies.

3. Specificity. The criterion of specificity requires that a cause lead to a single effect, not multiple effects. This argument has often been advanced, especially by those seeking to exonerate smoking as a cause of lung cancer. Causes of a given effect, however, cannot be expected to be without other effects on any logical grounds. In fact, everyday experience teaches us repeatedly that single events may have many effects. Hill's discussion of this standard for inference is replete with reservations, but even so, the criterion seems useless and misleading.

4. Temporality. Temporality refers to the necessity that the cause precede the effect in time.

5. Biologic Gradient. Biologic gradient refers to the presence of a dose-response curve. If the response is taken as an epidemiologic measure of effect, measured as a function of comparative disease incidence, then this condition will ordinarily be met. Some causal associations, however, show no apparent trend of effect with dose; an example is the association between DES and adenocarcinoma of the vagina. A possible explanation is that the doses of DES that were administered were all sufficiently great to produce the maximum effect, but actual development of disease depends on other component causes. Associations that do show a dose-response trend are not necessarily causal; confounding can result in such a trend between a noncausal risk factor and disease if the confounding factor itself demonstrates a biologic gradient in its relation with disease.

6. Plausibility. Plausibility refers to the biologic plausibility of the hypothesis, an important concern but one that may be difficult to judge. Sartwell [1960], emphasizing this point, cited the remarks of Cheever, in 1861, who

was commenting on the etiology of typhus before its mode of transmission was known:

> It could be no more ridiculous for the stranger who passed the night in the steerage of an emigrant ship to ascribe the typhus, which he there contracted, to the vermin with which bodies of the sick might be infested. An adequate cause, one reasonable in itself, must correct the coincidences of simple experience.

7. Coherence. Taken from the Surgeon General's report on Smoking and Health [1964], the term *coherence* implies that a cause and effect interpretation for an association does not conflict with what is known of the natural history and biology of the disease. The examples Hill gives for coherence, such as the histopathologic effect of smoking on bronchial epithelium (in reference to the association between smoking and lung cancer) or the difference in lung cancer incidence by sex, could reasonably be considered examples of plausibility as well as coherence; the distinction appears to be a fine one. Hill emphasizes that the absence of coherent information, as distinguished, apparently, from the presence of conflicting information, should not be taken as evidence against an association being considered causal.

8. Experimental Evidence. Such evidence is seldom available for human populations.

9. Analogy. The insight derived from analogy seems to be handicapped by the inventive imagination of scientists who can find analogies everywhere. Nevertheless, the simple analogies that Hill offers—if one drug can cause birth defects, perhaps another one can also—could conceivably enhance the credibility that an association is causal.

As is evident, these nine aspects of epidemiologic evidence offered by Hill to judge whether an association is causal are saddled with reservations and exceptions; some may be wrong *(specificity)* or occasionally irrelevant *(experimental evidence* and perhaps *analogy)*. Hill admitted that

> None of my nine viewpoints can bring indisputable evidence for or against the cause-and-effect hypothesis and none can be required as a sine qua non.

In describing the inadequacy of these standards, Hill goes too far. The fourth standard, the temporality of an association, is a sine qua non: If the "cause" does not precede the effect, that indeed is indisputable evidence that the association is not causal. Other than this one condition, which is part of the concept of causation, there are no reliable criteria for determining whether an association is causal.

In fairness to Hill, it must be emphasized that he clearly did not intend that these "viewpoints" be used as criteria for inference; indeed, he stated that he did not believe that any "hard-and-fast rules" could be posed for causal inference. If these viewpoints are used by some as a checklist for inference, we should recall that they were not proposed as such. Indeed, it is dubious that the inferential process can be enhanced by the rote consideration of checklist criteria [Lanes and Poole, 1984]. We know from Hume, Popper, and others that causal inference is at best tentative and is still a subjective process.

The failure of some researchers to recognize the theoretical impossibility of "proving" the causal nature of an association has led to fruitless debates pitting skeptics who await such proof against scientists who are persuaded to make an inference on the basis of existing evidence. The responsibility of scientists for making causal judgments was Hill's final emphasis in his discussion of causation:

All scientific work is incomplete—whether it be observational or experimental. All scientific work is liable to be upset or modified by advancing knowledge. That does not confer upon us a freedom to ignore the knowledge we already have, or to postpone the action that it appears to demand at a given time.

Recently, Lanes [1985] has proposed that causal inference is not part of science at all, but lies strictly in the domain of public policy. According to this view, since all scientific theories could be wrong, policy makers should weigh the consequences of actions under various theories. Scientists should inform policy makers about scientific theories, and leave the choice of a theory and an action to policy makers. Not many public health scientists are inclined toward such a strict separation between science and policy, but as a working philosophy it has the advantage of not putting scientists in the awkward position of being advocates for a particular theory [Rothman and Poole, 1985]. Indeed, history shows that skepticism is preferable in science.

REFERENCES

Brown, H. I. *Perception, Theory and Commitment. The New Philosophy of Science.* Chicago: University of Chicago Press, 1977.

Einstein, A. Letter to Max Born, 1924. Cited in A. P. French (ed.), *Einstein. A Centenary Volume.* Cambridge, Mass.: Harvard University Press, 1979.

Ephron, E. *The Apocalyptics. Cancer and the Big Lie.* New York: Simon and Schuster, 1984.

Fraiberg, S. *The Magic Years.* New York: Scribner's, 1959.

Higginson, J. Population studies in cancer. *Acta Unio. Internat. Contra Cancrum* 1960; 16:1667–1670.

Higginson, J. Proportion of cancer due to occupation. *Prev. Med.* 1980; 9:180–188.

Hill, A. B. The environment and disease: Association or causation? *Proc. R. Soc. Med.* 1965; 58:295–300.

Kuhn, T. S. *The Structure of Scientific Revolutions* (2nd ed.). Chicago: University of Chicago Press, 1962.

Lanes, S. Causal inference is not a matter of science. *Am. J. Epidemiol.* 1985; 122:550.

Lanes, S. F., and Poole, C. "Truth in packaging?" The unwrapping of epidemiologic research. *J. Occup. Med.* 1984; 26:571–574.

Mill, J. S. *A System of Logic, Ratiocinative and Inductive* (5th ed.). London: Parker, Son and Bowin, 1862. Cited in D. W. Clark and B. MacMahon (eds.), *Preventive and Community Medicine* (2nd ed.). Boston: Little, Brown, 1981. Chap. 2.

Popper, K. R. *The Logic of Scientific Discovery.* New York: Harper & Row, 1965.

Reichenbach, H. *The Rise of Scientific Philosophy.* Berkeley: University of California Press, 1951.

Rothman, K. J. Causes. *Am. J. Epidemiol.* 1976; 104:587–592.

Rothman, K. J. Causes and risks. In M. A. Clark (ed.), *Pulmonary Disease: Defense Mechanisms and Populations at Risk.* Lexington, Ky.: Tobacco and Health Research Institute, 1977.

Rothman, K. J. Induction and latent periods. *Am. J. Epidemiol.* 1981; 114:253–259.

Rothman, K. J. Causation and causal inference. In D. Schottenfeld and J. F. Fraumeni (eds.), *Cancer Epidemiology and Prevention.* Philadelphia: Saunders, 1982.

Rothman, K. J. and Poole, C. Science and policy making. *Am. J. Public Health* 1985; 75:340–341.

Sartwell, P. On the methodology of investigations of etiologic factors in chronic diseases—further comments. *J. Chron. Dis.* 1960; 11:61–63.

U.S. Department of Health, Education and Welfare. Smoking and Health: Report of the Advisory Committee to the Surgeon General of the Public Health Service. Public Health Service Publication No. 1103, Washington, D.C.: Government Printing Office, 1964.

Waldrop, M. M. String as a theory of everything. *Science* 1985; 229:1251–1253.

3. MEASURES OF DISEASE FREQUENCY

The clearest of many definitions of epidemiology that has been proposed has been attributed to Gaylord Anderson [Cole, 1979]. His definition is

Epidemiology: the study of the occurrence of illness

Other sciences are also directed toward the study of illness, but in epidemiology the focus is on the *occurrence* of illness. As a branch of science, epidemiology deals with the evaluation of scientific hypotheses. These hypotheses are often posed as qualitative propositions. The "null" form of such propositions is highly refutable and, as discussed in the previous chapter, derives its empirical content from this characteristic. Unlike the framing of hypotheses, scientific research, which comprises the activity of attempted refutation of hypotheses, is predicated on measurement. Qualitatively stated hypotheses about evolution, the formation of the earth, the effect of gravity on light waves, or the method by which birds find their way during migration are all tested by measurements of the phenomena that relate to the hypotheses. The physicist Kelvin aptly stated the importance of measurement in science [cited in Beiser, 1960]:

I often say that when you can measure what you are speaking about, and express it in numbers, you know something about it; but when you cannot express it in numbers, your knowledge is of a meagre and unsatisfactory kind; it may be the beginning of knowledge, but you have scarcely, in your thoughts, advanced to the stage of Science, whatever the matter may be.

From Hippocrates to Sydenham, physicians have considered the causes of disease, but it was only when measurement of the occurrence of disease replaced reflection about causation that scientific knowledge about causation made impressive strides. The fundamental task in epidemiologic research is thus to quantify the occurrence of illness. The goal is to evaluate hypotheses about the causation of illness and its sequelae and to relate disease occurrence to characteristics of people and their environment.

There are three basic measures of disease frequency. *Incidence rate* is a measure of the instantaneous force of disease occurrence. *Cumulative incidence* measures the proportion of people who convert, during a specified period of time, from nondiseased to diseased. *Prevalence* measures the proportion of people who have disease at a specific instant. These measures and their interrelation will be described in detail.

INCIDENCE

In attempting to measure the frequency of disease occurrence in a population, it is insufficient merely to record the number of people or the proportion of the population that is affected. It is also necessary to take into account the time elapsed before disease occurs. To understand this, con-

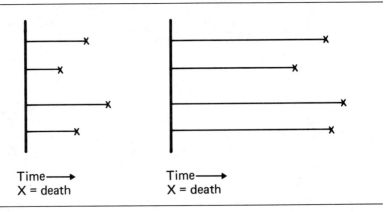

Fig. 3-1. *Two different patterns of disease occurrence.*

sider the frequency of a disease that ultimately affects all people, namely, death. Since all people are eventually affected, the time from birth to death becomes the determining factor in measuring the occurrence of death. Time differentiates between the two situations shown in Figure 3-1.

Thus, an incidence measure must take into account the number of individuals in a population that becomes ill and the time periods experienced by members of the population during which these events occur. *Incidence rate* is therefore defined as the number of disease onsets in the population divided by the sum of the time periods of observation for all individuals in the population:

$$\text{Incidence rate} = \frac{\text{no. disease onsets}}{\Sigma \text{ time periods}}$$

where Σ indicates the sum of time periods for all individuals.

For many epidemiologic applications, the possibility of a person getting a disease more than once is ruled out by either convention or biology. If the disease is rhinitis, we may simply wish to measure the incidence of "first" occurrence, even though disease can occur repeatedly; for cancer, heart disease, and many other illnesses, first occurrence is often of greater interest for study than subsequent occurrences in the same individual. For an outcome such as death or a disease such as diabetes, which is considered not to recur but to be a permanent state once diagnosed, only first occurrence can be studied. When the events tallied are first occurrences of disease, then the observation period for each individual who develops the disease terminates with the onset of disease.

Because incidence rate is a quotient with a frequency in the numerator and a measure of time in the denominator, its dimensionality is time^{-1}, that is, the reciprocal of time. The denominator of the rate can also be

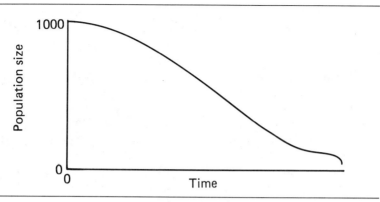

Fig. 3-2. Size of a fixed population of 1,000 people, by time.

considered a product of population size by the average time period of observation for a member of the population, although this product is, like any product, only a shorthand description of the appropriate summation. The denominator of the incidence rate is often referred to as a measure of "person-time" to distinguish the time summation from ordinary clock time. The person-time measure forms the observational experience in which disease onsets can be observed. Implicit in the measure is the concept that a given amount of person-time, say 100 person-years, can be derived from observing a variety of populations in a variety of circumstances. That is, the observations of 100 persons for 1 year, 50 persons for 2 years, 200 persons for 6 months, or one person for 100 years are assumed to be equivalent. One unit of person-time is assumed to be equivalent to and independent of another unit of person-time. This assumption, although generally a reasonable one, could be unwarranted in extreme situations—for example, observing one individual for 100 years to obtain 100 person-years. Usually the units of person-time are restricted by age, which eliminates extreme departures from independence of the person-time units. One could not obtain 100 person-years of experience in the age range 50 to 54 years with fewer than 20 individuals.

Conceptually we can imagine the person-time experience of two distinct types of populations, the *fixed population* and the *dynamic population.* A fixed population adds no new members, whereas a dynamic population does. Suppose we are measuring the *mortality rate,* defined as the incidence rate of death, in a fixed population of 1,000 people. After a period of sufficient time, the original 1,000 will have dwindled to zero. A graph of the size of the population with time might look like that in Figure 3-2.

The curve slopes downward because the 1,000 individuals eventually all die. The population is fixed in the sense that we consider the fate of only the 1,000 individuals initially identified. The person-time experience of these 1,000 individuals is represented by the area under the downward-sloping curve in the diagram. As each individual dies, the curve notches downward; that individual no longer contributes to the person-time observation pool of the fixed population. Each individual's contribution is exactly equal to the length of time that individual is followed from start to finish; in this example, since the entire population is followed until death, the finish is the individual's death. In other instances, the contribution to the person-time experience would continue until the onset of disease or some arbitrary cutoff time for observation, whichever came sooner.

Suppose we added up the total person-time experience of this fixed population of 1,000 and obtained a total of 75,000 person-years. The mortality rate would be $(1,000/75,000)\text{year}^{-1}$ since the 75,000 person-years represent the experience of all 1,000 people until their deaths. A fixed population facing a constant death rate would decline exponentially in size, but in practice "exponential decay" virtually never occurs. Because a fixed population ages steadily during the observation period, the death or disease rate in a fixed population generally changes with time because of the change in age. *Life-table* methodology is a procedure by which the mortality (or morbidity) of a fixed population is evaluated within successive small time intervals so that the time dependence of mortality can be elucidated.

A dynamic population differs from a fixed population in that we do not restrict the observations to any fixed group. Instead, we extend the observations to those entering the population as observation time proceeds. People enter a population in various ways. Some are born into it; others migrate into it. For a population of people of a specific age, individuals also enter the population by aging into it. Similarly, individuals can exit from the person-time observational experience by dying, aging out of a defined age group, emigrating, and becoming diseased, if only first bouts of a disease are being studied. If the number of people entering a population is exactly balanced by the number exiting the population in any period of time, the population is said to be in a *steady state*. Steady state is a property that applies only to dynamic populations, not to fixed populations.

The graph of the size of a dynamic population in steady state is simply a horizontal line. People are continually entering and leaving the person-time experience in a way that might be diagrammed as shown in Figure 3-3.

In the diagram, the symbol $>$ represents an individual entering the person-time experience, a line segment represents that individual's contribution to the person-time experience, the termination of a line segment indicates removal from the person-time experience, and X indicates removal from the person-time experience because of disease onset. In theory, if the incidence rate is constant during time, any portion of the population-time experience of a dynamic population in a steady state will

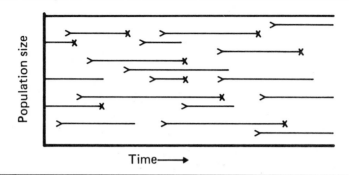

Fig. 3-3. Size of a dynamic population, by time, with an indication of population turnover.

provide a good estimate of disease incidence, The value of incidence will be the ratio of the number of cases of disease onset, indicated by X, to the two-dimensional (population × time) area. Because this ratio is equivalent to the density of disease onsets in the observational area, the incidence rate has also been referred to as *incidence density* [Miettinen, 1976]. Another synonym for the measure is *force of morbidity* (or *force of mortality* in reference to deaths).

The numerical range for incidence rate is zero to infinity, corresponding to the range of densities of points in two-dimensional space. How can disease incidence be infinite? Infinity is the theoretical upper limit for a disease that is universal and strikes quickly. If a population in a space colony were suddenly all exposed without protective gear to the environment of space, the incidence rate of death would be extremely high, though not quite at infinity, because death would not be instantaneous. The limiting value of infinity is approached only at the instant of some sudden holocaust. To some it may be surprising that an incidence rate can exceed the value of 1.0, which would seem to indicate that more than 100 percent of a population is affected. It is true that at most only 100 percent of a population can get a disease, but the incidence rate does not measure the proportion of a population with illness. The measure is not a proportion—recall that incidence rate is measured in units of the reciprocal of time. Among 100 people, no more than 100 deaths can occur, but those 100 deaths can occur in 10,000 person-years, in 1,000 person-years, in 100 person-years, or even in 1 person-year (if the 100 deaths occur after an average of 3.65 days each). An incidence rate of 100 cases (or deaths) per 1 person-year might be expressed as

$$100 \; \frac{\text{cases}}{\text{person-year}}$$

It might also be expressed as

$$10{,}000 \; \frac{\text{cases}}{\text{person-century}} \quad \text{or}$$

$$8.33 \; \frac{\text{cases}}{\text{person-month}} \quad \text{or}$$

$$1.92 \; \frac{\text{cases}}{\text{person-week}} \quad \text{or}$$

$$0.27 \; \frac{\text{cases}}{\text{person-day}}$$

The numerical value of an incidence rate in itself has no interpretability because it depends on the arbitrary selection of the time unit. It is essential in presenting incidence rates to give the appropriate time units, either as the examples given above or as in 8.33 month^{-1} or 1.92 week^{-1}. In epidemiologic writing, the units are often given only implicitly rather than explicitly, as in "an annual incidence of 50 per 100,000." The latter quantity is equivalent to

$$\frac{50}{100{,}000} \; \frac{\text{cases}}{\text{person-years}} \quad \text{or} \quad 5 \times 10^{-4} \; \text{year}^{-1}$$

It is preferable, however, not to use an expression such as "annual incidence of"; this description is analogous to describing a velocity of 60 miles/hr as "an hourly velocity of 60 miles." Aside from being clumsy, it makes an inappropriate implication about time, as if the measure applied to the entire stated interval of time when in fact it does not. A velocity of 60 miles/hr does not apply to an hour of time; one need not travel at the velocity for an hour nor spend an hour to measure it. The velocity of 60 miles/hr is an instantaneous concept: One can readily conceive of traveling at that velocity at a specific instant in time. Whether the velocity is expressed as 60 miles/hr or 88 feet/sec or 0.57 astronomical units/century makes no difference; the same speed is indicated, and the units of time used to express it have no bearing on the instantaneous nature of the measure. The same principle applies to incidence rate [Elandt-Johnson, 1975]. Like velocity, it is always an instantaneous concept, even with units of person-years or person-centuries. Thus, there is nothing annual about an "annual incidence," and it would be preferable not to use such terminology.

The dimensionality of incidence rate, that is, the reciprocal of time, makes it an awkward measure to absorb intuitively. The measure does, however, have an interpretation. Referring back to Figure 3-2, one can see that the area under the curve is equal to N(T), where N is the number of people in the fixed population and T is the average time until death. This is equivalent to saying that the area under the curve is equal to the area of a rectangle with height N and width T. Since T is the average time until death for N people, the total person-time experience is N(T). The time-averaged mortality rate at complete follow-up, then, is $N/[N(T)] = 1/T$; that is, the mortality rate equals the reciprocal of the average time until death, or, more generally, incidence rate equals the reciprocal of the average time until disease onset [Morrison, 1979]. Thus, a mortality rate of 0.04 yr^{-1} indicates an average time until death of 25 years. If the outcome is not death but either disease onset or death only from a specific cause, the interpretation above must be modified slightly. The time period at issue is then the average time until disease onset, assuming that a person is not at risk of other causes of death. That is, the measure is a time conditional on no other *competing risks* of death. This interpretation of incidence rates as the inverse of the average "waiting time" will not be valid unless the incidence rate can be used to describe a population in steady state or a fixed population with complete follow-up. For example, the mortality rate for the United States in 1977 was 0.0088 year^{-1}, suggesting a mean lifespan, or expectation of life, of 114 years. Other analyses indicate that the actual expectation of life in 1977 was 73 years. The discrepancy is due to the lack of a steady state.

CUMULATIVE INCIDENCE — *measure of average risk*

Despite the interpretation that can be given to incidence rate, it is occasionally more convenient to use a more readily interpretable measure of disease occurrence. Such a measure is the *cumulative incidence,* which may be defined as the proportion of a fixed population that becomes diseased in a stated period of time. If *risk* is defined as the probability of an individual developing disease in a specified time interval, then cumulative incidence is a measure of average risk. Like any proportion, the value of cumulative incidence ranges from zero to 1 and is dimensionless. It is uninterpretable, however, without specification of the time period to which it applies. A cumulative incidence of death of 3 percent may be low if it refers to a 40-year period, whereas it would be high if it applies to a 40-day period.

It is possible to derive estimates of cumulative incidence from incidence rate. Consider a fixed population (Fig. 3-4).

At time t, $CI_t = (P_0 - P_t)/P_0$; in words, the cumulative incidence at time t equals the number of people who have exited the fixed population by time t because of disease ($P_0 - P_t$) divided by the initial number of people

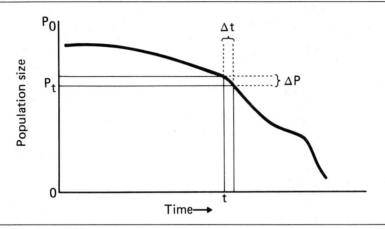

Fig. 3-4. Size of a fixed population, by time, indicating a small decrement at time t.

in the population. The incidence rate at time t is the ratio of new cases to the person-time observation experience; thus

$$I_t = \frac{-\Delta P}{P_t \Delta t}$$

or, written in terms of differential calculus,

$$I_t = \frac{-dP}{P_t dt} \qquad -I_t dt = \frac{dP}{P_t}$$

(The minus sign is used because the change in P is negative in relation to t; without the minus sign, the incidence measure would be negative.) Integrating both sides,

$$-\int_0^t I_t dt = \ln(P_t) - \ln(P_0)$$

Taking antilogs,

$$\exp\left(-\int_0^t I_t dt\right) = P_t/P_0$$

and since

$$CI_t = \frac{P_0 - P_t}{P_0}$$

we have

$$CI_t = 1 - \exp\left(-\int_0^t I_t dt\right)$$

This is estimated as

$$CI_t = 1 - \exp\left(-\sum_i I_i \Delta t_i\right)$$

where the summation of the index, i, is over categories of time covering the interval [0,t].

For a constant incidence rate,

$$CI_t = 1 - e^{-I\Delta t}$$

Because $e^x \doteq 1 + x$ for $|x|$ less than about 0.1, a good approximation for a small cumulative incidence (less than 0.1) is

$$CI_t \doteq \sum_i I_i \Delta t_i \quad \text{or} \quad CI_t \doteq I\Delta t$$

if the rate is constant with time. Thus, to estimate small risks, one can simply multiply the incidence rate by the time period. The above approximation offers another interpretation for the incidence rate; it can be viewed as the ratio of a short-term risk to the time period for the risk as the duration of the time period approaches zero.

The cumulative incidence measure is premised on the assumption that there are no competing risks of death. Thus, if an individual at age 40 faces a cumulative incidence, or risk, of 35 percent in 30 years for cardiovascular death, this is interpreted as the probability of dying from cardiovascular disease given that the individual is free from other risks of death. Because no one is actually free from competing risks, the cumulative incidence measure for any outcome other than death from all causes is a hypothetical measure. In principle, cumulative incidence for lengthy periods is unobservable and must be inferred because of the influence of competing risks.

A specific type of cumulative incidence is the *case fatality rate,* which is the cumulative incidence of death among those who develop an illness (it is therefore technically not a rate but a proportion). The time period for measuring the case fatality rate is often unstated, but it is always better to specify it. When unstated, presumably there is a short period of increased risk. For long periods of risk of death after disease onset, it is preferable to use the mortality rate among those with the illness rather than the case fatality rate, so that the actual time at risk for each individual can be taken into account. Because, in a steady state, the reciprocal of a rate is the average time elapsed until the event, the overall mortality rate of a disease in a population is related to the incidence rate and the mortality rate among cases as follows [Morrison, 1979]:

$$M_T = \frac{1}{T} = \frac{1}{T_1 + T_2} = \frac{1}{1/I + 1/M_c}$$

where M_T is the total population mortality rate, T is the life expectancy, T_1 is the average time until disease onset, T_2 is the average time from disease onset to death, I is the incidence rate of disease, and M_c is the mortality rate among cases.

PREVALENCE

Unlike incidence measures, which focus on events, *prevalence* focuses on disease status. Prevalence may be defined as the proportion of a population that is affected by disease at a given point in time. The term *point prevalence* is sometimes used to mean the same thing. An individual that dies from an illness is thereby removed from the group that constitutes the numerator of prevalence; consequently, mortality from an illness decreases prevalence. Diseases with large incidence rates may have low prevalences if they are soon fatal. People may also exit from the prevalence pool by recovering from disease.

Earlier it was stated that a population in steady state has an equal number of people entering and exiting during any unit of time. This concept can be extended to refer to a subpopulation of ill people, or a *prevalence pool* (i.e., the numerator of a prevalence). In a steady state, the number of people entering the prevalence pool is balanced by the number exiting from it:

Inflow (to prevalence pool) = outflow (from prevalence pool)

People enter the prevalence pool from the nondiseased population. If the total number of people in a population is N and the prevalence pool is P, then the size of the nondiseased population that "feeds" the prevalence pool is $N - P$. During any time interval, Δt, the number of people who enter the prevalence pool is

$$I\Delta t(N - P)$$

where I is the incidence rate. During the same time interval Δt, the outflow from the prevalence pool is

$$I'\Delta t P$$

where I' represents the incidence rate of exiting from the prevalence pool, that is, the number who exit divided by the person-time experience of those in the prevalence pool. Earlier we saw that the reciprocal of an incidence rate in a steady state equals the mean duration of time spent before the incident event. Therefore, the reciprocal of I' is the mean duration of illness, $\bar{D}$. Thus,

$$\text{Inflow} = I\Delta t(N - P) = \text{outflow} = (1/\bar{D})\Delta tP$$

$$I\Delta t(N - P) = (1/\bar{D})\Delta tP$$

$$P/(N - P) = I\bar{D}$$

$P/(N - P)$ is the ratio of ill to not-ill (we could call them healthy except that we mean they are not ill from a specific illness, which doesn't imply an absence of all illness) people in the population, or equivalently, the ratio of prevalence to the complement of prevalence $(1 - \text{prevalence})$. The ratio of a proportion to the quantity 1 minus the proportion is referred to as *odds*. In this case, $P/(N - P)$ is the *prevalence odds,* or odds of having a disease relative to not having the disease. Thus, the prevalence odds equals the incidence rate times the mean duration of illness. If the prevalence is small, say less than 0.1, then it follows that

$$\text{Prevalence} \doteq I\bar{D}$$

since prevalence will approximate the prevalence odds for small values of prevalence. More generally [Freeman and Hutchison, 1980],

$$\text{Prevalence} = \frac{I\bar{D}}{1 + I\bar{D}}$$

which can be obtained from the above expression for prevalence odds.

Prevalence, being a proportion, is dimensionless, with a range of zero to 1.0. The above equations are in accord with these requirements, because in each of them the incidence rate, with a dimensionality of the reciprocal of time, is multiplied by the mean duration of illness, giving a dimensionless product. Furthermore, the product has the range of zero to infinity, which corresponds to the range of prevalence odds, whereas the expression

$$\frac{I\bar{D}}{1 + I\bar{D}}$$

is always in the range zero to 1.0.

Seldom is prevalence of direct interest in etiologic applications of epidemiologic research. Since the probability of surviving with disease affects prevalence, studies of prevalence, or studies based on prevalent cases, yield associations that reflect the determinants of survival with disease just as well as the causes of disease. Better survival and therefore a higher prevalence might indeed be related to the action of preventives that somehow mitigate the disease once it occurs.

Nevertheless, for one class of diseases, namely, congenital malformations, prevalence is the measure usually employed. The proportion of babies born with some malformation is a prevalence, not an incidence rate. The incidence of malformations refers to the occurrence of the malformations among the susceptible populations of embryos. Many malformations lead to early embryonic or fetal death that is classified, if recognized, as a miscarriage rather than a birth. Thus, malformed babies at birth represent only those individuals who survived long enough with their malformations to be recorded as a birth. This is indeed a prevalence measure, the reference point in time being the moment of birth. Generally, it would be more useful and desirable to study the incidence than the prevalence of congenital malformations, but usually this is not possible. Consequently, in this area of research, prevalent rather than incident cases are studied.

Prevalence is sometimes used to measure the occurrence of nonlethal degenerative diseases with no clear moment of onset. In this and other situations, prevalence is measured simply for convenience, and inferences are made about incidence by using assumptions about the duration of illness. Of course, in epidemiologic applications outside of etiologic research, such as planning for health resources and facilities, prevalence may be a more germaine measure than incidence.

REFERENCES

Cole, P. The evolving case-control study. *J. Chron. Dis.* 1979; 32:15–27.

Beiser, A. *The World of Physics.* New York: McGraw-Hill, 1960.

Elandt-Johnson, R. C. Definition of rates: Some remarks on their use and misuse. *Am. J. Epidemiol.* 1975; 102:267–271.

Freeman, J., and Hutchison, G. B. Prevalence, incidence and duration. *Am. J. Epidemiol.* 1980; 112:707–723.

Miettinen, O. S. Estimability and estimation in case-referent studies. *Am. J. Epidemiol.* 1976; 103:226–235.

Morrison, A. S. Sequential pathogenic components of rates. *Am. J. Epidemiol.* 1979; 109:709–718.

4. MEASURES OF EFFECT

Epidemiologists use the term *effect* in two senses. In a general sense, any instance of disease may be the effect of a given cause. In a more particular and quantitative sense, an effect is the difference in disease occurrence between two groups of people who differ with respect to a causal characteristic; the characteristic is generally referred to as an *exposure*.

Absolute effects are differences in incidence rate, cumulative incidence, or prevalence. *Relative effects* involve ratios of these measures. An *attributable proportion* is the proportion of a diseased population for which the exposure is one of the component causes in the sufficient cause that caused the disease.

ABSOLUTE EFFECT

Suppose that all sufficient causes of a particular disease were divided into two sets, those that contain a specific cause and those that do not. We can summarize this situation with the following diagram (Fig. 4-1).

U and U′ represent different collections of causal factors. Note that disease can occur either with or without E, the exposure of interest. The absolute effect of exposure E corresponds biologically to the existence of sufficient causes that require E as a component. Epidemiologically, the effect of E can be assessed by measuring the incidence rate of sufficient causes that contain E. People who have the exposure can nevertheless develop the disease from a mechanism that does not include the exposure, so that it does not suffice to measure the incidence rate of disease among those exposed. The incidence rate among the exposed reflects the incidence of both sets of sufficient causes represented in the diagram. The incidence rate of sufficient causes containing E must be derived by subtraction of the incidence rate of the sufficient causes that lack E. This rate can be measured in a population that resembles the exposed population but lacks the exposure. Thus, if I_1 is the incidence rate of disease in an exposed population and I_0 is the rate in a comparable unexposed population, $I_1 - I_0$ represents the incidence rate of disease with the exposure as a component cause. The absolute effect is the difference in incidence rates between an exposed and an unexposed population.

This measure is also often referred to straightforwardly as *rate difference*. Synonyms include attributable risk [Walter, 1976], which derives from the closely related measure, *risk difference,* sometimes also used as a synonym for rate difference. Properly, however, risk difference should denote only a difference in risks or cumulative incidences rather than incidence rates. Thus, while rate difference has a range from minus infinity to plus infinity and the same dimensionality as the rate involved (time $^{-1}$ if incidence), risk difference has a range from -1 to $+1$ and is dimensionless.

The term *attributable risk* is unwarranted if no cause-effect relation exists between exposure and disease. If the exposure causes a change in

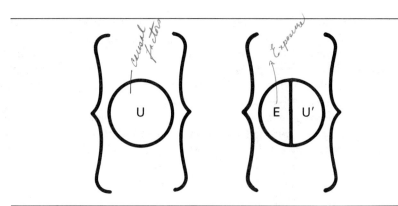

Fig. 4-1. Two types of sufficient cause of a disease.

incidence or risk, then the risk or rate difference observed may indeed be attributable to the exposure, but many scientists might reasonably object to the unnecessary causal implication inherent in the term attributable risk (or attributable rate). To the extent that a rate difference is indeed attributable to the exposure, however, the measure is a useful one for estimating the magnitude of the public health problem presented by the exposure. In this context it is noteworthy that the absolute effect is not affected by changes in the baseline incidence rate of disease.

RELATIVE EFFECT

Relative effect is based on the ratio of the absolute effect to a baseline rate. Analogous measures are used routinely whenever change or growth is measured. For example, if the investment of a sum of money has yielded a gain of $1,000 in 1 year, the absolute increase in value does not reveal how effective the investment was. If the initial investment was $5,000 and grew to $6,000 in 1 year, then we judge the investment by relating the gain, $6,000 − $5,000, to the initial amount. That is, we take the $1,000 gain and divide it by the $5,000 of the original principal, obtaining 20 percent as the relative, as opposed to the absolute, gain.

Analogously, we evaluate relative effect in epidemiology by taking the absolute effect, or rate difference, and dividing it by a reference value, which is usually the rate among the unexposed. Thus, if I_0 is the incidence rate among unexposed and I_1 is the incidence rate among exposed persons, the absolute effect is

$$I_1 - I_0$$

and the relative effect is

$$\frac{I_1 - I_0}{I_0} = \frac{I_1}{I_0} - 1 \qquad\qquad [4\text{--}1]$$

Compared with the absolute effect, the relative effect measure is often a clearer indicator of the strength of an association or, under the appropriate circumstances, causal role [Cornfield and Haenszel, 1960]. Consequently, it is the usual measure for etiologic research. The relative effect measure has two components, the ratio of incidence rates (I_1/I_0) and the constant (-1). Typically, the constant is omitted from the measure; epidemiologists usually refer only to the ratio component of the measure; it is known as the *incidence rate ratio* or *risk ratio,* which are purely descriptive terms, and also as *relative risk, relative rate,* or simply *rate ratio.* With the constant omitted from the measure, there is a translation of scale. When there is no effect, $I_1 = I_0$, and the full measure is $1 - 1 = 0$, whereas the rate ratio component of the measure is unity. It is important to remember this scale translation when interpreting rate ratio measures. For example, if one exposure has a rate ratio of 3, and a second exposure has a rate ratio of 2, the effect of the second exposure is only half as great as that of the first because the "baseline" value, that value corresponding to the absence of effect, is unity for the rate ratio measure alone.

Although epidemiologists usually use just the rate ratio measure, omitting the -1, occasionally they do not. Reference may be made, for example, to a "30 percent greater risk among exposed"; this implies that the ratio of I_1 to I_0 is 1.3, but the 30 percent comes after subtracting 1 from 1.3. Sometimes the full measure $(I_1 - I_0)/I_0$ is referred to as *excess relative risk* to distinguish it from I_1/I_0 [Cole and MacMahon, 1971].

Because relative effect involves the division of one rate by another, the measure is dimensionless. The value of relative effect ranges from -1 to plus infinity, or from 0 to infinity if the constant is omitted from the measure.

The value of risk is time-dependent. Similarly, the value of the ratio of two risks or two cumulative incidences depends on the time period over which the risks or cumulative incidences are computed. During a long period of time, risk or cumulative incidence will approach unity, and the ratio of two risks will also approach unity, no matter what the values of the underlying incidence rates are. (This is an epidemiologic manifestation of the aphorism, "In the long run, we are all dead.")

Over a short period of time, risk and cumulative incidence are approximately equal to the product of incidence rate with time, so that the ratio of two risks or two cumulative incidences is approximately equal to the ratio of the two underlying incidence rates. The approximation of the ratio of cumulative incidences to the ratio of incidence rates is better for smaller cumulative incidences, or, equivalently, shorter time intervals, approaching equality as the time interval approaches zero. Although both risk and cumulative incidence approach zero as the time interval becomes vanishingly small, the ratio of two such shrinking measures approaches the non-zero limiting value of the incidence rate ratio. These relationships can be summarized symbolically as follows:

$$CI = 1 - e^{-I\Delta t} \to 1 \quad \text{as} \quad \Delta t \to \infty$$

$$\frac{CI_1}{CI_0} \to 1 \quad \text{as} \quad \Delta t \to \infty$$

$$CI \doteq I\Delta t \to 0 \quad \text{as} \quad \Delta t \to 0$$

$$\frac{CI_1}{CI_0} \to \frac{I_1}{I_0} \quad \text{as} \quad \Delta t \to 0$$

Unlike the absolute effect, the magnitude of the relative effect depends on the magnitude of the baseline incidence rate. This dependence is one of the major difficulties in interpreting relative measures because the same absolute effect in two populations can correspond to greatly differing relative effects [Peacock, 1971]; conversely, the same relative effects for two populations could correspond to greatly differing absolute effects.

ATTRIBUTABLE PROPORTION

To obtain the relative effect, the absolute effect was divided by the rate among the unexposed, thereby measuring the absolute increment in disease occurrence in multiples of the rate of occurrence in the absence of exposure. If the absolute effect is divided by the rate of occurrence among the exposed rather than the unexposed, the result is a measure of the proportion of the disease among the exposed that is "related to" the exposure, the *attributable proportion.* This measure has also been termed the *etiologic fraction* [Miettinen, 1974] and *attributable risk percent* [Cole and MacMahon, 1971].

The attributable proportion (AP) for the exposed population is defined as

$$AP_E = \frac{I_1 - I_0}{I_1} = 1 - \frac{1}{RR} = \frac{RR - 1}{RR} \qquad [4\text{--}2]$$

where I_1 is the incidence among exposed, I_0 is the incidence among unexposed, and RR is the rate ratio, I_1/I_0. It can be interpreted as the proportion of exposed cases for whom the disease is attributable to the exposure. It conveys a sense of how much of the disease in an exposed population can be prevented by blocking the effect of the exposure or eliminating the exposure.

The proportion of all cases occurring in a mixed population of exposed and unexposed individuals that is attributable to exposure can be determined as

$$AP_T = \frac{I_T - I_0}{I_T} = \frac{P_0 I_1 + (1 - P_0)I_0 - I_0}{P_0 I_1 + (1 - P_0)I_0}$$

where I_T is the overall incidence rate in the combined population of exposed and unexposed individuals and P_0 represents the proportion of the total population that is exposed. Dividing the numerator and denominator of the above expression by $P_0 I_0$ gives

$$AP_T = \frac{RR - 1}{RR + 1/P_0 - 1}$$

Since the incidence rate ratio can be estimated by the exposure odds ratio, $P_1(1 - P_0)/[P_0(1 - P_1)]$, where P_1 is the proportion of cases that is exposed (see Chapter 6), we can also write the above expression as [Miettinen, 1974]

$$AP_T = \frac{(RR - 1)P_1}{RR} = AP_E \cdot P_1$$

If an exposure is preventive, so that $I_1 < I_0$, the absolute effect is negative and the rate ratio is less than 1.0. The attributable proportion is undefined for preventives, but an analogous measure, the *prevented fraction* (or proportion) was defined for preventives by Miettinen [1974] as

$$PF = \frac{I_0 - I_1}{I_0} = 1 - RR$$

This prevented fraction can be interpreted as the proportion of the potential cases (in the absence of exposure) that was prevented by exposure.

REFERENCES

Cole, P., and MacMahon, B. Attributable risk percent in case-control studies. *Br. J. Prev. Soc. Med.* 1971; 25:242–244.

Cornfield, J., and Haenszel, W. Some aspects of retrospective studies. *J. Chron. Dis.* 1960; 11:523–534.

Miettinen, O. S. Proportion of disease caused or prevented by a given exposure, trait or intervention. *Am. J. Epidemiol.* 1974; 99:325–332.

Peacock, P. B. The non-comparability of relative risks from different studies. *Biometrics* 1971; 27:903–907.

Walter, S. D. The estimation and interpretation of attributable risk in health research. *Biometrics* 1976; 32:829–849.

5. STANDARDIZATION OF RATES

The epidemiologic measures of effect described in the previous chapter all involve the comparison of incidence, risk, or prevalence measures. The comparison of rates using effect measures is conceptually straightforward, but in practice it is subject to a variety of distortions that should be avoided to the extent possible. The standardization of rates is an elemental and traditional method to reduce distortion in a comparison. The underlying issues will be defined and discussed in detail in subsequent chapters, but because standardization is such a basic tool for the comparison of rates, it is appropriate to introduce it now directly following measures of effect.

THE PRINCIPLE OF STANDARDIZATION

Suppose that we wish to compare the 1962 mortality in Sweden with that in Panama. Sweden, with a population of 7,496,000, had 73,555 deaths for a mortality rate of 0.0098 year^{-1}, whereas Panama, with a population of 1,075,000, had 7,871 deaths for a mortality rate of 0.0073 year^{-1}. Apparently the mortality rate in Sweden was a third greater than that in Panama. Before concluding that life in Sweden in 1962 was considerably more risky than life in Panama, we should examine the mortality rates according to age. For our purposes, the following age-specific mortality data suffice (Table 5-1).

For people under age 60, the mortality rate was greater in Panama; for people age 60 or older, it was 10 percent greater in Sweden than in Panama. The age-specific comparisons, showing less mortality in Sweden until age 60, after which mortality in the two countries is similar, presents an extremely different impression than the comparison of the overall mortality without regard to age. It is evident from the data in the table that the age distributions of Sweden and Panama are strikingly different; the mortality experience of Panamanians in 1962 was dominated by the 69 percent of them who were under age 30, whereas in Sweden only 42 percent of the population was under 30. The lower mortality rate for Panama can be accounted for by the fact that Panamanians were younger than Swedes, and younger people tend to have a lower mortality rate than older people.

When the total number of cases in a population is divided by the total person-time experience, the resulting incidence rate is described as the *crude rate*. A crude rate measures the actual experience of a population. As we saw in the above example, a comparison of crude rates can be misleading because the comparison can be distorted by differences in other factors that can affect the outcome, such as age. A comparison of the crude mortality rates in Sweden and Panama suggests that mortality is 34 percent greater in Sweden, but we know that this comparison is influenced by the fact that Swedes are older than Panamanians. *Standardization* is one way to remove the distortion introduced by the different age distributions.

The principle behind standardization is to calculate hypothetical crude

Table 5-1. Mortality in Sweden and Panama in 1962, by age

	Age		
	0–29	30–59	60+
Population			
Sweden	3,145,000	3,057,000	1,294,000
Panama	741,000	275,000	59,000
Deaths			
Sweden	3,523	10,928	59,104
Panama	3,904	1,421	2,456
Mortality rate			
Sweden	0.0011 yr^{-1}	0.0036 yr^{-1}	0.0457 yr^{-1}
Panama	0.0053 yr^{-1}	0.0052 yr^{-1}	0.0416 yr^{-1}

rates for each compared group using an identical artificial distribution for the factor to be standardized; the artificial distribution is known as the *standard*. To compare the 1962 mortality in Sweden and Panama, standardized for age, we must choose an age standard; it may be the age distribution of one of the populations to be compared (e.g., either Sweden or Panama), it may be the combined age distribution, or it can be any other age distribution that is of potential interest. Choice of the standard should generally be guided by the target of inference. For example, when comparing a single group exposed to a specific agent with an unexposed group, the distribution of the exposed group is often the most reasonable choice for a standard because the effect of interest occurs among the exposed.

The *standardized rate* is defined as a weighted average of the category-specific rates, with the weights taken from the standard distribution. Suppose we wished to standardize the mortality rates from Sweden and Panama to the following standard age distribution:

	Weight
Age	*(percent)*
0–29	0.35
30–59	0.35
60+	0.30

We would multiply each of the above weights by the mortality rate for the corresponding age category; the sum over the age categories would give the standardized rate. For Sweden, we would get

Age	Mortality Rate	Weight (percent)	Product
0–29	0.0011 yr^{-1}	0.35	0.00039 yr^{-1}
30–59	0.0036 yr^{-1}	0.35	0.00126 yr^{-1}
60+	0.0457 yr^{-1}	0.30	0.01371 yr^{-1}
			0.01536 yr^{-1}

The age-standardized mortality rate for Sweden, standardized to the age distribution above, is 0.01536 yr^{-1}. Does this mortality rate have any direct interpretability? It can be conceptualized as the overall mortality rate that Sweden would have had if the age distribution of Swedes were shifted from what it actually was in 1962 to the age distribution of the standard. Because the standard distribution is more heavily weighted toward the oldest age category than the actual population, the standardized mortality rate is greater than the crude mortality rate. The standardized rate is the hypothetical value of the crude rate if the age distribution had been that of the standard.

Standardizing the age-specific 1962 mortality rates for Panama to the same age standard gives the following result:

Age	Mortality Rate	Weight (percent)	Product
0–29	0.0053 yr^{-1}	0.35	0.00186 yr^{-1}
30–59	0.0052 yr^{-1}	0.35	0.00182 yr^{-1}
60+	0.0416 yr^{-1}	0.30	0.01248 yr^{-1}
			0.01616 yr^{-1}

A comparison of the standardized rates indicates a standardized mortality difference of 0.0008 yr^{-1} favoring the Swedes, or, to put it in relative terms, the Panamanians have a standardized mortality that is 5 percent greater (the standardized rate ratio is 1.05).

The choice of standard can affect the comparison. If the mortality data were standardized to the age distribution of Panama, the weights would be

Age	Weight (percent)
0–29	0.69
30–50	0.26
60+	0.05

.01616
.01536
———
.00080

Applying this standard, the standardized rates would be 0.0040 yr^{-1} for Sweden and 0.0073 yr^{-1} for Panama. Now the standardized rate difference is 0.0033 yr^{-1} in favor of the Swedes, or an 82 percent greater mortality for the Panamanians (the standardized rate ratio is 1.82). Unlike the previous standard, which gives nearly equal emphasis to the different age categories, the Panamanian age distribution is heavily weighted toward the youngest age category, the one in which the Swedes do considerably better than the Panamanians. This difference is reflected in the comparison of the standardized mortality rates.

Note that when the age standard is the age distribution of Panama, the standardized rate for Panama is equal to the crude rate for Panama. Like a standardized rate, the crude rate is a weighted average of the category-specific rates, with the weights equal to the age distribution of the actual population.

Let's examine this idea more closely. The formula for a standardized rate is

$$SR = \frac{\Sigma \, w_i R_i}{\Sigma \, w_i}$$

where R_i is the category-specific rate in category i, and w_i is the weight for category i, derived from the standard. Dividing by Σw_i converts any set of weights $\{w_i\}$ into a set of proportions that add to unity. If weights are chosen so that their sum is unity, as in the examples above, it is unnecessary to include Σw_i as a divisor in the formula because it would be division by unity. Each R_i has a numerator, the number of cases, and a denominator, typically an amount of person-time experience. Let us refer to the numerator of R_i as y_i and the denominator as n_i. Then the standardized rate is calculated as

$$SR = \frac{\Sigma \, w_i \cdot \dfrac{y_i}{n_i}}{\Sigma \, w_i}$$

Now suppose that we are standardizing to the actual population distribution. Thus, the standard, which is the set of weights $\{w_i\}$, is identical to the actual population distribution of person-time experience, which is the set of denominators $\{n_i\}$. If $w_i = n_i$ for all i, we can write the formula as

$$SR = \frac{\Sigma \, n_i \cdot \dfrac{y_i}{n_i}}{\Sigma \, n_i} = \frac{\Sigma \, y_i}{\Sigma \, n_i} = \text{crude rate}$$

Thus, we can confirm the validity of the earlier assertion that a standardized rate can be interpreted as the hypothetical crude rate if the population had the distribution of the standard; if the standard is the actual distribution, then the "hypothetical" crude rate is the actual crude rate.

"INDIRECT" VERSUS "DIRECT" STANDARDIZATION

The definition for standardization given in the preceding section has long been referred to as "direct" standardization to distinguish it from alternative approaches, the most popular of which has been referred to as "indirect" standardization [Wolfenden, 1923]. Whereas "direct" standardization is a process involving weighting a set of observed category-specific rates according to a standard distribution, "indirect" standardization is supposed to be a different process, in which the standard, instead of supplying the weighting distribution, supplies a standard set of rates, which are then weighted to the distribution of the population under study. This process alone cannot characterize any disease experience in the population under study because it so far involves no information on the occurrence of disease in the study population. The process is used, therefore, to generate an "expected" rate or an expected number for the crude rate or total number of cases in the population. The comparison between the study population and the standard is generally presented as a *standardized morbidity* (or mortality) *ratio* or, simply, an SMR. The hallmark of an SMR is the ratio of an "observed" number of cases to an expected number.

For convenience, let us refer to the study population as "exposed." The observed number is the total number of cases in this exposed population. The expected number is obtained by multiplying the category-specific rates of the unexposed population by the denominators in each category of the exposed population. If the exposed rate in category i is R_{1i}, with numerator y_{1i} and denominator n_{1i}, and the unexposed rate in category i is R_{0i}, with numerator y_{0i} and denominator n_{0i}, then the SMR is obtained as follows:

$$\text{SMR} = \frac{\Sigma \, y_{1i}}{\Sigma \, n_{1i} \cdot \dfrac{y_{0i}}{n_{0i}}} = \frac{\text{observed}}{\text{expected}}$$

This is equivalent to taking the ratio of the crude rate in the exposed population to the "indirectly" standardized rate or expected rate; the standardization weights the unexposed population category-specific rates by the weights from the corresponding categories of the exposed population:

$$\text{SMR} = \frac{\dfrac{\Sigma \, y_{1i}}{\Sigma \, n_{1i}}}{\dfrac{\Sigma \, n_{1i} \cdot \dfrac{y_{0i}}{n_{0i}}}{\Sigma \, n_{1i}}}$$

The above formula is identical to the previous one except that both the numerator and the denominator of the SMR have been divided by Σn_{1i}. Written in this way, the SMR is clearly seen to be the ratio of two standardized rates that have been standardized to the exposed distribution. The numerator of the SMR is the crude rate in the exposed population, and the denominator is a weighted average of the category-specific rates in the unexposed population, weighted by the distribution of the exposed population. Thus, both sets of category-specific rates, in exposed and unexposed populations, are weighted to the distribution of the exposed population.

There is nothing in this standardization process that warrants a methodologic distinction from the standardization described previously. So-called indirect standardization is, like so-called direct standardization, simply the process of taking a weighted average of category-specific rates. With an SMR, the weights for averaging the rates always derive from the exposed population, the group that gives rise to the observed cases, so the standard is always the exposed population. But only a single, unified concept exists for standardization, despite the fact that two different "methods" have been taught for the standardization process.

Unfortunately, a common misconception exists that with "indirect" standardization, the standard is the unexposed group, which provides a standard set of rates. This misconception has been the source of a common methodologic error: a comparison of SMRs that have different standards. Suppose workers in a factory are classified into two degrees of exposure to a potentially toxic agent according to the part of the plant in which they work. If mortality is evaluated using SMRs with nonexposed rates supplied from general population data, as is often done, the incorrect view of SMRs would generate the belief that the SMR for each type of exposure was standardized to the same standard, because the standard, under this misconception, is taken to be the general population that supplies the rates used to calculate the expected number for each SMR. In fact, however, although each SMR has the same unexposed group, each is standardized to a different exposed group of workers. The two SMRs actually use different standards; therefore, the SMRs are not comparable to one another and should not be compared to evaluate the relative effect of the two exposures. This is not to say that such an evaluation cannot be done; it can be done easily by using a common standard for the three sets of rates involved, the general population and the two exposed groups.

Consider an example. Suppose we have two age categories, young and old, and the rates as given in Table 5-2.

The rates for exposures 1 and 2 are identical in each age category; for young people they are 10 times the rate in the general population (unexposed), and for old people they are twice the rate in the general population.

Table 5-2. Hypothetical incidence rates, by age,
for two exposure groups and a general population

Age category	General population	Exposure 1	Exposure 2
Young			
Cases	50	50	5
Person-yrs	100000	10000	1000
Incidence	2,000 0.0005 yr^{-1}	0.005 yr^{-1}	0.005 yr^{-1}
Old			
Cases	400	4	40
Person-yrs	200000	1000	10000
Incidence	0.002 yr^{-1}	0.004 yr^{-1}	0.004 yr^{-1}

First let us standardize all the rates properly to the age distribution of the general population. For the general population itself, this gives the crude rate of 450/(300,000 person-years) = 0.0015 yr^{-1}. For exposure 1 this gives C

$$\frac{1}{3}(0.005 \text{ yr}^{-1}) + \frac{2}{3}(0.004 \text{ yr}^{-1}) = 0.0043 \text{ yr}^{-1}$$

and for exposure 2 we get the identical result because the category-specific rates are identical to those of exposure 1. The ratio of standardized rates, referred to as the *standardized rate ratio* (SRR), for exposure 1 relative to the general population is

$$\text{SRR}_1 = \frac{0.0043 \text{ yr}^{-1}}{0.0015 \text{ yr}^{-1}} = 2.87$$

and the identical result is obtained for SRR_2. With standardization to a common standard, the standardized rate ratios for this example must be equal because the category-specific rates for populations exposed to factors 1 and 2 are identical.

Now let us examine what happens when the SMRs are calculated for exposures 1 and 2. For exposure 1, the SMR is calculated as

$$\text{SMR}_1 = \frac{\text{observed}}{\text{expected}} = \frac{50 + 4}{\dfrac{50}{100,000}(10,000) + \dfrac{400}{200,000}(1,000)}$$

$$= \frac{54}{5 + 2} = \frac{54}{7} = 7.71$$

For exposure 2, the SMR is

$$\text{SMR}_2 = \frac{\text{observed}}{\text{expected}} = \frac{5 + 40}{\dfrac{50}{100,000}(1,000) + \dfrac{400}{200,000}(10,000)}$$

$$= \frac{45}{0.5 + 20} = 2.20$$

The two SMRs are drastically different, not because the effect of exposure 1 is any greater than the effect of exposure 2 (the effects are equal), but because the population with exposure 1 is mostly young and the population with exposure 2 is mostly old. Among young people the relative effect is much greater, and consequently SMR_1 is much greater than SMR_2. The only reason for the difference between the two SMRs is the differing age distribution of the two exposed populations. Though a standardization process has been employed to standardize for age, the process involves applying a different age standard to each exposed group, namely, the age distribution of the exposed population itself. This example points out the danger of the misconception that with "indirect" standardization the group supplying the rate from which the expected numbers are generated is the standard. Under this misconception, one might falsely believe that the rates in both populations with exposures 1 and 2 have been standardized for age ("indirectly") using a common standard (the general population) and that therefore SMR_1 and SMR_2 are comparable. To avoid this error, it is important to appreciate that there is a unique concept of standardization that corresponds to what has been described as "direct" standardization. The calculation of SMRs is not a different approach—it is simply the same process using the exposed population of the SMR as the standard. Comparing SMRs amounts to comparing measures with different standards and is therefore invalid, even if the same set of unexposed rates is used in the computation of the SMRs. It is a simple matter to use a common standard and obtain standardized rate ratios that can be compared validly.

Since many epidemiologic studies, especially those dealing with occupational exposures, present a comparison of SMRs, it may seem surprising that the invalidity of such comparisons has been well known for decades. More than 60 years ago Wolfenden [1923] noted that "although in most cases the indirect method will give a close approximation . . . nevertheless it should be substituted for the direct method—especially in important cases—only after due examination." A decade later, Yule [1934] took a firmer position, declaring that the "indirect" method, which he preferred to call the "changing base method" (as contrasted with the "direct" method, which he referred to as the "fixed base method"), "is not fully a method of standardization at all, but is only safe for the comparison of single pairs of populations."

Why has an invalid method remained in popular use? Aside from the inertia of tradition, which after many decades must be a strong influence, there are two reasons, both of which were cited as advantages of the "changing base method" by Yule in 1934: (1) The SMR can be calculated without specific knowledge of the values for the standardizing factor for the exposed cases. For example, an age-standardized SMR requires no knowledge of the ages of the exposed cases. (2) The SMR is usually subject to less random error than a standardized rate ratio computed using a standard other than the exposed group. The greater statistical stability derives from the lack of dependence of the SMR on category-specific rates in the exposed population; to get the SMR the crude rate in the exposed population is compared with a standardized rate from the reference population. The first advantage is seldom important, since the information, if not already on hand, is usually readily obtainable, and furthermore, the denominator figures for the exposed population, which require much more extensive effort to obtain, are still necessary. The second advantage, a reduction in random error, comes at the expense of a possible bias. Despite these small advantages, Yule emphasized that "the non-comparability, strictly speaking, of these rates should always be borne in mind." Except in circumstances in which the advantages of using SMRs in a comparison of several groups clearly outweigh the disadvantages of the shifting standard that results, a common standard should be employed, and comparison of SMRs should be avoided.

REFERENCES

Wolfenden, H. H. On the methods of comparing the mortalities of two or more communities, and the standardization of death rates. *J. R. Stat. Soc.* 1923; 86:399–411.

Yule, G. U. On some points relating to vital statistics, more especially statistics of occupational mortality. *J. R. Stat. Soc.* 1934; 97:1–84.

6. TYPES OF EPIDEMIOLOGIC STUDY

The paradigm of the scientific process is the controlled observation achieved through an experiment. In a broad sense, a scientific experiment is a set of observations, conducted under controlled circumstances, in which the scientist manipulates the conditions to ascertain what effect such manipulation has on the outcome. Some might enlarge this definition to include controlled observations without manipulation of the conditions; thus, the astronomic observations during the solar eclipse of 1919 that confirmed Einstein's general theory of relativity might be considered an experiment. Nevertheless, the word *experiment* usually connotes manipulation of conditions. Loosely, experiment is used to describe tentative changes introduced even in the absence of controlled observation, such as might be the case with experimental teaching procedures tried by a professor.

The objective of experimentation is the creation of duplicate sets of circumstances in which only one factor that is relevant to the outcome varies, making it possible to observe the effect of variation in that factor. Achievement of this objective requires an ability to control all the relevant conditions that would affect the outcome under study. For experiments in the physical sciences, the objective may be achievable by controlling temperature, pressure, and electromagnetic field, or even a subset of these. In the biologic sciences, however, the conditions affecting the outcome are often so complex and occult that they cannot be made uniform. In studying the causes of cancer, for example, it is impossible to create conditions that will invariably give rise to cancer after a fixed time interval, even if the population is a group of cloned laboratory mice. Inevitably there will be what is called "biologic variation," which refers to variation in the set of conditions that produces the effect.

In biologic experimentation, then, the objective of creating duplicate sets of circumstances in which only one relevant factor varies is unrealistic (it could be argued that this objective is unrealistic in the physical sciences also). Instead, the objective is attenuated by attempting to create circumstances in which the extent of variation of extraneous factors that affect the outcome is kept small in relation to the variation of the factor under study. When the effect follows the cause under study after a lengthy induction period, the sources of variation that might modify the effect are potentially more numerous and more difficult to control.

Epidemiologic study types have their roots in the concepts of scientific experimentation. When epidemiologic experiments are feasible, their design is guided by principles that reduce variation by extraneous factors in comparison with the study factors. Epidemiologic experiments include *clinical trials* (with patients as subjects), *field trials* (with healthy subjects), and *community intervention trials* (with the intervention assigned to groups of healthy subjects). When experiments are not feasible, nonexperimental studies are designed to simulate what might have been learned if an experiment had been conducted. Nonexperimental studies include *follow-up* studies (in which subjects are selected with reference to their exposure status), *case-control* studies (in which subjects are selected in reference to their disease status), *cross-sectional* and *proportional mortality* studies, which are varieties of case-control studies, and *ecologic studies,* in which the unit of observation is a group of people.

EXPERIMENTAL STUDIES

In an experiment, those who are exposed to the agent or putative cause are exposed because the investigator has assigned the exposure to the subject. Furthermore, the assignment of the exposure must be part of the study protocol—that is, it must be intended to achieve the scientific objective of the study. For example, suppose that a physician treating headache had prescribed a patented drug to his wealthy patients and a generic counterpart to his indigent patients because the presumed greater reliability of the patented version was, in his judgment, not worth the greater cost for those of modest means. Should the physician later conduct research to evaluate the two medications, he could not consider himself to be conducting an experiment, despite the fact that the investigator had assigned the exposures. To conduct a proper experiment, he would have to assign the drugs according to a protocol that would reduce variation between the two groups with respect to other potential causes of headache. Assignment of exposure in experiments is intended to help the study rather than the individual subject.

Because the goals of the study rather than the subject's needs determine the exposure assignment, ethical constraints limit the circumstances in which epidemiologic experiments are feasible to those situations in which the subject's best interests are met by the scientific protocol; specifically, there should be reasonable assurance that the subject could not be treated better than the possibilities that the protocol provides. An obvious constraint is that exposures assigned to subjects should be limited to potential preventives of disease or disease consequences. This limitation alone confines most etiologic research to the nonexperimental variety. A second constraint is that the exposure alternatives should be equally acceptable under present knowledge. A third constraint is that subjects admitted to the study should not be thereby deprived of some preferable form of treatment or preventive not included in the study. For example, it is unethical to include a placebo therapy in circumstances for which an accepted remedy or preventive already exists. Additionally, subjects must be fully informed of their participation in an experiment and of the possible consequences.

Even with these limitations, many epidemiologic experiments are conducted. Most fall into the specialized area of clinical trials, which are epidemiologic studies of different treatments for patients who already have some disease *(trial* is used as a synonym for *experiment).* Epidemiologic experiments with primary preventives, intended to prevent disease onset in the first place, are less common; these are referred to either as field trials or as community intervention trials.

Clinical Trials

A clinical trial is an experiment with patients as subjects. The goal is to evaluate one or more new treatments for a disease or condition. The exposures in a clinical trial are not primary preventives, since they do not prevent occurrence of the initial disease, but they are preventives of the sequelae of the initial disease. For example, a modified diet after myocardial infarction may prevent reinfarction and subsequent death, or chemotherapeutic agents may prevent recurrence of cancer.

Subjects in clinical trials must be diagnosed as having the disease in question and must be admitted to the study soon enough following diagnosis to permit the treatment assignment to occur in timely fashion. Subjects whose illness is too mild or too severe to permit the form of treatment or alternative treatment being studied must be excluded. Treatment assignment should be designed to minimize variation of extraneous factors that might affect the comparison. For example, if some physicians participating in the study favored the new therapy, they could conceivably influence assignment of their patients, or the more seriously afflicted patients, to the new treatment. If, indeed, the more seriously afflicted patients tended to get the new treatment, then valid evaluation of the new treatment would be compromised. To avoid this and related problems, it is customary to assign treatments in clinical trials in a way that promotes comparability among treatment groups with respect to "baseline" characteristics and is also unpredictable and beyond the control of study personnel. It is almost universally agreed that a random assignment scheme is the best way to accomplish these objectives [Byar et al., 1976; Peto et al., 1976]. The validity of the trial ultimately depends on the extent to which the random process achieves identity of distribution for relevant baseline characteristics.

Field Trials

Field trials differ from clinical trials in that they deal with subjects who have not yet gotten disease and therefore are not patients. Whereas the complications of a given disease may occur with high probability during a relatively short time, typically the risk of a disease occurring among people who are free of the disease is small. Consequently, field trials usually require a greater number of subjects than clinical trials and therefore are more expensive. Furthermore, since the subjects are not patients, who usually come to a central location for treatment, a field trial typically necessitates visiting subjects in the "field" (at work, home, or school) or establishing centers from which the study can be conducted and to which subjects are urged to report. These design features add to cost.

The expense of field trials limits their use to the study of preventives of either extremely common or extremely serious diseases. Several field trials were conducted to determine the efficacy of large doses of vitamin C in preventing the common cold [Karlowski et al., 1975; Dykes and Meier, 1975]. Poliomyelitis, a rare but serious illness, was a sufficient public health concern to warrant what may have been the largest formal human experiment ever attempted, the Salk vaccine trial, in which the vaccine or a placebo were administered to more than 1,000,000 school children [Francis et al., 1955]. When the disease outcome occurs rarely, it is more efficient to study subjects thought to be at higher risk. Thus, the trial of hepatitis B vaccine was carried out in a population of New York City homosexuals, among whom hepatitis B infection occurs with much greater frequency than is usual among New Yorkers [Szmuness, 1980]. Similar reasoning is often applied to clinical trials, in which patients at low risk of complications are often excluded. Analogously, several clinical trials of the effect of lowering serum cholesterol levels on the risk of myocardial infarction have been undertaken with subjects who have already experienced a myocardial infarction because such patients are at high risk for a second infarction [Leren, 1966; Detre and Shaw, 1974]. It is much more costly to conduct a trial designed to study the effect of lowering serum cholesterol on the first occurrence of a myocardial infarction because many more subjects must be included to provide a reasonable number of outcome events to study. The MRFIT field trial (Multiple Risk Factor Intervention Trial) was a study of several primary preventives of myocardial infarction, including diet; although it admitted only high-risk individuals and endeavored to reduce risk through several simultaneous interventions, the study involved 12,866 subjects and cost $115 million [Kolata, 1982].

As in clinical trials, exposures in field trials should be assigned in a way that promotes comparability of groups and removes any discretion in assignment from the study's staff. A random assignment scheme is again an ideal choice, but the difficulties of implementing such a scheme in a large-scale field trial can outweigh the advantages. For example, it may be convenient to distribute vaccinations to groups receiving a single "batch" of vaccine, especially if storage and transport of the vaccine is difficult. Because such choices can seriously affect the interpretation of experimental findings, the advantages and disadvantages need to be carefully weighed.

Community Intervention Trials

The community intervention trial is an extension of the field trial that involves intervention on a community-wide basis. Conceptually, the distinction hinges on whether the intervention could be implemented separately for each individual or not. Whereas a vaccine is administered singly to individual people, water fluoridation to prevent dental caries is not: it is administered to individual water supplies rather than to individual people. Consequently, water fluoridation could not be studied with a conventional field trial. Instead, it was evaluated by community intervention trials, in which entire communities were selected, and exposure was assigned on a community basis. Other examples of preventives that might be implemented on a community-wide basis include fast-response emergency resuscitation programs and educational programs conducted using mass media, such as Project Burn-Prevention in Massachusetts [MacKay and Rothman, 1982].

Some interventions are implemented most conveniently with groups of subjects smaller than entire communities. Dietary intervention may be made most conveniently by family or household; environmental interventions may affect an entire office, plant, or residential building. Protective sports equipment may have to be assigned to an entire team or league. Intervention groups may be army units, classrooms, vehicle occupants, or any other group whose members are simultaneously exposed to the intervention. The scientific foundation of experiments using such interventions is identical to that of community intervention trials; what sets all these studies apart from ordinary field trials is that individual assignment of exposure is impossible or impractical. Random assignment of exposure to groups of individuals may be feasible, but the larger the group relative to the total study size, the less that is accomplished by random assignment. If only two communities are involved, one of which will receive the intervention and the other of which will not, such as in the Newburgh-Kingston water fluoridation trial, it cannot matter whether the community that receives the fluoride is assigned randomly or not; differences in baseline characteristics will have the same magnitude whatever the method of assignment—only the direction of the difference will be affected. The closer to individualized assignment permitted by the study design, the closer to identity of distribution of baseline characteristics that can be achieved by randomization.

NONEXPERIMENTAL STUDIES

The limitations imposed by ethics and cost restrict epidemiologic research to nonexperimental studies in most circumstances. Whereas it is unethical for an investigator to expose a person to a potential cause of disease simply to learn about etiology, people often willingly or unwillingly expose themselves to many potentially harmful factors. The extent of such exposures has been eloquently described by MacMahon [1979]:

They choose a broad range of dosages of a variety of potentially toxic substances. Consider the cigarette habit to which hundreds of millions of persons have exposed themselves at levels ranging from almost zero (for those exposed only through smoking by others) to the addict's three or four cigarettes per waking hour, and the consequent two million or more deaths from lung cancer in the last half century in this country alone. Consider the fact that fewer than half of American women pass through menopause without either having their uterus surgically removed, being liberally dosed with hormones that are known to increase cancer risk in animals, or both. Consider the implications of the fact that more than fifty million women worldwide take regularly for contraceptive purposes a combination of hormones that essentially cuts off the function of their own ovaries.

The goal of nonexperimental research is to simulate the results of an experiment, had one been possible. Whereas in an experiment the investigator has the power to assign exposures in a way that enhances the validity of the study, in nonexperimental research the investigator cannot control the circumstances of exposure. Nevertheless, the investigator is not doomed to accept a murky and unreliable system of observation from which invalid inferences would readily emerge. Since the investigator cannot assign exposure in nonexperimental studies, he or she must rely heavily on the primary source of discretion that remains, the selection of subjects.

If the paradigm of scientific observation is the experiment, then the paradigm of nonexperimental epidemiologic research is the "natural experiment." When experimentation is not possible, the ideal circumstances for the epidemiologist are those in which nature contrives to produce the conditions that would have been achievable if an experiment had been conducted. By far the most renowned example, the prototype of all natural experiments, is the elegant study of cholera in London conducted by John Snow. In London during the mid-nineteenth century there were several water companies that piped drinking water to residents. Snow's natural experiment consisted of comparing the cholera mortality rates for residents subscribing to two of the major water companies, the Southwark and Vauxhall Company, which piped impure Thames water contaminated with sewage, and the Lambeth Company, which in 1852 changed its collection from opposite Hungerford Market to Thames Ditton, thus obtaining a supply of water free of the sewage of London. As Snow [1860] described it,

> ... the intermixing of the water supply of the Southwark and Vauxhall Company with that of the Lambeth Company, over an extensive part of London, admitted of the subject being sifted in such a way as to yield the most incontrovertible proof on one side or the other. In the subdistricts ... supplied by both companies, the mixing of the supply is of the most intimate kind. The pipes of each company go down all the streets, and into nearly all the courts and alleys. A few houses are supplied by one company and a few by the other, according to the decision of the owner or occupier at the time when the Water Companies were in active competition. In many cases a single house has a supply different from that on either side. Each company supplies both rich and poor, both large houses and small; there is no difference in either the condition or occupation of the persons receiving the water of the different companies ... it is obvious that no experiment could have

been devised which would more thoroughly test the effect of water supply on the progress of cholera than this.

The experiment, too, was on the grandest scale. No fewer than three hundred thousand people of both sexes, of every age and occupation, and of every rank and station, from gentle folks down to the very poor, were divided into two groups without their choice, and, in most cases, without their knowledge; one group being supplied with water containing the sewage of London, and amongst it, whatever might have come from the cholera patients, the other group having water quite free from impurity.

To turn this experiment to account, all that was required was to learn the supply of water to each individual house where a fatal attack of cholera might occur . . . .

There are two primary types of nonexperimental studies: *follow-up* (or *cohort*) studies and *case-control* studies. The follow-up study is a direct analogue of the experiment, differing only in that the investigator does not assign the exposure. In case-control studies, although parallels with follow-up studies can be drawn, the conceptual basis of the study design differs enough from the scientific paradigms that a methodologically separate set of concerns emerges for design, analysis, and interpretation.

Follow-Up (Cohort) Studies

A follow-up study is one in which two or more groups of people that are free of disease and that differ according to extent of exposure to a potential cause of the disease are compared with respect to incidence of the disease in each of the groups. The follow-up study, defined in this way, comprises all experimental studies as well as natural experiments such as Snow's study of cholera. The essential element of a follow-up study is that incidence rates are calculable for each study group. (The study groups are sometimes referred to as *cohorts,* from the Latin word for one of the ten divisions of an ancient Roman legion.)

In Snow's natural experiment on drinking water and cholera, he was able to derive the approximate relative mortality from cholera, using households as the denominator, separately for the Lambeth Company and the Southwark and Vauxhall Company [Snow, 1860]:

According to a return which was made to Parliament, the Southwark and Vauxhall Company supplied 40,046 houses from January 1 to December 31, 1853, and the Lambeth Company supplied 26,107 houses during the same period; consequently, as 286 fatal attacks of cholera took place, in the first four weeks of the epidemic, in houses supplied by the former company, and only 14 in houses supplied by the latter, the proportion of fatal attacks to each 10,000 houses was as follows: Southwark and Vauxhall 71, Lambeth 5. The cholera was therefore fourteen times as fatal at this period, amongst persons having the impure water of the Southwark and Vauxhall Company, as amongst those having the purer water from Thames Ditton.

THE DEFINITION OF COHORTS AND FOLLOW-UP PERIOD

It is a simple matter to classify individuals into two or more groups and then measure the frequency of disease occurrence in these groups. Nevertheless, the most meaningful inferences are possible only when cohorts and the period of follow-up are strictly defined according to basic principles and biologic understanding.

An important axiom is that a cause always precedes the effect. Therefore, exposed individuals should not be considered as entering the follow-up period until after the exposure has occurred. This obvious restriction is a theoretical boundary that must be further restricted to accommodate a biologically appropriate induction time—the period during which the sufficient cause becomes complete—and the latent period—the period after causation before the disease is detected [Rothman, 1981]. Thus, for survivors of the atomic bombs in Japan, the effect of their exposure to radiation on subsequent cancer risk should not be evaluated with a follow-up period that begins the day after exposure. Allowance for a minimum induction time and a latent period would call for beginning the follow-up period some months or years after the bomb explosion, the exact value depending on the specific cancer risk to be evaluated.

If the appropriate minimum induction and latent period is unknown, this ignorance does not warrant starting the follow-up period immediately after exposure. In the absence of specific knowledge, an assumption must be made about the length of the minimum induction period; beginning follow-up immediately after exposure corresponds to assuming that the minimum period for disease induction and latency is zero, an extreme and probably incorrect assumption. Varying the assumption may provide information about the length of the induction and latent periods [Rothman, 1981], since the closer the assumption is to the truth, the larger will be the measured effect (see the discussion in Chapter 7 on nondifferential misclassification). Analogous assumptions must be addressed about the maximum duration of the induction and latent periods.

If the exposure is itself chronic, as opposed to occurring at a point in time, the definition of exposure is more complicated. We must conceptualize a period during which the exposure accumulates to a sufficient extent to trigger a step in the causal process; this accumulation of exposure experience may be a complex function of the intensity of the exposure and time. The induction period begins only after the exposure has reached this hypothetical triggering point. Occupational epidemiologists have often measured the induction time for occupational exposure from the time of first exposure, but this procedure involves the extreme assumption that the first contact with the exposure amounted to a biologically effective exposure. Whatever assumption is adopted, it should be made an explicit part of the definition of the cohort and the period of follow-up.

A subject who meets the definition for entry into a cohort should not be excluded from the cohort on the basis of exposure experience after entry. Suppose that the objective for a follow-up study is to evaluate the effect on mortality of smoking two or more packs of cigarettes a day for 10 continuous years. Assume that the minimum induction period is zero (for death from myocardial infarction) and that the maximum induction period is 50 years (for death from lung cancer). People who smoke two or more packs daily for their adult lifetimes will be eligible as study subjects exactly 10 years after beginning to smoke. A person who smoked for 5 years and then quit for 1 year in repeating cycles would never be eligible, since cohort entry requires 10 continuous years of smoking. Subjects who enter the cohort should not be excluded if they later quit smoking: Change in exposure may presage a change in disease status, or change in exposure may simply be a function of time. In either situation, bias would result from making an ex post facto exclusion. In randomized trials it is standard advice that all subjects, once randomized, should be included in the assigned groups whatever happens subsequent to randomization [Peto et al., 1976]. This rule can be generalized to all follow-up studies: Once a subject is entered into a cohort, the subject should not be excluded from that cohort on the basis of subsequent exposure experience. It is reasonable, however, to exclude part of the potential follow-up experience of a subject if that experience is outside the relevant time window defined by the induction and latent period assumptions. Such experience excluded from the follow-up related to exposure can either be disregarded or, if appropriate, considered as experience related to nonexposure.

Defining nonexposure can also be complicated. Potentially, it includes the experience of exposed subjects before exposure or, more generally, the experience of exposed subjects outside the time window defined by the assumptions about induction and latent periods. When several exposures are being evaluated, nonexposure should correspond to absence of all exposures. A common error, one perhaps more likely to occur in case-control studies than in follow-up studies, is to compare each exposed group with the complementary set of nonexposed, eschewing a single well-defined reference group. This use of a shifting reference group for exposure is easily seen to be incorrect when the compared groups are categorized by different levels of a single exposure. For example, it would clearly be a mistake to compare light smokers with non–light smokers (comprising both nonsmokers and heavy smokers). It is similarly incorrect to compare each of several different exposures to a shifting reference group that comprises the complement of each: Doing so may result in causes appearing to be preventives and will generally lead to underestimates of effects.

EXPENSE

Follow-up studies are generally large enterprises. Most diseases affect only a small proportion of a population, even if the population is followed for many years. To obtain steady estimates of incidence requires a substantial number of cases of disease, and therefore the person-time experience giving rise to the cases must also be substantial. Person-time experience can be accumulated by following cohorts for a long span of time. Some cohorts with special exposures (such as Japanese victims of atomic bombs [Beebe, 1979]) or with detailed medical and personal histories (such as the Framingham, Massachusetts study cohort [Kannel, 1984]) have indeed been followed for decades. If a study is intended to provide more timely results, however, the requisite person-time experience can be attained by increasing the size of the cohorts. Of course, lengthy studies of large populations are expensive; it is not uncommon for follow-up studies to expend millions of dollars, and price tags in excess of $100 million have occurred. Most of the expense derives from the need to establish a continuing system for monitoring disease occurrence in a large population.

The expense of follow-up studies often limits feasibility. The lower the disease incidence, the poorer the feasibility of a follow-up study. Feasibility is further handicapped by a long induction period between the hypothesized cause and its effect. A long induction time ipso facto contributes to a low overall incidence because of the additional person-time in the denominator, but it also imposes the burden of a study that must span, to detect any effect, an interval at least as long, and in practice considerably longer, than the minimum induction period. Follow-up studies are ill-suited for rare diseases with long induction periods in relation to the exposure of interest, which is only to say that such follow-up studies are expensive in relation to the amount of information returned.

The expense of follow-up studies can be reduced in a variety of ways. One way is to use an existing system for monitoring disease occurrence. For example, a regional cancer registry may be used to ascertain cancer occurrence among cohort members. If the expense of case ascertainment is already being borne by the registry, the study will be considerably cheaper.

Another way to reduce cost is to rely on historical cohorts. Rather than identifying cohort members concurrently with the initiation of the study and planning to have the follow-up period occur during the study, the investigator may choose to identify cohort members based on records of previous exposure. The follow-up period until the occurrence of disease may be wholly or partially in the past. If wholly in the past, then the investigators must also rely on records to ascertain disease in cohort members. If the follow-up period begins before the period during which the study is conducted but extends into the study period, then active surveillance or a new monitoring system to ascertain disease can be devised. When both exposure and disease are historical, the study is described as a *retrospective cohort* study, *retrospective follow-up* study, or *historical cohort* study. To the extent that follow-up is retrospective, that is, covers a

time period before the study, the study costs less than an equivalent prospective study.

A third way to reduce cost is to replace one of the cohorts, specifically
the unexposed cohort, with general population information. Rather than
collecting new information on a large unexposed population, existing data
on the general population is used for comparison. This procedure has
obvious drawbacks. First, it is reasonable only if there is some assurance
that only a small proportion of the general population is exposed to the
agent under study. To the extent that part of the general population is
exposed, there is misclassification error that will introduce a bias into the
comparison in the direction of underestimating the effect (see Chap. 7).
Second, the outcome information obtained in the study should be comparable in quality to that already existing for the general population. If
mortality data are used, then the cause of death listed on death certificates
should be used to classify study subjects, since the death certificate is also
the source of information for mortality data for the general population. If
additional medical information were to be used only for the exposed cohort, the data thus obtained would not be comparable to the general population data.

A fourth way to reduce the cost of a follow-up study is to conduct a case-
control study within the cohort rather than including the entire cohort
population in the study. Such "nested" case-control studies can often be
conducted at a fraction of the cost of a follow-up study and yet produce
the same findings with nearly the same level of precision. The case-control
approach, discussed below, is becoming increasingly popular even in occupational epidemiology, which has long been a holdout for the tradition
of follow-up studies [Paddle, 1981].

TRACING OF SUBJECTS

Follow-up studies that span many years present logistic problems that can
adversely affect validity. The core problem is to trace the study subjects.
Whether the study is retrospective or prospective, it is often difficult to
locate people or their records many years after they have been enrolled
into study cohorts. In prospective studies it may be possible to maintain
periodic contact with study subjects and thereby keep current information
on their location. Such tracking adds to the costs of prospective follow-up
studies, but the increasing mobility of society warrants stronger efforts to
trace subjects. A substantial number of subjects lost to follow-up can raise
serious doubts about the validity of the study. Follow-ups that trace less
than about 60 percent of subjects are generally regarded with skepticism,
but even follow-up of 70 or 80 percent or more can be too low to provide
sufficient reassurance against bias if there is reason to believe that loss to
follow-up may be correlated with both exposure and disease [Greenland,
1977].

SPECIAL EXPOSURE AND GENERAL POPULATION COHORTS

An attractive feature of follow-up studies is the capability they provide to study a range of possible health effects stemming from a single exposure. A mortality follow-up can be accomplished just as easily for all cases of death as for any specific cause. Health surveillance for one disease end point can usually be expanded to include many or all end points without much additional work. A follow-up study can provide a comprehensive picture of the health effect of a given exposure. Attempts to derive such comprehensive information about exposures motivate the identification of "special exposure" cohorts, which are identifiable groups with exposure to agents of interest. Examples of such special exposure cohorts include occupational cohorts exposed to workplace exposures, soldiers exposed to "Agent Orange" in Vietnam, residents of the Love Canal area of Niagara, New York, exposed to chemical wastes, Seventh Day Adventists exposed to vegetarian diets, and atomic bomb victims exposed to ionizing radiation. These exposures are not common and require the identification of exposed cohorts to provide enough information for study.

Common exposures are sometimes studied through follow-up studies that survey a segment of the population that is identified without regard to exposure status. Such "general population" cohorts have been used to study the effects of smoking, oral contraceptives, diet, and hypertension. A successful general population cohort study should aim to evaluate exposures that a substantial proportion of people have experienced; otherwise, the nonexposed cohort will be inefficiently large relative to the size of the exposed cohort. General population follow-up studies offer the advantage of allowing investigators to study a range of disease outcomes for more than one exposure. A surveyed population can be classified according to smoking, alcoholic beverage consumption, diet, drug use, medical history, and many other factors of potential interest. A disadvantage is that usually the exposure information must be obtained by interviews with each subject, as opposed to obtaining information from records as is often done with special exposure cohorts.

Case-Control Studies

The sophisticated use and understanding of case-control studies is the most outstanding methodologic development of modern epidemiology. Conceptually there are clear links from experimental studies to nonexperimental follow-up studies to case-control studies, but case-control studies nevertheless differ enough from the scientific paradigm of experimentation that a casual approach to their conduct and interpretation invites misconception and possibly serious error.

RATIONALE FOR THE CASE-CONTROL STUDY DESIGN

Imagine a dynamic steady-state population of exposed and unexposed individuals. The relevant data on disease incidence for a time period of length t might be summarized as

$$I_1 = \frac{a}{P_1 t}$$

and

$$I_0 = \frac{b}{P_0 t}$$

where I_1 and I_0 are the incidence rates among exposed and unexposed, respectively, a and b are the respective numbers of individuals who developed disease during time interval t, and P_1 and P_0 are the respective population sizes. In a follow-up study the numerator and denominator of each rate are measured; doing so requires enumerating the entire population and keeping it under surveillance. A case-control study is an attempt to render the observations made on the population more efficient. The cases in a case-control study are the individuals who became ill during the time period, that is, a total of (a + b) individuals. The controls are a sample of the combined cohorts that gave rise to the cases. If a proportion, k, of the combined exposed and unexposed cohorts is taken as controls, and the number of such controls is c for exposed and d for unexposed, then the incidence rates among exposed and unexposed could be estimated as

$$I_1 = k \frac{a}{ct}$$

and

$$I_0 = k \frac{b}{dt}$$

If k, the sampling fraction for controls, is known, then estimates of disease incidence are obtainable for both exposed and unexposed groups, just as in a follow-up study. Even if k is unknown, however, which is usually the situation, the relative incidence, or rate ratio (RR, often referred to as *relative risk*), is obtained as

$$RR = \frac{I_1}{I_0} = \frac{ad}{bc} \qquad [6\text{-}1]$$

Since the sampling fraction, k, is identical for both exposed and unexposed, it divides out, as does t. The resulting quantity, ad/bc, is the exposure odds ratio (ratio of exposure odds among cases to exposure odds among controls), often referred to simply as the *odds ratio*. This cancellation of the sampling fraction for controls in the odds ratio thus provides an unbiased estimate of the incidence rate ratio from case-control data [Sheehe, 1962; Miettinen, 1976]. The central condition for conducting valid case-control studies is that controls be selected independently of exposure status to guarantee that the sampling fraction can be removed from the odds ratio calculation.

The case-control design can be conceptualized as a follow-up design in which the person-time experience of the denominators of the incidence rates is sampled rather than measured outright. The sampling must be independent of exposure; by revealing the relative size of the person-time denominators for the exposed and unexposed incidence rates, the sampling process allows the calculation of the relative magnitude of incidence rates. Viewed in this way, the case-control study design can be considered a more efficient form of the follow-up study, in which the cases are the same as those that would be included in a follow-up study and the controls provide a fast and inexpensive means of inferring the distribution of person-time experience according to exposure in the population that gave rise to the cases.

SELECTION OF CASES AND CONTROLS

The above discussion presumes that all cases from the population are included as subjects in the case-control study. This argument can be turned around to make it less restrictive: The cases that are included in a case-control study represent the totality of cases from some hypothetical population that produced the cases that were selected. A case not selected is thus presumed to arise from a different source population. Then the objective in selecting controls is to choose individuals representative of those who, had they developed disease, would have been selected as cases and, of course, to choose these controls independently of exposure. Thus, case-control studies need not include all cases occurring within a recognizable population, such as within a geographic boundary; the cases identified in a single clinic or even by a single medical practitioner are possible case series as long as it is understood that the population from which the cases derive is restricted to those people who would have been included as cases had they developed the disease. Controls must be selected to represent such a population.

Some textbooks have stressed the need for representativeness in the selection of cases and controls; the advice has been that cases are supposed to be representative of all persons with the disease and that controls should be representative of the entire nondiseased population. Such advice is clearly wrong.

A case-control study may be restricted to any type of case that may be of interest: female cases, old cases, severely ill cases, cases that died soon after disease onset, mild cases (often of greater interest than severe cases when studying congenital malformations if the severe cases die in utero), cases from Philadelphia, cases among factory workers, and so on. In none of these examples would the cases be representative of all persons with the disease, and yet perfectly valid case-control studies are possible using such unrepresentative case series [Cole, 1979]. It is true that cases must be selected independently of exposure, but the prevalence of exposure among cases may nevertheless be higher or lower than the prevalence among other persons with disease if the cases differ by such factors as age, sex, or severity from other persons with disease.

It is equally wrong to seek controls that are representative of the entire nondiseased population. The main objective in selecting controls is to select subjects who represent those who might have become cases in the study; if cases are selected from one hospital out of many in a city, the controls should represent those people who, had they developed the disease under study, would have gone to the same hospital. Such people may differ vastly from the general population by age, race, sex (e.g., if the cases come from a Veterans Administration Hospital), socioeconomic status, occupation, and so on, and consequently they may also differ from the general population with regard to exposure.

There have been epidemiologic studies that were population-based in the geographic sense, including in the case series every case of illness occurring in a geographic area and a representative sample of the base population as controls (though usually with some age restriction). Such studies are few in number because they are expensive. Most case-control studies are based on series of subjects who have been ascertained only from specific selection factors operating outside the control of the investigator such as, for example, attendance at one or more designated clinics. Such studies are reasonable and valid provided that the investigator selects subjects independently of exposure and chooses controls who would have navigated the same pathway of selection forces as the cases had they been ill. The challenge in such studies is to convert this conceptual definition of control subjects into a control-selection protocol.

One of the reasons for emphasizing the similarities rather than the differences between follow-up and case-control studies is that numerous principles apply to both types of study but are more evident in the context of follow-up studies. Since a case-control study is always conceptualized within the framework of a hypothetical follow-up study, many principles relating to subject selection apply identically to both types of study. For example, it is widely appreciated that follow-up studies can be based on special cohorts rather than on the general population. It follows that case-control studies can be conducted by sampling controls from within those special cohorts. The utility of such focused case-control studies belies the proposition that in case-control studies the controls need to be representative of all persons in the population without disease.

Another illustration of this general idea, that principles applicable to case-control studies can often be best understood by applying principles from follow-up studies, relates to the concept of "exposure opportunity." The issue is whether the opportunity for exposure should be controlled in a case-control study [Poole, 1985]. Excluding sterile women from a case-control study of oral contraceptives and matching for duration of employment within an industry in a study of occupational exposure are examples of attempts to control for exposure opportunity. In a follow-up study there is no preoccupation with whether a given subject has had an opportunity to become exposed; the interest is in the fact of exposure rather than the opportunity for exposure. (On the other hand, if a factor that enhances or decreases the opportunity for exposure is also a risk factor for disease, then it is a confounding factor and should be controlled.) The irrelevance of exposure opportunity in case-control studies, like many other principles, becomes clear when the question is translated to the setting of a follow-up study.

We have seen that in a dynamic population a case-control study can produce the same estimate of the ratio of incidence rates that would be obtained if a follow-up study had been conducted. A conceptually important feature of the selection of controls is their continuous eligibility to become cases. Suppose the study period spans 3 years. An individual free of disease in year 1 is a potential control and might go on to develop the disease in year 3, thus becoming a case. How is such an individual treated in the analysis? Practically speaking, of course, it will matter little, since a study is unlikely to have many subjects eligible to be both a case and a control, but the question is of interest because it is targeted at the theoretical underpinnings of the purpose of a control group in case-control studies. Since the individual in question did develop disease during the study period, many investigators would be tempted to count the person as a case, but not a control. Recall, however, that if a follow-up study were being conducted, each person who develops disease would contribute to the person-time experience in the denominator of the incidence rate until the time of disease onset. The control group in case-control studies is intended to provide estimates of the relative size of the denominators of the incidence rates for the compared groups. Therefore, each case in a case-control study should be eligible as a control until the time of disease onset, and each control should be eligible to become a case later during the study period. An individual selected as a control who later develops the disease should be counted as both a control and a case [Lubin and Gail, 1984]. This surprising conclusion is more readily digested if one considers a case-control study of death from any cause; since every person will eventually become a case were the study to run sufficiently long, there is no alternative but to accept that cases are eligible to be controls at any time before disease onset.

To the extent that exposure information may change with time, the inclusion of the same person in a study at different times may lead to different exposure information for the separate ascertainments. For example, if poisoning victims are the cases in a case-control study, one might ask them about food ingested within the previous day or days; if a contaminated food item was a cause of the illness for some cases, then the exposure history for these individuals might well differ from what would have been elicited from the same individuals weeks before, when they might have been included as controls in the same study.

Occasionally a research study involves a limited period of risk that has ended before the study begins. For example, a case-control study of an epidemic of diarrheal illness after a social gathering may begin after all the potential cases have occurred (because the maximum induction time has elapsed). If controls are selected from among those who were free of disease at the end of the epidemic, an unbiased estimation of the ratio of incidence rates is not achievable. Nevertheless, the odds ratio (equation 6-1) will provide a reasonable approximation of the ratio of incidence rates, provided that the cumulative incidences during the risk period are low, that is, less than about 20 percent, and that the prevalence of exposure remains reasonably steady during the study period [Greenland and Thomas, 1982]. If the investigator prefers to estimate the risk ratio rather than the incidence rate ratio, which is a reasonable preference when the period of risk is well defined, the odds ratio estimator can still be used (since the incidence rate ratio approximates the risk ratio for small risks), but because two approximations are now involved the accuracy is not as good. (Direct estimation of the risk ratio is generally preferable, but the statistical properties of the odds ratio parameter are attractive in some applications, as discussed in Chapter 11.) Table 6-1 illustrates the accuracy of the approximations involved for different values of risk.

Case-control studies can also be based on prevalent cases rather than incident cases. Instead of including as cases only those who develop the illness during a specified time period (i.e., incident cases), it is possible to select as cases any existing cases of illness at a point in time. If the duration of illness is unrelated to exposure, then a case-control study based on prevalent cases and controls who are selected during the risk period will provide an odds ratio that is an unbiased estimator of the incidence rate ratio. If exposure affects the duration of illness, then a case-control study based on prevalent cases will be unable to distinguish an etiologic role for the exposure from its effect on duration unless the effect on duration is known. Consequently, it is strongly preferable, whenever possible, to select incident rather than prevalent cases. As discussed in Chapter 3, the most common study situation in which prevalent cases are usually drawn is the study of congenital malformations. In such studies, cases ascertained at birth represent prevalent cases because they have survived with the malformation from the time of its occurrence until birth. It would be etiologically more useful to ascertain all incident cases, including affected abortuses that do not survive until birth. Many of these, how-

Table 6-1. *Accuracy of the odds ratio approximation*
to the ratio of incidence rates and to the ratio of risks
for case-control studies in which controls are selected after a
defined period of risk (modified from Greenland and Thomas [1982]).

Risk in unexposed	Risk in exposed	Odds ratio	Ratio of incidence rates*	Ratio of risks
0.5	0.6	1.50	1.32	1.20
0.4	0.6	2.25	1.79	1.50
0.3	0.6	3.50	2.57	2.00
0.2	0.6	6.00	4.11	3.00
0.1	0.6	13.5	8.70	6.00
0.1	0.4	6.00	4.85	4.00
0.1	0.2	2.25	2.19	2.00
0.05	0.2	4.75	4.35	4.00
0.05	0.1	2.11	2.05	2.00
0.02	0.05	2.58	2.54	2.50

*The ratio of incidence rates can be calculated from the risks for exposed (R_1) and unexposed (R_0) as $[\ln(1 - R_1)]/[\ln(1 - R_0)]$

ever, do not survive until ascertainment is feasible, and thus it is virtually inevitable that case-control studies of congenital malformations are based on prevalent cases. Another situation in which prevalent cases are commonly used is the study of nonlethal chronic conditions such as obesity.

STRENGTHS AND WEAKNESSES
Whereas follow-up studies are useful for evaluating the range of effects related to a single exposure, case-control studies can only provide information about the one effect that afflicts the cases selected. It is possible, of course, to select multiple series of cases with various diseases, but such an approach amounts to launching several simultaneous case-control studies (the different case series might or might not require separate control series depending on the conditions of ascertainment of the case series). On the other hand, a case-control study can conveniently provide information on a wide range of potentially etiologic exposures that might relate to a specific disease, whereas typically a follow-up study focuses on only one exposure (general population cohort studies are an exception, providing information on a wide range of exposures and diseases).

Some strengths and weaknesses of follow-up studies have symmetric weaknesses and strengths in case-control studies. Already mentioned is the ability of follow-up studies to evaluate a range of effects related to the exposure, whereas a case-control study can evaluate a range of exposures related to the disease. Whereas the evaluation of effects on rare diseases is problematic in follow-up studies, rare diseases are well suited to case-control studies; on the other hand, case-control studies are inefficient for the evaluation of the effects of exposures that are rare in the source population for the cases. A concern in follow-up studies is the tracing of subjects to avoid loss to follow-up. In case-control studies the analogous concern is determining the correct exposure for all subjects to avoid the loss of subjects with unknown exposure. In follow-up studies, because exposure status is determined before the presence of disease is known either to the subject or to the investigator, there is no possibility of the disease outcome influencing the exposure classification; in case-control studies, if the exposure information comes from the subject after disease onset, knowledge of the disease could affect exposure data. This possibility for bias in case-control studies has no counterpart in follow-up studies. Of course, knowledge of exposure can affect the determination of disease status for subjects in follow-up studies, but this difficulty exists for any type of study. Offsetting the drawback of an additional potential source of bias in case-control studies is the important advantage that follow-up studies are usually large and expensive, whereas case-control studies are smaller and less expensive. The greater efficiency of case-control studies is a strength that may compensate for the greater possibility of bias.

Case-control studies have endured a poor reputation, sometimes serving as the "whipping boy" of epidemiologic research. Those who denigrate case-control research often refer disparagingly to "retrospective" studies without making the distinction made by epidemiologists between retrospective follow-up studies and case-control studies; the bulk of suspicion of so-called retrospective studies, however, is reserved for case-control studies. It is undeniable that case-control studies present more opportunities for bias and mistaken inference than other types of research. One reason is the possibility of recall bias in classifying exposure. The primary reason for error, however, has nothing to do with the validity of the information obtainable from case-control studies; it relates to the relative ease with which a case-control study can be mounted. Because it need not be extremely expensive nor time-consuming to conduct a case-control study, many studies have been conducted by would-be investigators who lack even a rudimentary appreciation for epidemiologic principles. A typical instance might be a study based on a series of patients seen by a single physician or a group of practitioners, with or without a control series. Occasionally such haphazard research can produce fruitful or even extremely important results, but often the results are wrong because basic research principles have been violated. The poor reputation suffered by case-control studies stems more from their inept conduct than from any inherent weakness in the conceptual approach. It is encouraging to observe the steady increase in case-control studies that have been designed, reported, and analyzed with respect for the principles of good study design, thereby minimizing the possibility for bias to distort the findings.

Cross-Sectional Studies versus Longitudinal Studies

The essential differentiating characteristic between follow-up and case-control studies is the identifying characteristic on the basis of which subjects are ascertained. For follow-up studies this characteristic is some potentially etiologic antecedent of disease (the exposure), and for case-control studies it is the disease. Occasionally a study is undertaken in which individuals are included as subjects without regard either to exposure or to disease.

If a population is enrolled in a study and then those individuals who are free of disease are followed to measure disease occurrence, the study is a general population follow-up study. A study that includes as subjects all persons in the population at the time of ascertainment, including those who have the disease, is usually referred to as a *cross-sectional study*. A cross-sectional study, although often presented as different from both follow-up and case-control designs, can usually be conceptualized as the case-control analogue of the general population follow-up study. The cases are a prevalence series of individuals with the disease, and the controls are the remainder of the studied population. Usually the exposure information is ascertained simultaneously with the disease information; the contemporaneous classification of people with respect to both exposure and disease is thought to be the essence of the cross-sectional approach. Nevertheless, research is usually more meaningful when the investigator considers the exposure categorization with reference to the period of time that might be etiologically relevant to current disease, that is, with reference to a meaningful induction period.

Cross-sectional studies often deal with exposures that cannot change, such as blood type or other invariable personal characteristics. For such exposures, current information is as useful as any. For variable exposures, however, current information may be less desirable than etiologically more relevant information from the past. In a study of the etiology of respiratory cancer that compares smoking information on cases and noncases, the current smoking habits of subjects are not nearly as relevant as their smoking histories. The cross-sectional approach to such a question could well be viewed as a case-control study with an excessively large control group (because few people in a population would have respiratory cancer) and with smoking information from an inappropriate time period.

Although current information is often too recent to be etiologically meaningful, occasionally there is adequate justification for its use. If there is reason to believe that a good correlation exists between current exposure and the relevant past exposure, and if recall of previous exposure is likely to be unreliable, it may be reasonable to ascertain current exposure status as a proxy for the relevant exposure. Studies on dietary preferences, for example, often extract detailed current information because precise information on food consumption can thus be obtained, whereas recall of dietary information is likely to be vague and unreliable. Studies dependent on current exposure when previous exposure is relevant obviously suffer in validity to the extent that the previous exposure of subjects differs from current exposure.

Ideally, then, etiologic research should always be *longitudinal* rather than cross-sectional; that is, there should always be an allowance for a time interval between exposure and disease onset that corresponds to a meaningful induction period. In follow-up studies, the interval is accommodated by restricting the accumulation of person-time experience in the denominator of incidence rates for the exposed to that period of time following exposure that corresponds to the limits of the possible induction period. In case-control studies, the interval is accommodated by relating to the disease the exposure status at a time that antecedes the disease onset by an amount that again corresponds to the limits of the possible induction period. Suppose one were studying whether exposure to canine distemper in one's pet caused multiple sclerosis, and the induction period (to the time of diagnosis) was assumed to be 10 to 25 years. In a follow-up study, exposed individuals would not contribute to person-time at risk until 10 years from the time that the pet had distemper. Such contribution to the risk experience would begin at 10 years and would last 15 years (the duration of the induction-time interval) or less if the subject were removed from follow-up (because he or she died, was lost, or was diagnosed with multiple sclerosis). Only if multiple sclerosis were diagnosed during this same interval would it be considered to be potentially related to exposure. In a case-control study, cases of multiple sclerosis would be classified as exposed if their pet dog had distemper during the interval between 10 and 25 years before the diagnosis of multiple sclerosis. If exposure to distemper occurred outside of this time window, the case would be considered unexposed. Controls would be questioned in reference to a comparable time period and similarly classified.

An example of this technique was a case-control study of pyloric stenosis that examined the role of Bendectin exposure during early gestation [Aselton et al., 1984]. Different time windows of 1 week's duration during early pregnancy were assumed. The data indicated that exposure during week 5 of pregnancy or after week 12 led to a relative risk estimate of less than 2.0, whereas an estimate equal to or greater than 3.0 was obtained for exposure to Bendectin during weeks 6 to 12. The maximum effect, a relative risk of 3.7, was estimated for exposure during weeks 8 and 9 after conception. This example illustrates how epidemiologic analyses can be used to define a narrow period of causal action, even if little is known about the period a priori. If, instead of this approach, only one analysis using a single definition of exposure had been conducted, little or no information about the time relation between exposure and disease would have resulted, and the maximum effect estimate would probably have been underestimated.

As was mentioned earlier in discussing the definition of cohorts, even if there is no specific knowledge about the induction period, the issue must nevertheless be addressed. It is important for an investigator to realize that no epidemiologic study can be conducted or epidemiologic data analyzed to evaluate cause and effect without making some assumptions, explicit or implicit, about the timing between exposure and disease.

Any system that classifies individuals as diseased or not diseased in relation to some exposure is based on some assumption about induction time. If a case-control study includes as relevant exposure any history of exposure from birth (or conception) until diagnosis, surely some period irrelevant to meaningful exposure would be included, diluting the effect of relevant exposure. If a cross-sectional study relates current exposure to disease (the onset of which may even have antedated the exposure), this too involves an assumption about induction period. Often the assumption about induction period is implicit and obscure. Good research practice dictates making such assumptions explicit and evaluating them to the extent possible. One step to this end is to view cross-sectional studies of exposures that vary with time as case-control studies with a specific assumption of zero induction time.

Whatever assumption is made about the induction period will affect the study results, since inaccurate assumptions cause a type of misclassification that tends to reduce the magnitude of associations and underestimate effects. This phenomenon can be used to learn about the induction period, as the study on pyloric stenosis demonstrates; by repeating the analysis of the data while varying the assigned limits for the induction period, it is possible to determine which assumption about induction period leads to the largest effect estimate. The assumed induction period giving the largest effect estimate is the one that best describes, on the basis of the data in the study at hand, the timing of the etiologic relation under study, presuming, of course, that there is an etiologic relation [Rothman, 1981].

Proportional Mortality Studies

A *proportional mortality study* includes only dead subjects. The proportion of dead exposed subjects who have been assigned one or more specific causes of death is compared with a corresponding proportion of dead unexposed subjects. The resulting *proportional mortality ratio,* often abbreviated PMR, is taken as a measure of the effect of the exposure. Superficially, the comparison of proportions of subjects dying from a specific cause for an exposed and an unexposed group resembles a cohort study measuring cumulative incidence. The resemblance is deceiving, however, because a proportional mortality study does not involve the identification of cohorts. All subjects are dead at the time of entry into the study, so there is no follow-up period.

The premise of a proportional mortality study is that if the exposure causes (or prevents) a specific fatal illness, there should be proportionately more (or fewer) deaths from that cause among dead people who have been exposed than among dead people who have not been exposed. It is well recognized that this reasoning suffers an important flaw. The PMR measure cannot distinguish between the effect of an exposure that prevents deaths in some categories from that of an exposure that causes deaths in other categories, or some mixture of these actions [McDowall, 1983]. For example, a proportional mortality study could find a proportional excess of cancer deaths among heavy aspirin takers compared with nonusers of aspirin, but this finding might be attributable to a preventive effect of aspirin on cardiovascular deaths, which compose the great majority of noncancer deaths. An implicit assumption of a proportional mortality study is that the overall death rate for categories other than the ones under study is not related to the exposure.

The ambiguity in interpreting a PMR is not necessarily a fatal flaw, since the measure will often provide leads worth pursuing about causal relations. In many situations it may be only one or a few narrow categories of death that are of interest, and it may be judged implausible that an exposure would substantially affect the remaining categories that form the reference group. Some epidemiologists have argued that it may even be desirable to evaluate departures from the relative frequency of death rather than absolute differences in mortality [Kupper et al., 1978], but the rationale for such a view is not based on biologic considerations.

Many of the difficulties attendant on interpreting proportional mortality studies can be mitigated by considering a proportional mortality study as a variant of the case-control study. To do so requires conceptualizing a combined population of exposed and unexposed individuals in which the cases occurred; the cases are those deaths, both exposed and unexposed, in the specific category or categories of interest. Thus far this description could be that of an ordinary case-control study based on fatal cases. The distinction stems from the control series. The principle of control series selection is to choose individuals representing the base population from which the cases came, to learn the distribution of exposure within that population. Instead of sampling controls directly from the base population, we can sample deaths occurring in the base population provided that the exposure distribution among the deaths sampled is the same as the distribution in the base population—that is, the exposure should not be related to the control causes of death [McLaughlin et al., 1985]. This provision is the source of the interpretation problems for the PMR, but if we keep the objectives of control selection in mind, it becomes clear that we are not bound to select as controls all deaths other than those in the categories designated as cases. We can instead select one specific category or a set of categories of death, chosen on the basis of a presumed lack of association with the exposure. In this way, other causes of death for which a relation with exposure is known, suspected, or merely plausible can be excluded. The principle behind selecting the control categories of death for inclusion in the study is identical to the principle of selecting a control series for any case-control study. Deaths in categories not included as part of the control series should be excluded from the study or possibly treated as alternative case groups.

Treating a proportional mortality study as a case-control study can thus enhance the validity of the comparisons made. In addition, by analyzing the data as ordinary case-control data and focusing on the odds ratio, the usual epidemiologic measures of effect that can be derived from case-control studies can be the object of inference [Wang and Miettinen, 1982]. The conceptual clarity that results from considering such studies as case-control studies warrants dropping the term proportional mortality study from the epidemiologist's lexicon and the use of the inelegant proportional mortality ratio along with it.

Ecologic Studies

All the study types described thus far share the characteristic that the observations made pertain to individual people. It is possible to conduct research in which the unit of observation is a group of people rather than an individual; such studies are called *ecologic studies*. The groups may be classes in a school, factories, cities, counties, or nations. The only requirement is that information on the populations studied is available to measure each population with respect to exposure and disease. Incidence or mortality is the preferable measure by which to quantify disease occurrence in populations. Exposure is also measured by some overall index; for example, county data on alcohol consumption may be available from alcohol tax data, information on socioeconomic status is available for census tracts from the decennial census, and environmental data (temperature, air quality, and so on) may be available locally or regionally.

Because the data in ecologic studies are based on measurements averaged over populations, the degree of association between exposure and disease is usually more tenuous. In addition, proxy measures for exposure (e.g., alcohol tax data rather than consumption data) and disease (mortality rather than incidence) further attenuate the associations. The greatest difficulty with ecologic studies, however, usually stems from the unavailability of data necessary for control of confounding in the analysis. Inadequate control of confounding coupled with associations that are attenuated to begin with produces results that may be of questionable validity. The problem of inappropriate inferences from ecologic data has been referred to as the "ecologic fallacy" [Morgenstern, 1982] (see also Chap. 14). Despite such problems, ecologic studies have been useful in describing differences in populations; even if confounded by unknown or uncontrollable factors, such differences at least signal the presence of effects worthy of further investigation.

REFERENCES

Aselton, P., Jick, H., Chentow, S. J., et al. Pyloric stenosis and maternal Bendectin exposure. *Am. J. Epidemiol.* 1984; 120:251–256.

Beebe, G. W. Reflections on the work of the Atomic Bomb Casualty Commission in Japan. *Epidemiol. Rev.* 1979; 1:184–210.

Byar, D. P., Simon, R. M., Friedewald, W. T., et al. Randomized clinical trials. Perspectives on some recent ideas. *N. Engl. J. Med.* 1976; 295:74–80.

Cole, P. The evolving case-control study. *J. Chron. Dis.* 1979; 32:15–27.

Detre, K. M., and Shaw, L. Long-term changes of serum cholesterol with cholesterol-altering drugs in patients with coronary heart disease. *Circulation* 1974; 50:998–1005.

Dykes, M. H. M., and Meier, P. Ascorbic acid and the common cold. Evaluation of its efficacy and toxicity. *J.A.M.A.* 1975; 231:1073–1079.

Francis, T. F., Korns, R. F., Voight, R. B., et al. An evaluation of the 1954 poliomyelitis vaccine trials. *Am. J. Public Health* 1955; 45[May Suppl.]:1–63.

Greenland, S. Response and follow-up bias in cohort studies. *Am. J. Epidemiol.* 1977; 106:184–187.

Greenland, S., and Thomas, D. C. On the need for the rare disease assumption in case-control studies. *Am. J. Epidemiol.* 1982; 116:547–553.

Kannel, W. B., and Abbott, R. D. Incidence and prognosis of unrecognized myocardial infarction. An update on the Framingham study. *N. Engl. J. Med.* 1984; 311:1144–1147.

Karlowski, T. R., Chalmers, T. C., Frenkel, L. D., et al. Ascorbic acid for the common cold. A prophylactic and therapeutic trial. *J.A.M.A.* 1975; 231:1038–1042.

Kolata, G. Heart study produces a surprise result. *Science* 1982; 218:31–32.

Kupper, L. L., McMichael, A. J., Symons, M. J., et al. On the utility of proportional mortality analysis. *J. Chron. Dis.* 1978; 31:15–22.

Leren, P. The effect of plasma cholesterol lowering diet in male survivors of myocardial infarction. *Acta Med. Scand.* [Suppl.] 1966; 466:5–92.

Lubin, J. H., and Gail, M. H. Biased selection of controls for case-control analyses of cohort studies. *Biometrics* 1984; 40:63–75.

MacKay, A. M., and Rothman, K. J. The incidence and severity of burn injuries following Project Burn Prevention. *Am. J. Public Health* 1982; 72:248–252.

MacMahon, B. Strengths and limitations of epidemiology. In National Academy of Sciences, *The National Research Council in 1979.* Washington, D.C.: National Academy of Sciences, 1979.

McDowall, M. Adjusting proportional mortality ratios for the influence of extraneous causes of death. *Stat. Med.* 1983; 2:467–475.

McLaughlin, J. K., Blot, W. J., Mehl, E. S., et al. Problems in the use of dead controls in case-control studies. I. General results. *Am. J. Epidemiol.* 1985; 121:131–139.

Miettinen, O. S. Estimability and estimation in case-referent studies. *Am. J. Epidemiol.* 1976; 103:226–235.

Morgenstern, H. Uses of ecologic analysis in epidemiologic research. *Am. J. Public Health* 1982; 72:1336–1344.

Paddle, G. M. A strategy for the identification of carcinogens in a large, complex chemical company. In R. Peto and M. Schneiderman [eds.] (Banbury Report No. 9), *Quantification of Occupational Cancer.* New York: Cold Spring Harbor Laboratory, 1981.

Peto, R., Pike, M. C., Armitage, P. et al. Design and analysis of randomized clinical trials requiring prolonged observation of each patient. I. Introduction and design. *Br. J. Cancer* 1976; 34:585–612.

Poole, C. Exposure opportunity in case-control studies. *Am. J. Epidemiol.* 1986; 122. In press.

Rothman, K. J. Induction and latent periods. *Am. J. Epidemiol.* 1981; 114:253–259.

Sheehe, P. R. Dynamic risk analysis in retrospective matched pair studies of disease. *Biometrics* 1962; 18:323–341.

Snow, J. *On the Mode of Communication of Cholera* (2nd ed.). London: John Churchill, 1860. (Facsimile of 1936 reprinted edition by Hafner, New York, 1965.)

Szmuness, W. Hepatitis B vaccine. Demonstration of efficacy in a controlled clinical trial in a high-risk population in the United States. *N. Engl. J. Med.* 1980; 303:833–841.

Wang, J., and Miettinen, O. S. Occupational mortality studies: principles of validity. *Scand. J. Work Environ. Health* 1982; 8:153–158.

Every epidemiologic study should be viewed as a measurement exercise. This simple view in itself provides firm guidance in planning, carrying out, and interpreting epidemiologic studies. The specific objectives of an epidemiologic study should always involve obtaining estimates of one of the measures of disease occurrence or effect described previously or some derivative of these measures. Sometimes the objectives of a study are expressed qualitatively, for example, "to learn whether moderate daily alcohol consumption during pregnancy causes low birthweight." Some scientists are reluctant to speak so blatantly about cause and effect, but in statements of hypothesis and in describing study objectives such boldness serves to keep the real goal firmly in focus and is therefore highly preferable to insipid statements about "association" instead of "causation." Still, an objective that begins "to learn whether . . ." is a qualitative one and is weaker than a statement such as "to determine the proportion of babies born with weight under 2,500 grams to women who consume moderate daily amounts of alcohol." Greater detail could further enhance this statement of objectives, but the essential distinction here is between a qualitative objective (e.g., to answer a question "yes" or "no") and a quantitative one (to measure something).

The specific parameter to be measured should be made clear, explicitly or implicitly, from the statement of study objectives. For some studies, the object of measurement may be just an incidence rate or some other measure of disease frequency in a population. For many studies, the object of measurement is the effect of some agent or characteristic, and the parameter of interest is either the difference or ratio of incidence between those exposed and those unexposed to the study factor. If the study is a complicated one for which the objectives are, for example, to evaluate the extent to which the carcinogenic action of tobacco smoke on the oral mucosa is influenced by chronic consumption of alcohol, it is necessary to mention explicitly the parameter to be used (some index of interaction), since epidemiologists have not yet reached accord on how such interactions are ideally measured. If the study objectives are more straightforward, perhaps to evaluate the extent to which daily aspirin intake decreases risk for a first myocardial infarction, it is safe to presume that the object of measurement will be some comparison (by difference or ratio) of either incidence rate or cumulative incidence. The initial premise that something is being measured programs the analysis of the study and the presentation of the data to proceed along specific lines.

As a reviewer or reader of an epidemiologic study, one's first priority is to scrutinize the statement of study objectives to learn the object of measurement of the study. As an epidemiologic author, one's first priority is to state the objectives of the study clearly and quantitatively so that the parameter to be measured is certain. Any study with poorly conceptualized objectives is ipso facto a poor study. The process of refining a statement of objectives that has been vaguely cast sharpens not only the statement of objectives itself but the insights of the investigator or reader.

The overall goal of an epidemiologic study is accuracy in measurement: to estimate the value of the parameter that is the object of measurement with little error. Sources of error in measurement may be classified as either *random* or *systematic*. The principles of study design emerge from consideration of approaches to reducing both types of measurement error.

PRECISION (LACK OF RANDOM ERROR)

Precision in epidemiologic measurements corresponds to the reduction of random error. Precision can be improved in two ways: The primary means is to increase the size of the study; precision can also be improved by modifying the design of the study to increase the efficiency with which information is obtained from a given number of study subjects.

What exactly is random error? Many people believe that chance plays a fundamental role in all physical and, by implication, biologic phenomena. For some the belief in chance is so dominant that it vaults random occurrences into an important role as component causes of all we experience. Others believe that causality may be viewed as deterministic, meaning that a full elaboration of the relevant factors in a given set of circumstances leads unwaveringly, on sufficient analysis, to a perfect prediction of effects resulting from these causes. Under the latter view, all experience is predestined to unravel in a theoretically predictable way that follows inexorably from the previous pattern of actions. Even with this extreme deterministic view, however, the possibility of acquiring sufficient knowledge to predict effects perfectly in any but trivial cause-effect patterns is negligible. Unpredictability of determined outcomes makes them indistinguishable from random occurrences. A unifying description of unpredictability can be forged that equates random error with ignorance about determinants. In short, random error is that part of our experience that we cannot predict. In principle, predicting the outcome of a tossed coin represents a physical problem the solution of which is feasible through the application of physical laws. Inadequate information usually makes the result of such predictions indistinguishable from random guesswork. Whether the sources of variation that we cannot explain are actually due to chance or not makes little difference: We treat such variation as being due to chance until we can explain it, and thereby reduce it, by relating it to known factors.

In an epidemiologic study, random error has many components, but a major contributor is the process of selecting the specific study subjects. This process is usually referred to as *sampling;* the attendant random error is known as *sampling error.* Case-control studies literally involve a sampling process, but all epidemiologic studies, including follow-up studies, which do not involve actual sampling of subjects, are said to have sampling error. The explanation is that the subjects in a study, whether literally sampled or not, are viewed as a figurative sample of possible people who could have been included in the study. The study subjects are a sampling of the biologic experience of a broader conceptual population. For this reason, the statistical dictum that there is no sampling error if an entire population, as opposed to a sample of it, is studied does not apply to epidemiologic studies, even if an entire population is included in the study. Conceptually, the actual subjects are always a sample.

Study Size

The primary way to reduce random error, or increase precision, in an epidemiologic study is to enlarge the size of the study. One method used to assess the adequacy of the size of a study is to calculate study size based on statistical "sample size" formulas [Schlesselman, 1974; Rothman and Boice, 1982]. These formulas relate the size of study to the following variables:

1. Level of "statistical significance" (alpha-error)
2. Chance of missing a real effect (beta-error)
3. Magnitude of effect
4. Disease rate in the absence of exposure (or exposure prevalence in the absence of disease)
5. Relative size of the compared groups (i.e., ratio of exposed to unexposed subjects, or of cases to controls)

Study size formulas specify the size necessary to detect an effect of postulated magnitude at a given significance level, beta-error, and so on. The quantitative allure of such calculations bestows on them a false rigor that can be misleading. Investigators may be too easily enticed into believing that the precise appearance of a size calculation pinpoints the demarcation between study sizes worth contemplating and those that are insufficiently large. In reality, no such demarcation exists. The significance level is completely arbitrary; so is the beta-error. Even if these are set at conventional values, how is the magnitude of effect determined? It is determined by an arbitrary judgment unless research on the study question is already quite solid, in which case the study will not add much. Similarly, estimating the exposure prevalence or disease rate is often a matter of guesswork. With all these arbitrary decisions and estimates, the number arrived at by calculation from formulas is subject to considerable manipulation, as all shrewd investigators know.

A slightly more informative method for assessing desirable study size is by the use of *power* calculations. Power is the complement to the beta-error: It is the probability of detecting (as "statistically significant") a postulated level of effect. For a nonzero effect, the power of a study increases toward 1.0 as the study size increases. Power curves, plotting power versus size, may easily be constructed for different levels of postulated effect.

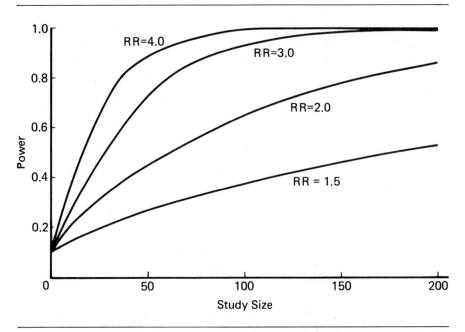

Fig. 7-1. Power curves for a case-control study with an equal number of cases and controls (Alpha = 0.1; exposure prevalence = 0.3).

Such curves give an indication of the informativeness of a contemplated study of a specific size and are thereby more useful in planning a study than a sample size calculation, although the same equation, with algebraic manipulation, can be used to calculate either power or size.

A family of power curves used in planning a study to detect different values of relative risk might look like that shown in Figure 7-1. These curves indicate the power of a study of a given size to detect (as "statistically significant") the effect values indicated. The curves in Figure 7-1 also show graphically the extent to which the study size must be increased to achieve greater power at various levels of relative risk. The use of power curves, while more informative than mere study size calculations, shares some of the same drawbacks. Examining families of curves rather than a single number for a specified power and level of effect reduces much of the arbitrariness in the planning process, but the arbitrariness of the reliance on a given level of "statistical significance" is still present. The superficiality of the concept of "statistical significance" in epidemiologic application will be examined later; for now, it is sufficient to emphasize that, whereas in a power or size calculation a study is classified as either "successful" or "unsuccessful" in determining that an effect is "statistically significant," it is inappropriate to consider "nonsignificant" studies to be totally uninformative or even in "error" (as in beta-error). Many oversimplications are inherent in this calculational approach to planning: Issues of dose-response, confounding, misclassification, interaction, and others are generally ignored in any size or power calculation, and yet such issues can greatly affect the informativeness of a study, rendering the judgments based on size calculation or even power curves superficial.

The essential deficiency in study size or power considerations can be viewed as a sidestepping of the issue that is the focus of this section, namely, precision. The fundamental interest of the scientist is in measurement, and precision in measurement implies an ability to obtain replicate values that differ little because the random error that affects them is small. Concern about precision is concern about the random variability of one's measure. It is well known that one can increase precision by increasing study size, but the concept of reducing variability in measurement is obscured in power or study size calculations, which focus on detection and statistical testing rather than on precision in measurement. These concepts are only indirectly related to precision. For example, power calculations cannot be performed when there is no relation postulated between exposure and disease (and therefore there is nothing to "detect"); nevertheless, the issue of precision is no less important to the investigator in planning a study when the investigator anticipates the possibility that the effect may be zero.

A more satisfactory approach to estimating study precision is to postulate the study data and calculate the precision of effect estimates just as one would in the data analysis, by using confidence intervals. This approach, like power or sample size calculations, requires some arbitrary assumptions about the magnitude of the effect and the level of confidence, but it has some clear advantages. First, it is feasible even for zero effects. Second, it liberates the investigator from thinking about "statistical significance" in study planning.

There is, in addition, a deeper sense in which all judgments in planning study size are arbitrary. The considerations in determining study size discussed so far are all technical ones that fail to take into account the value of the information obtained. The focal decision in planning study size, and consequently study precision, is determining how to balance the value of greater precision in study results against the greater cost. The decision amounts to a cost-benefit analysis of expending greater effort or funds to gain greater precision. The greater precision has a value to the beneficiaries of the research, but the value is indeterminate, since it is always uncertain how many beneficiaries there will be, now and later. Consequently, the cost-benefit problem is not soluble; only informal guesses as to a cost-efficient size for an epidemiologic study are feasible. Such guesses may incorporate information from power curves about the planned study but also involve intricacies of many social, political, and biologic factors that are not mere technical considerations that can be plugged into an equation. In the final analysis, the question of the most appropriate study size is not a technical decision to be determined by calculation but a judgment to be determined by experience, intuition, and insight.

Study Efficiency

A follow-up study of 100,000 men to determine the magnitude, if any, of the reduction in cardiovascular mortality due to daily aspirin consumption might be considered a study with good precision because it is so large. If we learn, however, that only 100 of the men take aspirin daily, we must revise this view, because the information from these 100 exposed subjects will not be substantial, despite the fact that there are 99,900 comparison subjects. If we learned that all the men were between the ages of 30 and 39, we would also revise our view of the study's precision because little information on cardiovascular disease is obtainable from men under 40 years of age. If those taking aspirin were all 40 to 49 years old but the others were all over age 50, then the efficiency of the study might be severely handicapped, depending on how the nonoverlapping age distributions were handled in the analysis.

A variety of design aspects affect study efficiency and in turn affect the precision of study results. These factors include the proportion of subjects exposed, the proportion of subjects who have or will develop disease, and the distributions of subjects according to key variables that must be controlled in the analysis.

Study efficiency can be judged on two different scales. One relates the total information content of the data to the total number of subjects (or amount of person-time experience) in the study. The other relates the total information content to the costs of acquiring that information. Some options in study design improve the information content per subject studied but only at an increased cost; individual matching is an example of this. The question of efficiency is addressed better by judging the information against its cost rather than against the number of subjects studied, which is in itself not of primary interest.

VALIDITY (LACK OF SYSTEMATIC ERROR)

The validity of a study is usually separated into two components: the validity of the inferences drawn as they pertain to the actual subjects in the study *(internal validity)*; and the validity of the inferences as they pertain to people outside the study population *(external validity* or *generalizability)*. Under such a scheme, internal validity is clearly a prerequisite for external validity. The dichotomization of validity in this way may have infelicitous implications for the inferential process, since it seems to emphasize a mechanical approach of "applying" study results to "target populations" for the process of scientific generalization. A more appropriate view, described below, is one in which the essence of scientific generalization is the formulation of abstract concepts relating the study factors, concepts that are not themselves tied to specific populations. Internal validity in a study is still a prerequisite for the study to contribute usefully to this process of abstraction, but the generalization process is otherwise separate from the concerns of internal validity and the mechanics of the study design. The terminology of internal and external validity is used here, but this separateness in the two processes should be borne in mind.

Internal Validity

Internal validity implies validity of inference for the study subjects themselves. Specifically, it implies an accurate measurement apart from random errors. Various types of biases can detract from internal validity; Sackett [1979] has listed dozens of possible biases that can distort the estimation of an epidemiologic measure. The distinction among these biases is occasionally difficult to make, but three general types can be identified: selection bias, information bias, and confounding. These categories are not always clearly demarcated; factors that appear to be responsible for a selection bias can also be viewed, under some circumstances, as confounding factors. Information biases can also be construed as confounding. A useful practical distinction between confounding and other biases is to consider a bias confounding if it can be controlled in the data analysis; methods used to deal with biases are discussed in Chapter 8..

SELECTION BIAS

The essential feature of an epidemiologic study is a comparison of two or more groups for disease or exposure frequency. A selection bias is a distortion of the effect measured; it results from procedures used to select subjects that lead to an effect estimate among subjects included in the study different from the estimate obtainable from the entire population theoretically targeted for study.

One form of such bias is *self-selection* bias. When the Centers for Disease Control (CDC) investigated subsequent leukemia incidence among troops who had been present at the Smoky Atomic Test in Nevada [Caldwell et al., 1980], 76 percent of the troops identified as members of that cohort were traced. Of those traced, 82 percent were tracked down by the investigators, but 18 percent of the subjects "traced" contacted the investigators on their own initiative in response to publicity about the investigation. This self-referral of subjects is ordinarily considered a threat to validity, since the reasons for self-referral may be associated with the outcome under study [Criqui et al., 1979]. In the Smoky study, there were four leukemia cases among the 18 percent of subjects who referred themselves and four among the 82 percent of subjects traced by the investigators, indicating that self-referral was indeed a problem in the study.

Self-selection can also occur before subjects are identified for study. For example, it is routine to find that the mortality of active workers is less than that of the population as a whole [McMichael, 1976; Fox and Collier,

1976]. This "healthy-worker effect" presumably derives from a screening process, perhaps largely self-selection, that allows relatively healthy people to become or remain workers, whereas those who remain unemployed, retired, disabled, or otherwise out of the active worker population are as a group less healthy.

Another type of selection bias occurring before subjects are identified for study is *diagnostic bias* [Sackett, 1979]. When the relation between oral contraceptives and venous thromboembolism was first investigated with case-control studies of hospitalized patients, there was concern that some of the women had been hospitalized with a diagnosis of venous thromboembolism because their physicians suspected a relation between this disease and oral contraceptives and had known about oral contraceptive use in patients who presented with suggestive symptoms [Sartwell et al., 1969]. A study of hospitalized patients with thromboembolism could lead to an exaggerated estimate of the effect of oral contraceptives on thromboembolism if the hospitalization and determination of the diagnosis were influenced by the history of oral-contraceptive use.

Many varieties of selection bias could be described. The common element of such biases is that the relation between exposure and disease is different for those who participate and those who would be theoretically eligible for study but do not participate [Greenland, 1977]. The central issue was aptly summarized by Greenland:*

Selection bias is a theoretical possibility whenever correlates of the outcome capable of influencing study participation are existent in some individuals at the beginning of the study. These correlates may be unmeasured or even unrecognized by the investigator. The question then arises, what is the actual likelihood of an important bias effect existing in a given study situation? Answering this question involves using subject matter knowledge to derive an epidemiologic judgment of the "reasonableness" of the existence of such a bias.

INFORMATION BIAS

Once the series to be compared have been identified, the information to be compared must be obtained. Bias in evaluating an effect can occur from errors in obtaining the needed information. Information bias can occur whenever there are errors in the classification of subjects, but the consequences of the bias are different depending on whether the classification error on one axis of classification (either exposure or disease) is independent of the classification on the other axis. The existence of classification errors that are not independent of the other axis is referred to as *differential misclassification,* whereas the existence of classification errors for either exposure or disease that are independent of the other axis is considered *nondifferential misclassification.*

*Greenland was writing about follow-up studies, but if the "outcome" in case-control studies is considered to be exposure, then the point applies equally well to case-control studies.

Suppose a follow-up study were undertaken to compare incidence rates of emphysema among smokers and nonsmokers. Emphysema is a disease that may go undiagnosed without unusual medical attention. If smokers, because of concern about health-related effects of smoking or as a consequence of other health effects of smoking (such as bronchitis), seek medical attention to a greater degree than nonsmokers, then emphysema might be diagnosed more frequently among smokers than among nonsmokers simply as a consequence of the greater medical attention. Unless steps were taken to ensure comparable follow-up, an information bias would result: An "excess" of emphysema incidence would be found among smokers compared with nonsmokers that is unrelated to any biologic effect of smoking. This is an example of differential misclassification, since the underdiagnosis of emphysema, a misclassification error, occurs more frequently for nonsmokers than for smokers. Sackett [1979] has described it as a diagnostic bias, but unlike the diagnostic bias in the studies of oral contraceptives and thromboembolism described earlier, it is not a selection bias, since it occurs among subjects already included in the study. Nevertheless, the similarities between some selection biases and differential misclassification biases are worth noting.

In case-control studies of congenital malformations, the etiologic information may be obtained at interview from mothers of malformed babies, with mothers of healthy babies as controls. Another variety of differential misclassification, referred to as *recall bias,* can result if the mothers of malformed infants recall exposures more thoroughly than mothers of healthy infants. It is supposed that the birth of a malformed infant serves as a stimulus to a mother to recall all events that might have played some role in the unfortunate outcome. Presumably such women will remember exposures such as infectious disease, trauma, and drugs more accurately than mothers of healthy infants, who have not had a comparable stimulus. Consequently, information on such exposures will be ascertained more frequently from mothers of malformed babies, and an apparent effect, unrelated to any biologic effect, will result from this recall bias. Recall bias is a possibility in any case-control study that uses an anamnestic response, since the cases and controls by definition are people who differ with respect to their disease experience, and this difference may affect recall. Klemetti and Saxen [1967] found that the amount of time lapsed between the exposure and the recall was a more important indicator of the accuracy of recall; studies in which the average time since exposure was different for interviewed cases and controls would thus suffer a differential misclassification.

Differential misclassification can result in an information bias that exaggerates or underestimates an effect. In the examples above, the misclassification serves to exaggerate the effects under study, but examples to the contrary are not hard to imagine.

Another type of misclassification problem can occur when an exposure

Table 7-1. The effect of nondifferential misclassification
of alcohol consumption on the estimation of the incidence
rate difference and ratio for laryngeal cancer (hypothetical data)

	Incidence rate ($\times 10^5$ yr)	Rate difference ($\times 10^5$ yr)	Rate ratio
No misclassification			
1,000,000 drinkers	50		
500,000 teetotalers	10	40	5.0
Half of drinkers classed with teetotalers			
500,000 drinkers	50		
1,000,000 "teetotalers" (50 percent are actually drinkers)	30	20	1.7
Half of drinkers classed with teetotalers and one-third of teetotalers classed with drinkers			
666,667 "drinkers" (25 percent are actually teetotalers)	40		
833,333 "teetotalers" (60 percent are actually drinkers)	34	6	1.2

or disease classification is incorrect for equal proportions of subjects in the compared groups. Such *nondifferential* misclassification has generally been considered a lesser threat to validity than differential misclassification, since the bias introduced by nondifferential misclassification is always in a predictable direction: toward the null condition [Bross, 1954; Copeland et al., 1977]. As an example, consider a follow-up study comparing the incidence of laryngeal cancer among drinkers of alcohol with the incidence among teetotalers. Assume that drinkers actually have an incidence of 0.00050 yr^{-1}, whereas teetotalers have an incidence of 0.00010 yr^{-1}, only one-fifth as great. Let us assume that two-thirds of the study population consists of drinkers, but only 50 percent of them acknowledge it. The result is a population in which one-third of subjects are identified (correctly) as drinkers and have an incidence of disease of 0.00050 yr^{-1}, but the remaining two-thirds of the population consists of equal numbers of drinkers and nondrinkers, among whom the average incidence would be 0.00030 yr^{-1} rather than 0.00010 yr^{-1} (Table 7-1). The effect, if estimated in absolute terms, has been reduced by misclassification from 0.00040 yr^{-1} to 0.00020 yr^{-1}; in relative terms the incidence ratio has been reduced from 5 to 1.7. This bias toward the null value results from nondifferential misclassification of some alcohol drinkers as nondrinkers. The misclassification can occur simultaneously in both directions; that is, teetotalers might also be incorrectly classified as drinkers. In the example, if in addition to half of the drinkers being misclassified as teetotalers, one-third of the teetotalers were also misclassified as drinkers, the resulting incidence rates would be 0.00040 yr^{-1} for the "drinkers" and 0.00034 yr^{-1} for the "teetotalers." The additional misclassification has almost completely wiped out the difference between the groups.

When an effect exists, bias from nondifferential misclassification of exposure always is in the direction of the null value. Nondifferential misclassification of disease is slightly more complicated. In case-control studies, in which subjects are selected initially according to whether or not they have disease, nondifferential misclassification of disease status again introduces a bias toward the null value. In follow-up studies, however, the effect of nondifferential misclassification depends on which measure of effect is being estimated and in which direction the misclassification occurs—that is, overascertainment or underascertainment. Underascertainment is more usual. If only a proportion of actual cases are ascertained, but this proportion is equal for exposed and unexposed groups and there is no overascertainment, the rate ratio measure is unaffected. The rate difference measure, however, will be biased toward the null value; specifically, the estimate will be equal to the unbiased value multiplied by the proportion of cases ascertained. With overascertainment, the cases of interest are diluted with additional subjects who do not have disease. If such subjects are added proportionally to the size of the total exposed and unexposed denominators, this should in principle result in no change in the estimate of rate difference but in a bias toward the null value for the rate ratio.

Since the bias from nondifferential misclassification is always in the direction of the null value, historically it has not been a great source of concern to epidemiologists, who have generally considered it more acceptable to underestimate effects than to overestimate effects. Nevertheless, nondifferential misclassification is a serious problem: The bias it introduces possibly accounts for many discrepancies among epidemiologic studies. Many studies ascertain information in a way that guarantees substantial misclassification. For example, suppose aspirin transiently reduces risk of myocardial infarction. The word *transiently* implies a brief induction period. Any study that considered as exposure aspirin use outside of a narrow time interval before the occurrence of a myocardial infarction would be misclassifying aspirin use: There is relevant use of aspirin, and there is use of aspirin that is irrelevant because it does not allow the exposure to act causally under the causal hypothesis with its specified induction period. Many studies ask about "ever use" (use at any time during an individual's life) of drugs or other exposures. Such cumulative indices over an individual's lifetime inevitably augment possibly relevant exposure with irrelevant exposure, thus introducing a bias toward the null value through nondifferential misclassification.

In follow-up studies in which there are disease categories with few subjects, investigators are occasionally tempted to combine outcome categories to increase the number of subjects in each analysis, thereby gaining precision. This collapsing of categories is a serious mistake. The gain in precision comes at the cost of an almost guaranteed bias in rate ratio estimation, a bias that may make study results uninterpretable or lead to misinterpretations. For example, Smithells and Shepard [1978] investigated the teratogenicity of the drug Bendectin, a drug indicated for nausea of pregnancy. Because only 35 babies in their follow-up study were born with a malformation, their analysis was focused on the single outcome, "malformation." But no teratogen causes all malformations; if such an analysis fails to find an effect, the failure may simply be the result of the grouping of many malformations not related to Bendectin with those that are. In fact, despite the authors' claim that "their study provides substantial evidence that Bendectin is not teratogenic in man," their data indicated a strong (though imprecise) relation between Bendectin and cardiac malformations. Unwarranted assurances of a lack of effect can easily emerge from studies in which a wide range of etiologically unrelated outcomes are grouped.

To some extent, nondifferential misclassification introduces a bias toward the null value in virtually every epidemiologic study. Such bias is a greater concern in interpreting studies that seem to indicate the absence of an effect. Consequently, in studies that indicate little or no effect, it is crucial for the researchers to consider the problem of nondifferential misclassification to determine to what extent a real effect might have been obscured. On the other hand, in studies that describe a strong nonzero effect, preoccupation with nondifferential misclassification is unwarranted. Occasionally critics of a study will argue that poor exposure data (or a poor disease classification) invalidate the results, but this argument is incorrect if the results indicate a nonzero effect. True, such misclassification can introduce a bias, but the bias is always in the direction of underestimating the effect.

The importance of appreciating the direction of bias from nondifferential misclassification was illustrated by the interpretation of a study on spermicides and birth defects [Jick et al., 1981]. This study reported an increased prevalence of several types of congenital disorder among women who were identified as having filled a prescription for spermicides during a specified interval before the birth. The exposure information was only a rough correlate of the actual use of spermicides during a theoretically relevant time period, but the misclassification that resulted was nondifferential, since the prescription information was recorded on a computer log before the outcome was known. One of the criticisms raised about the study was that inaccuracies in the exposure information cast doubt on the validity of the findings [Felarca et al., 1981; Oakley, 1982]. Whatever bias was present on this account, however, led to an underestimation of any real effect, so this criticism is inappropriate [Jick et al., 1981a].

Generally speaking, it is incorrect to dismiss a study reporting an effect simply because there is substantial nondifferential misclassification, since an estimate of effect without the misclassification would be even greater, provided that the misclassification applies uniformly to all subjects. Thus, the implications of nondifferential misclassification depend heavily on whether the study is perceived as "positive" or "negative." Emphasis on measurement instead of on a qualitative description of study results lessens the likelihood for misinterpretation, but even so it is important to bear in mind the direction and likely magnitude of a bias.

CONFOUNDING

The concept of confounding is a central one in modern epidemiology. Although confounding occurs in experimental research, it is a considerably more important issue in nonexperimental research. Consequently, the understanding of the concept has developed only recently in parallel with the growth of nonexperimental research. It will be convenient to describe confounding first in respect to its main features and then gradually lead into a more refined definition.

On the simplest level, confounding may be considered a mixing of effects. Specifically, the estimate of the effect of the exposure of interest is distorted because it is mixed with the effect of an extraneous factor. The distortion introduced by a confounding factor can be large, and it can lead to overestimation or underestimation of an effect depending on the direction of the associations that the confounding factor has with exposure and disease. Confounding can even change the apparent direction of an effect.

The notion of an extraneous factor changing the direction of an association has been noted as "Simpson's Paradox." Suppose a man enters a shop to buy a hat and finds a table of 30 hats, 10 black and 20 gray. He discovers that 9 of the 10 black hats fit, but only 17 of the 20 gray hats fit. Thus, he notes that the proportion of black hats that fit is 90 percent compared with 85 percent of the gray hats. At another table in the same shop, he finds another 30 hats, 20 black and 10 gray. At this table, 3 (15 percent) of the black hats fit, but only 1 (10 percent) of the gray hats fit. Before he chooses a hat, the shop closes for the evening, so he returns the following morning. Overnight the clerk has piled all the hats on the same table: Now there are 30 of each color. The shopper remembers that yesterday the proportion of black hats that fit was greater at each of the two tables. Today he finds that, though all the same hats are displayed, when mixed together only 40 percent (12 of 30) of the black hats fit, whereas 60 percent (18 of 30) of the gray hats fit. Though this curious reversal is referred to as Simpson's Paradox, the phenomenon is not really a paradox; neither logic nor any of the premises are contravened. The phenomenon is analogous to confounding, which can distort an association even to the extent that its direction is reversed [Rothman, 1975].

For an extraneous factor to be a confounder, it must have an effect, that is, the factor must be predictive of the occurrence of disease. The effect need not be causal; frequently only a correlate of a causal factor is identified as a confounding factor. A common example is social class, which itself is presumably causally related to few if any diseases but is a correlate of many causes of disease. Similarly, some would claim that age, which is related to nearly every disease, is itself only an artificial marker of more fundamental biologic changes. In this view, age is not a causal risk factor but nevertheless is a potential confounding factor in many situations.

An extraneous risk factor is confounding only if its effect becomes mixed with the effect under study. (Confounding can occur even if the factor under study has zero effect. "Mixing of effects" is not intended to imply that the exposure under study has a nonzero effect. On the other hand, if the extraneous factor has no effect—that is, if it is not associated with the disease, it will not cause any distortion in the estimate of the effect of exposure.) The mixing of the effects comes about from an association between the exposure and the extraneous factor. For example, consider a study to determine whether alcohol drinkers experience a greater incidence of oral cancer than teetotalers. Smoking is an extraneous factor that is related to the disease (smoking has an effect on oral cancer incidence); it is also associated with alcohol drinking, since there are many people who are general "abstainers," refraining from alcohol consumption, smoking, and perhaps other habits. Consequently, alcohol drinkers include among them a greater proportion of smokers than would be found among nondrinkers. Since smoking increases the incidence of oral cancer, alcohol drinkers will have a greater incidence than nondrinkers quite apart from any influence of alcohol drinking itself but simply as a consequence of the greater amount of smoking among alcohol drinkers. Thus, the apparent effect of alcohol drinking is distorted by the effect of smoking; the two effects are intermixed in the single comparison of alcohol drinkers with nondrinkers. The degree of bias or distortion depends on the magnitude of the smoking effect as well as on the strength of association between alcohol and smoking. Either absence of a smoking effect on oral cancer incidence or absence of an association between smoking and alcohol would lead to no confounding. Smoking must be associated with both oral cancer and alcohol drinking for it to be a confounding factor.

To put it in general terms, a confounding factor must be associated with both the exposure under study and the disease under study to be confounding. It is necessary, however, to make some restrictions on this broad characterization of the two defining associations of a confounding factor.

If the exposure under study has an effect, then any correlate of that exposure will also be associated with the disease as a consequence of its association with a risk factor for the disease. For example, suppose frequent beer consumption is associated with the consumption of pizza, and suppose that frequent beer consumption is a risk factor for rectal cancer. Would consumption of pizza be a confounding factor? At first it might seem that the answer is yes, since consumption of pizza is associated both with beer drinking and with rectal cancer. But if pizza consumption is associated with rectal cancer only secondarily to its association with beer consumption, it would not be confounding. A confounding factor must be predictive of disease occurrence apart from its association with exposure; that is, even among nonexposed individuals, the potentially confounding variate should be related to disease risk. If consumption of pizza were predictive of rectal cancer among nondrinkers of beer, then it would be confounding. If it is associated with rectal cancer only from its association with beer drinking, it is not confounding. (The situation in which a variate is a risk factor for disease only among exposed individuals is one of interaction between the exposure and the other variable. This topic is addressed in Chapter 15; it does not produce a bias.)

Analogously with this restriction on the association between a potential confounder and disease, the potential confounder should be associated with the exposure among the source population for cases, not merely among cases of the disease as a consequence of both variables being risk factors for disease.

It is also important to clarify what is meant by the term *extraneous* in the phrase "extraneous risk factor." This term implies that the predictiveness for disease risk involves a mechanism other than the one under study. Specifically, consider a causal mechanism where

$$[\text{exposure}] \xrightarrow{\text{causes}} [\text{altered physiology}] \xrightarrow{\text{causes}} [\text{disease}]$$

Is a variable measuring the altered physiologic state a confounding factor? It is certainly a risk factor for disease, and it is also correlated with exposure, since it results from exposure. It is even a risk factor for disease among nonexposed individuals, presuming that the altered physiology can result from causes other than the exposure in question. Nevertheless, it should not be considered confounding, since the effect of the exposure is mediated through the effect of the altered physiology. In this example, there is no mixing of effects: There is only the one effect. (Other causes of altered physiology, however, if correlated with the exposure, would be confounders.) Any factor that represents a step in the causal chain between exposure and disease is not a confounding factor.

Usually, an explicit mechanism for the causal action of the exposure has not been postulated. How, then, can an investigator decide if a factor is confounding or not? Such decisions must be made on the basis of the best available information seasoned by expert judgment. Profound uncertainties about mechanism can justify the handling of a potential confounding factor as both confounding and not confounding in different analyses. For example, in evaluating the effect of a fatty diet on cancer risk, it is unclear how to treat serum cholesterol levels. It seems to be a risk factor for cancer, and it is associated with a fatty diet, but possibly it mediates the action of a fatty diet on cancer risk; that is, perhaps it is an intermediate factor in the same etiologic sequence. In the face of uncertainty, one might consider serum cholesterol levels as confounding and evaluate the effect of a fatty diet on cancer risk mediated other than by serum cholesterol (by controlling confounding by serum cholesterol), in addition to considering it as an intermediate cause and consequently evaluating the effect of a fatty diet ignoring serum cholesterol in the analysis.

At this point we can consider a more refined definition of confounding. The essential concept is the superimposition of the effect of an extraneous risk factor on the estimated relation between the exposure under study and the disease outcome. To be confounding, the extraneous variable must have the following three characteristics:

1. A confounding variable must be a risk factor for the disease.

The potential confounding variable need not be an actual cause of the disease, but if it is not it must be a marker for an actual cause of the disease or the diagnosis of the disease. The association between the potential confounder and the disease should not derive only secondarily from an association with the exposure, which may be a cause of the disease. Therefore, a confounding variable should be a risk factor even among people who lack the exposure under study. Furthermore, a confounding factor should be a risk factor for disease among nonexposed individuals even after controlling for other known confounders.

It has been suggested that the certainty with which a variable is considered a risk factor for disease should, in principle, be based on a priori knowledge [Miettinen and Cook, 1981]. According to this view, the data may serve as a guide to the relation between the potential confounder and the disease, but it is the actual relation between the potentially confounding variate and disease, not the relation observed in the data, that determines whether confounding can occur. In large studies, the data will more closely reflect the underlying relation, but in small studies the data are a less reliable guide.

The following examples illustrate the role that prior knowledge is proposed to play in evaluating confounding. In a study of occupational exposures and lung cancer, if the data indicate no relation between smoking and lung cancer, this absence of a relation does not mean that smoking was not confounding the effect of occupational exposures in the study. Similarly, if in a study of sunlight exposure and melanoma, a priori knowledge suggests that there is no relation between gum chewing and melanoma occurrence, gum chewing should not be considered a confounding factor regardless of its association with melanoma in the study. In practice, investigators usually rely heavily on their data to infer the relation of a potential confounding factor to disease, since prior knowledge is often inadequate. For example, a cause of disease will be unrelated to disease in populations that lack complementary component causes. A discordance between the data and prior knowledge about a suspected or known risk factor may therefore signal an inadequacy in the detail of prior knowledge rather than in the data. Similarly, prior knowledge about the absence of an effect for a possible risk factor may be inadequate if based on studies with considerable nondifferential misclassification, or on studies conducted in populations lacking essential complementary component causes (i.e., susceptibility factors). On the other hand, it is also conceivable that prior knowledge about the absence of an effect could be based upon convictions firm enough to override any evidence to the contrary in the data. Thus, those selected in the draft lottery would presumably have the same risk for disease as those not selected, since the selection was a random sampling; based on this prior knowledge, selection in the draft lottery would not confound any exposure-disease relation even if it appeared to do so in a body of data.

2. A confounding variable must be associated with the exposure under study in the population from which the cases derive.

The association between a potential confounding variable and the exposure must not derive secondarily from the association between the exposure and disease. In a follow-up study measuring risk, this proviso implies only that the association between the potential confounding variable and the exposure must be present among subjects followed. In a follow-up study measuring incidence rates, the association must be present with respect to the person-time experience of the subjects. Thus, in follow-up studies the exposure-confounder association can be evaluated from the data in hand and does not even theoretically depend on prior knowledge.

In a case-control study, the proviso implies that the association must be present in the source population or person-time experience that gave rise to the cases and from which the controls were sampled. If the control series is large, it should provide a reasonable guide to the existence of the association between the potential confounding variable and the exposure. Nevertheless, the ultimate concern focuses on the degree of association between the potential confounder and the exposure in the source population that produced the study cases, of which the controls are only a sample. In principle, a priori knowledge about the source population determines whether confounding exists in a case-control study [Miettinen and Cook, 1981]. Unfortunately, reliable a priori information about the association between risk factors in specific populations is seldom available. Thus, in practice, even in case-control studies, the data in hand will usually have to serve for the evaluation of the association between the exposure and the potentially confounding variable.

In a follow-up study of occupational exposure and lung cancer, if smoking were unassociated with the occupational exposure in the study cohorts, then it would not be confounding. Neither would it be confounding in a nested case-control study conducted within the same population, even if the control series evinced an association between smoking and the occupational exposure. Since the source population did not have an association between smoking and the occupational exposure, exposed subjects did not face a greater risk for lung cancer because of smoking, and smoking was not confounding. As another example, consider a randomized experiment: Every risk factor has, as an expectation, zero association with the exposure. Nevertheless, if in the actual randomization it happens that an identified risk factor is, despite the randomization, associated with the exposure, it will be a confounding factor in the experiment.

3. A confounding variable must not be an intermediate step in the causal path between the exposure and the disease.

This criterion requires information outside the data. The investigator must decide whether the causal mechanism that might follow from exposure to disease would include the potentially confounding factor as an intermediate step. If so, the variable is not a confounder.

It is important to remember that confounding is a bias and therefore must be considered and dealt with as a quantitative problem. It is the amount of confounding rather than mere presence or absence that is important to evaluate. Methods to evaluate confounding quantitatively are described in Chapter 12.

Misclassification can affect confounding variables. If a confounding variable is misclassified, the ability to control confounding in the analysis is hampered [Greenland, 1980]. Nondifferential misclassification of exposure or disease will bias study results in the direction of the null hypothesis, but nondifferential misclassification of a confounding variable attenuates the degree to which confounding can be controlled and thus causes a bias in either direction, depending on the direction of the confounding. For this reason, misclassification of confounding factors can be a serious problem. If the confounding is strong and the exposure-disease relation is weak or zero, misclassification of the confounding factor can lead to extremely misleading results. For example, a strong causal relation between smoking and bladder cancer, coupled with a strong association between smoking and coffee drinking, makes smoking a strong confounder of any possible relation between coffee drinking and bladder cancer. Since the control of confounding by smoking depends on accurate smoking information, and since some misclassification of the relevant smoking information is inevitable no matter how smoking is measured, some residual confounding is inevitable [Morrison, 1982]. The problem of residual confounding would be even worse if the only available information on smoking were a simple dichotomy such as "ever smoked" versus "never smoked," since the lack of detailed specification of smoking prohibits adequate control of confounding. The resulting confounding is especially troublesome because to many investigators and readers it may appear that confounding by smoking has been controlled.

External Validity

The process of generalizing beyond a set of observations requires a judgment about what features of the observations may be extrapolated. Such judgments require an understanding of which conditions are relevant and which are irrelevant to the generalization. The essence of scientific generalization was nicely described by Reichenbach [1951]:

> The essence of knowledge is *generalization*. That fire can be produced by rubbing wood a certain way is a knowledge derived by generalization from individual experiences; the statement means that rubbing wood in this way will *always* produce fire. The art of discovery is therefore the art of correct generalization. What is irrelevant, such as the particular shape or size of the piece of wood used, is to be excluded from the generalization; what is relevant, for example, the dryness of the wood, is to be included in it. The meaning of the term *relevant* can thus be defined: that is relevant which must be mentioned for the generalization to be valid. The separation of relevant from irrelevant factors is the beginning of knowledge.

To consider an epidemiologic example, from a study of smoking and lung cancer in men, one might generalize the results to a target population of women. To do so presumes that being male is irrelevant to the carcinogenic action that smoking has on lung tissue, a judgment based on knowledge about the likely mechanism of carcinogenesis and the biologic similarity between male and female lungs. On the other hand, a study of diet and myocardial infarction in men might not be considered generalizable to women because physiologic difference between the sexes may play a role in the causal process. Determining the validity of a generalization is ultimately a matter of informed judgment.

Some epidemiologists have taught that generalization from a study group depends on the study group being a representative subgroup of the target population, in the sense of a sample. Whereas Reichenbach considered scientific generalization to be an art, others have considered it a mechanical aspect of sampling. Confusion over this point is deeply rooted, as indicated by the use of the term "sample-size" to refer to the number of subjects in a study. If scientific generalization were simply a matter of statistical generalization, it would be limited literally to those individuals who might have been included, through sampling, as study subjects. This misconception has influenced the design of many epidemiologic studies. If the notion were valid, there would be no application to humans of any results obtained from animal research. In addition, every population would require its own set of epidemiologic studies, and these studies would have to be repeated for every new generation.

The tendency to use "representative" study groups probably derives from early experience with surveys for which the inferential process ought to be purely statistical and not scientific. Social scientists often rely on statistical inference because decisions about what is relevant and what is irrelevant for generalization are more difficult in the social sciences, and populations are considerably more diverse in sociologic phenomena than in biologic phenomena. In the biologic sciences, however, investigators conduct experiments using animals with characteristics selected to enhance the validity of the experimental work rather than to represent the target population. Epidemiologic study designs are usually stronger if subject selection is guided by the need to make a valid comparison, which may call for severe restriction of admissible subjects to a narrow range of characteristics, rather than by a futile attempt to make the subjects representative, in a sampling sense, of the potential target populations.

Ultimately, the scientific goal of a study is to contribute to scientific knowledge. The inductive process of synthesizing knowledge from observations is, after centuries of examination, not yet well understood (see Chap. 2). It is clear, however, that the process involves moving from the particulars of a set of observations to the abstraction of a scientific hypothesis or theory. Scientific theories, such as Reichenbach's example about igniting wood, are divorced from time and place: They are abstractions that are, in the philosophic sense, universal statements. The essence of scientific generalization, then, is the process of moving from time- and place-specific observations to an abstract universal statement. This process is neither mechanical nor statistical, nor does it involve specific target populations. In this sense, the term external validity is a misnomer, and the term generalization must be interpreted as abstraction. Study groups that are representative of larger populations in the statistical sense will generally not enhance the ability to abstract universal statements from observations, but study groups selected for characteristics that enable a study to distinguish effectively between competing scientific hypotheses will do so.

REFERENCES

Bross, I. Misclassification in 2 × 2 tables. *Biometrics* 1954;10:478–486.

Caldwell, G. G., Kelley, D. B., and Heath, C. W., Jr. Leukemia among participants in military maneuvers at a nuclear bomb test: A preliminary report. *J.A.M.A.* 1980;244:1575–1578.

Copeland, K. T., Checkoway, H., McMichael, A. J., et al. Bias due to misclassification in the estimation of relative risk. *Am. J. Epidemiol.* 1977;105:488–495.

Criqui, M. H., Austin, M., and Barrett-Connor, E. The effect of non-response on risk ratios in a cardiovascular disease study. *J. Chron. Dis.* 1979;32:633–638.

Felarca, L. C., Wardell, D. M., and Rowles, B. Vaginal spermicides and congenital disorders. *J.A.M.A.* 1981;246:2677.

Fox, A. J., and Collier, P. F. Low mortality rates in industrial cohort studies due to selection for work and survival in the industry. *Br. J. Prev. Soc. Med.* 1976;30:225–230.

Greenland, S. Response and follow-up bias in cohort studies. *Am. J. Epidemiol.* 1977;106:184–187.

Greenland, S. The effect of misclassification in the presence of covariates. *Am. J. Epidemiol.* 1980;112:564–569.

Jick, J., Walker, A. M., Rothman, K. J., et al. Vaginal spermicides and congenital disorders. *J.A.M.A.* 1981;245:1329–1332.

Jick, J., Walker, A. M., Rothman, K. J., et al. Vaginal spermicides and congenital disorders—reply. *J.A.M.A.* 1981a;246:2677–2678.

Klemetti, A., and Saxen, L. Prospective versus retrospective approach in the search for environmental causes of malformations. *Am. J. Public Health* 1967;57:2071–2075.

McMichael, A. J. Standardized mortality ratios and the "healthy worker effect": Scratching beneath the surface. *J. Occup. Med.* 1976;18:165–168.

Miettinen, O. S., and Cook, E. F. Confounding: Essence and detection. *Am. J. Epidemiol.* 1981;114:593–603.

Morrison, A. S., Buring, J. E., Verhoek, W. G., et al. Coffee drinking and cancer of the lower urinary tract. *J. Nat. Cancer Inst.* 1982;68:91–94.

Oakley, G. P., Jr. Spermicides and birth defects. *J.A.M.A.* 1982;247:2405.

Reichenbach, H. *The Rise of Scientific Philosophy.* New York: Harper & Row, 1965.

Rothman, K. J. A pictorial representation of confounding in epidemiologic studies. *J. Chron. Dis.* 1975;28:101–108.

Rothman, K. J., and Boice, J. D., Jr. *Epidemiologic Analysis with a Programmable Calculator* (2nd ed.). Chestnut Hill, Mass.: Epidemiology Resources Inc., 1982.

Sackett, D. L. Bias in analytic research. *J. Chron. Dis.* 1979;32:51–63.

Sartwell, P. E., Masi, A. T., Arthes, F. G., et al. Thromboembolism and oral contraceptives: An epidemiologic case-control study. *Am. J. Epidemiol.* 1969;90:365–380.

Schlesselman, J. J. Sample size requirements in cohort and case-control studies of disease. *Am. J. Epidemiol.* 1974;99:381–384.

Smithells, R. W., and Shepard, S. Teratogenicity testing in humans: A method demonstrating the safety of Bendectin. *Teratology* 1978;17:31–36.

8. STRATEGIES IN THE DESIGN OF EPIDEMIOLOGIC STUDIES

An epidemiologic study is properly viewed as an exercise in measurement, with accuracy as the goal. Design strategies are intended to reduce the sources of error, both systematic and random. Reduction of random error improves the precision of the measurement, whereas reduction of systematic error improves the validity of the measurement.

IMPROVING PRECISION

As described in Chapter 7, the primary way to improve the precision of a study is to study more subjects. Apart from the size of the study, the major design feature affecting study precision is the apportionment of subjects (or person-time units of observation) into study groups. The *efficiency* of a study may be assessed as the amount of information about the effect divided by the number of study subjects (note that *information* is defined in statistics as the reciprocal of variance). When the study factor has no effect, equal apportionment into groups is the most efficient design [Walter, 1977]: For example, in the absence of an effect it is more efficient to have 200,000 person-years of observation apportioned as 100,000 to an exposed group and 100,000 to an unexposed group than to have an apportionment ratio other than unity. Similarly, in a case-control study, in the absence of an effect it is most efficient to have an equal number of cases and controls. In the presence of an effect, the apportionment that is optimum for efficiency differs from equal apportionment by an amount that is a function of the parameters under study [Walter, 1977].

Another view of study efficiency relates the amount of information attained about the effect to the cost of obtaining it regardless of the number of subjects in the study. Often the acquisition cost is disparate for the information in different study groups. For example, retrospective follow-up studies often rely on population data for comparison. Such population data are acquired for a price that is orders of magnitude lower than the information on the exposed cohort. Similarly, in case-control studies, cases may be scarce and therefore expensive to ascertain, whereas controls may be plentiful. In such situations, more information is obtained per unit cost by expanding the comparison series in relation to the index series. The optimal apportionment ratio for cost efficiency has been shown to be approximately equal to the reciprocal of the square root of the cost ratio [Miettinen, 1969]. Thus, if cases cost four times as much as controls, the investigator should plan to include twice as many controls as cases. The "square root" rule has been shown to be strictly applicable only for small or null effects; a more generalized approach to improving cost efficiency that takes into account the conjectured magnitude of the effect and the type of data has been proposed by Morgenstern and Winn [1983]. Their

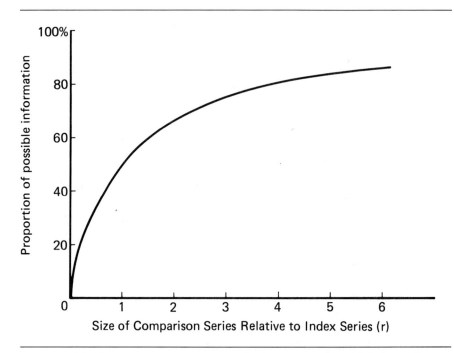

Fig. 8-1. The approximate proportion of information achievable [r/(r + 1)] in a crude comparison for an index series of fixed size according to the size of the comparison series relative to the index series (r).

formulas enable the investigator to optimize the precision of the estimation of effect in a study for a given expenditure.

Occasionally the index series cannot be expanded indefinitely, usually because practical constraints limit the feasibility of extending the study period or area. For such a series, the cost of acquiring additional subjects is essentially infinite, and the only available strategy for acquiring more information is to expand the comparison series. As the size of the comparison series increases relative to that of the index series, the amount of information in the study does not increase proportionally. If *r* is the ratio of the size of the comparison series relative to the index series, the proportion of the theoretically achievable information to be drawn from the index series with varying size comparisons is approximately r/(r + 1) for a crude comparison. Figure 8-1 illustrates the diminishing returns with increasing r.

The figure makes it clear that for a crude comparison there is little point in expending resources to achieve a ratio above 4 or 5, since nearly all the information achievable is already "extracted" from the index series using a comparison series four or five times as big. The only justification for achieving ratios higher than 4 or 5 would be in those circumstances in which the cost of obtaining the additional information was negligible, as it would be, for example, if all the data were already accessible on a computer file that must be read in toto; in such circumstances, there is no reason to ignore usable information that has no real cost, although it should be appreciated that an apportionment ratio of 500 is not much better than 5 with regard to the amount of information that can be obtained.

These arguments apply to crude comparisons in data analysis. What effect does stratification of the data have on efficiency and thus on precision? When data are analyzed according to strata, the essential comparisons are made within the strata. The preceding arguments then apply to the ratio of group sizes within each stratum. A stratum that contains a comparison series 10 times as large as the index series (or vice versa) is likely to be wasteful of information. A study that has a favorable apportionment ratio overall, say 1.0, may have apportionment ratios within strata that vary severely from low to high values: It is not uncommon to see some strata with the extreme apportionment ratios of 0 and infinity. The smaller the numbers within strata, the more extreme the variation in the apportionment ratio is likely to be (the extreme values result from zero subjects or person-time units for one group in a stratum). Small numbers within strata result from having too few subjects relative to the number of strata created; this problem can develop even with large studies, since the number of strata required in the analysis increases geometrically with the number of variables stratified on. Indeed, this problem is the major limitation of stratified analysis.

When stratification is anticipated, it may be sensible to seek an apportionment ratio that is larger than it would be otherwise. If the overall ratio is, say, 2, then stratum-specific values for the ratio may vary from low values, below unity, to high values much greater than 2. Thus, there would be some strata in which many of the index series observations are compared with few of the comparison series observations, whereas in other strata many comparison observations are squandered on few observations in the index series. This poor efficiency can reduce precision considerably. If the overall ratio chosen is 4 or 5, it may shift the stratum-specific ratios so that they all tend to be above unity, making for a considerably more efficient design. An overall ratio of 10 or even greater may be justifiable if considerable variation in the apportionment ratio across strata is anticipated.

Alternatively, precision can be maintained in a stratified analysis by designing the study to guarantee that the apportionment ratio does not vary severely across strata. This goal can be accomplished by selecting comparison subjects, individually or in groups, who have the same distribution with respect to the stratification variables as do the index subjects. This

102

process is known as "matching"; stratification and matching are treated in detail in Chapters 12 and 13.

IMPROVING VALIDITY

Choice of Comparison Groups

In a follow-up study, the comparison group serves to provide an estimate of what the disease incidence would have been in the exposed group had the exposure been absent or without effect. To accomplish this goal, it is not necessary to find an unexposed group that is exactly like the exposed group in every regard except exposure. It is sufficient to find a comparison group that is similar to the exposed group with respect to the important predictors of disease incidence. The comparison group can differ with respect to factors unrelated to disease incidence. In fact, the comparison group can differ even in respect to factors that affect disease incidence if the factors can be measured and adequately adjusted in the data analysis. Some argue that the closer the identity of the compared groups with respect to all measurable factors, the greater the validity, since some factors may affect disease incidence without the investigator's awareness. This view is not really contradictory to the view that the compared groups should be identical for all important predictors of incidence, but it supposes pessimistically that the investigator cannot have sufficient insight into disease etiology to rely on such insight in study design. As a practical matter, groups identical apart from an exposure of interest are not found outside the laboratory and perhaps not even inside one. In nonexperimental research, the investigator must be satisfied with considering only the factors thought to be relevant to disease occurrence. Thus, if it were known that gender did not influence risk for a disease under study, it would be acceptable to compare exposed and unexposed groups with differing distributions by gender.

Typically, the concerns about choice of a comparison group focus on factors that might lead to selection bias. Although confounding factors are also a problem, they can be controlled in the analysis if they are measured. Indeed, a useful conceptual distinction between selection bias and confounding is whether or not the bias can be removed in the analysis. For example, a follow-up study comparing mortality among lumberjacks with mortality among the general population would be subject to the criticism that lumberjacking is an occupation that involves self-selection of fit individuals, who would be expected to have a mortality lower than that of the general population. Such a study could not be considered a valid assessment of the effect of lumberjacking on mortality because of the selection bias. But what if the fitness of an individual who becomes a lumberjack could be measured and compared with the fitness of subjects drawn from the general population? If such a measurement were feasible and if difference in fitness could be controlled in the analysis, the problem of selection bias would be better viewed as one of confounding, which is removable. Since measurements on fitness at entry into a profession are generally unavailable, the investigator's efforts in such a situation would be focused on the choice of a comparison group that would avoid the selection bias. One possibility would be the approach taken by Paffenbarger and Hale [1975] in their study of longshoremen, in which they compared cardiovascular mortality among groups of longshoremen who engaged in different levels of physical activity on the job, on the presumption that the selection factors for entering the occupation were similar for the subgroups who engaged in tasks demanding high or low activity because work assignments are made after entering the profession.

In case-control studies, the control group provides an estimate of the exposure distribution in the source population from which the cases originate. As with follow-up studies, it is not necessary for the comparison group to be identical to the index group with respect to all factors apart from the exposure, but only the relevant factors. To the extent that case selection is influenced by factors that are related to the exposure, the control group should be subject to the same selection factors. Selection factors unrelated to exposure need not be identical for the two series, but again, there is often difficulty in determining which factors are relevant. Since completely identical groups will never be found, the process of determining which factors are relevant in choosing a comparison group is a critical feature of epidemiologic study design.

Selection bias was the central issue in the controversy about the role of exogenous estrogens in causing endometrial cancer. Several case-control studies had reported a strong association, with about a 10-fold increase in risk for women taking estrogens regularly for a number of years [Smith et al., 1975; Ziel and Finkle, 1975; Mack et al., 1976; Antunes et al., 1979]. Most investigators interpreted this increase in risk as a causal relation, but others suggested that estrogens were merely causing the cancers to be diagnosed rather than to occur [Horwitz and Feinstein, 1978]. The argument is premised on the knowledge that estrogens induce uterine bleeding, and therefore administration of estrogens would presumably lead many women to seek medical attention, thus causing a variety of gynecologic conditions to be detected. The resulting bias was referred to as "detection" bias. The remedy that was proposed was to use a control series of women with benign gynecologic diseases that would also be subject to the detection bias rather than a control series of women with other malignant disease, nongynecologic disease, or no disease, as earlier studies had done. The flaw in this reasoning was the incorrect assumption that estrogens caused a substantial proportion of endometrial cancers to be diagnosed that would otherwise have remained undiagnosed. Even if the administration of estrogens advances the date of diagnosis for endometrial cancer, such an advance in the time of diagnosis would not in itself lead to any substantial bias. Presumably a small proportion of pre-existing endometrial cancer cases that otherwise would not have been diagnosed did come to attention, but there is considerable evidence that, like any cancer, endometrial cancer usually progresses to cause symptoms leading to diagnosis. Although a permanent, nonprogressive early stage of endometrial cancer is a possibility, the studies that excluded such in situ cases from the case series still found a strong effect of estrogen administration on cancer risk [Horwitz and Feinstein, 1978; Antunes et al., 1979]. The proposed alternative comparison group, comprised of women with benign gynecologic conditions that generally would not in themselves cause symptoms leading to diagnosis, would provide an overestimate of the proportion of the source population of cases exposed to estrogens, since administration of estrogens would indeed cause the diagnosis of a substantial proportion of the benign conditions [Hutchison and Rothman, 1978]. The use of the control series with benign gynecologic conditions would lead to a selection bias that severely underestimated the effect of exogenous estrogens on risk of endometrial cancer [Greenland and Neutra, 1981]. The main lesson to be learned from this controversy is the importance of considering selection biases quantitatively as much as possible rather than qualitatively. Without appreciation for the magnitude of potential selection biases, the choice of a comparison group can result, as it did in this instance, in a bias so great that an intensely strong association is occluded; alternatively, a negligible association could as easily be exaggerated.

It is not always possible to prevent selection bias by an astute choice of a comparison group. Consider the selection bias inherent in the case-control study of oral contraceptives and thromboembolism. Women with symptoms consistent with thromboembolism were presumably more likely to be referred to a hospital for evaluation if their physicians determined that they were taking oral contraceptives. This selection bias would exaggerate the association between oral contraceptives and thromboembolic disease or falsely produce a positive association. To prevent such bias, one might first consider enrolling into the study a comparison group that was subject to equal selection forces as a consequence of oral contraceptive use. Even if such a group could be conjured up, however, we have already seen the difficulty in attempting to negate selection bias by finding a comparison group for which the selection forces are of the correct magnitude. The easiest way to achieve the goal is to eliminate as much as possible the selection forces related to oral contraceptive use. In this example, one approach would be to define the case series by including only those women whose symptoms and signs met a set of objective diagnostic criteria for thromboembolic disease. By reformulating the diagnostic criteria, cases who might otherwise be included simply because of their history of oral contraceptive use, as opposed to their disease manifestations, would not be included. Then the comparison group could be chosen to determine oral contraceptive use in the source population of cases without regard to selection forces based on the oral contraceptive history elicited by the physician. Of course, if the cases to whom the objective diagnostic criteria were applied included women who had been referred because they used oral contraceptives, the selection bias could not be eliminated in this way.

The identification of controls to be sampled in case-control studies often depends on the availability of a roster such as a directory of residents in a geographic area. Other approaches involve referral by cases, such as friends or neighbors (these approaches are equivalent to matched selection and require a matched analysis), or general sampling such as door-to-door solicitation (also usually on a matched basis). An increasingly popular method of identifying controls is the survey method of random digit dialing [Waksberg, 1978]. This method is reasonably suitable for identifying general population controls in areas where the prevalence of telephones among households is high. Telephone interviews are often nearly as effective as personal interviews and considerably easier to conduct. The response rate to telephone interviews has not been substantially worse than that obtained in other approaches to the ascertainment of controls from the general population [Ward et al., 1984]. The efficiency of random digit dialing can be especially beneficial in offsetting the high cost of individual matching, thus offering a relatively efficient method of finding matched controls from the general population [Robison and Daigle, 1984; Ward et al., 1984]. Computer-assisted telephone interview (CATI) software that controls the interview by computer and records the responses as the interview proceeds can be combined with random digit dialing to enhance the efficiency of telephone methods for data collection.

Some epidemiologists have recommended the routine use of two or more comparison groups drawn in different ways. Their premise is that no single comparison can control adequately for all possible biases, and sufficient confidence in the validity of the results cannot be achieved unless comparisons between the index series and several different comparison groups all indicate approximately the same result. Others argue contrarily that the possibility is remote that an investigator would place equal confidence in the validity of comparisons based on two or more different groups and that with different comparison groups one would expect different results to emerge. What would an investigator do if a lengthy and costly study produced discrepant results with two comparison groups? If the investigator had greater confidence in one of the groups, the results from the other would detract from the findings. Thus, some epidemiologists advocate choosing only one comparison group, the group in which one places greatest confidence. An intermediate position seems sensible; it seems reasonable to choose only one comparison group unless an additional group can add something unique that is important to control. For example, to control for environmental influences during adulthood, it might be reasonable to choose a spouse as a control, but to control for childhood environment (and gender) it might be reasonable to choose siblings as controls [Gutensohn et al., 1975].

Source of Information

Acquisition of information on disease, exposure, and auxiliary variables each presents different problems.

Information on disease occurrence is derivable through a variety of means. These include questioning subjects about symptoms before a diagnosis is made, examining subjects to make a diagnosis, asking subjects about medical diagnoses at interview or on questionnaires, and consulting medical record systems or vital statistics registries to determine the diagnoses or fact of death for study subjects. Existing records can provide cost-efficient information when they are available; the cost savings derives from the double benefit of not having to trace the healthy subjects in follow-up studies to determine that they are healthy and not having to conduct the medical workups. On the other hand, for follow-up studies one must be confident that the available records provide information on the complete cohorts under study. It is good practice to verify diagnoses whenever possible at least for a sample, if not for all cases. Pathologic confirmation for cancer, for example, is desirable to reduce misclassification in diagnosis. This step is not mandatory, however; excellent studies can be based on data in which the diagnoses are only presumptive as long as the magnitude and direction of the resulting misclassification are properly interpreted. As discussed in Chapter 7, if a study shows a strong positive association, misclassification of the diagnosis is a small concern, since such misclassification, if it occurs nondifferentially for exposed and unexposed subjects, only causes an underestimation of the magnitude of the association. If a study were to show no association, however, the use of presumptive diagnoses would be a greater concern, since the possibility then exists that misclassification obliterated an association. Unfortunately, the magnitude of the association is not known during the planning stage when decisions about diagnostic criteria must be made. Thus, it is generally preferable to use stringent diagnostic criteria. Nevertheless, for some diseases, such as multiple sclerosis, it may be difficult to establish a definitive diagnosis, so that nearly any set of criteria is presumptive in such situations.

Information on exposure derives less frequently from records than does information on disease, since recorded information on exposure is not often available. Exposures for which information is seldom recorded include factors such as smoking, alcohol, dietary items, and contact with sources of infection. Some exposures, such as the use of prescription drugs, are recorded but rarely in a format that is of any help to epidemiologists. Pharmacy records in the United States, for example, are usually not accessible in any way that would permit useful record linkage. Occupational exposures are recorded to the extent that information describing workplace activities exists. Actual exposure information for employees often must be inferred based on the nature of their jobs. Although recorded occupational information is thus extremely useful, there is usually considerable misclassification in determining the actual exposure to workplace agents for employees based on occupational records. Such misclassification becomes tolerable if studies are otherwise infeasible, especially if study results demonstrate a strong nonzero association despite misclassification.

When exposure information cannot be obtained from written or computer records, it is necessary to rely on human memories through interviews. In case-control studies, exposure information obtained from interviews is subject to recall bias (see Chap. 7). When this problem is an important concern, it may be addressed by using prerecorded exposure information, if this is available, or by choosing controls who, although they lack the disease under study, nevertheless have had an equal recall stimulus. An example of the latter approach would be, in a study of congenital malformation, a control series of infants with malformations other than the one under study. Only malformations thought to be unrelated to the exposures under study should be allowed as eligibility criteria for control infants.

One method often used to obtain interview information about subjects who are incapacitated or dead is to obtain the information from spouses or other family members. Agreement between the information obtainable from actual subjects and from surrogate respondents can be reasonably good for some factors such as dietary variables [Humble et al., 1984] but may be poor for other factors such as history of psychopathologic symptoms [Mendlewicz et al., 1975]. The type of respondent seems to be the most important determinant of the validity of surrogate information: Siblings provide the most accurate information about family details and events during early life, whereas spouses and offspring provide more accurate information about adult life [Pickle et al., 1983]. Like any misclassification, the magnitude of the bias from surrogate data depends on the degree of unreliability [Kupper, 1984].

Some misclassification of exposure is unavoidable in epidemiologic studies if one presumes to measure the exposure that relates most strongly to disease occurrence. To an extent, every variable measured in an epidemiologic study can be considered only a surrogate variable for some more appropriate measure of the underlying phenomenon. Consider measuring cigarette smoking as a cause of lung cancer. Assume for discussion purposes that it is the inhaled amount of benzpyrene that best predicts lung cancer risk. Even in a follow-up study, and certainly in a case-control study, one cannot hope to measure the inhaled amount of benzpyrene. What can be measured? Perhaps the daily consumption of cigarettes.

But then one needs to know what type of tobacco is used, how far down each cigarette is smoked, whether there is a filter on the cigarette, and how deeply the individual inhales, among other things. Generally, none of this can be determined with any reasonable accuracy. Even if it could be, the ideal measure of exposure must integrate this information over a period of time and allow for a reasonable but usually unknown induction period. In studying cigarette smoking and lung cancer, one would theoretically need accurate cigarette-smoking information for some period of time long before the lung cancer occurs or might occur. Since the exact time is uncertain and a variety of possibilities might have to be tried in a given analysis, in principle one needs accurate exposure information for a period covering many decades, including the details of how the exposure varied by time during this period. Since historical information of such accuracy is not attainable, some misclassification of exposure is unavoidable. One strong advantage of interview information is that interviews can provide information on exposure at different times in the past, whereas recorded information generally does not. Recorded exposure information can be distinctly inaccurate with respect to timing. For example, an individual may fill a prescription for a drug and not take any of it until some date well into the future. Recorded information might seem to suggest the individual was exposed at the time of filling the prescription but not at the later time, exactly the reverse of what occurred. It must be emphasized that these misclassification errors in exposure information, though pervasive and to some extent biasing the results of every epidemiologic study, are generally nondifferential errors that reduce associations but do not exaggerate them.

It is an unusual study that can be based on already recorded information for both exposure and disease, but even less often does sufficient recorded information exist to control adequately for confounding factors in the analysis. As discussed in the previous chapter, accuracy in determining confounding factors is as important as accuracy for the main variables under study. To the extent that a confounding factor is misclassified or that a surrogate variable is used in place of a factor of more direct interest, control of confounding by that factor will be impeded [Greenland, 1980; Kupper, 1984]. For example, in the extreme case in which the confounding information obtained is uncorrelated with the actual values of the confounding factor, adjustment according to the measured confounding factor would be an empty exercise without any effect on the results; no confounding would be removed from the data by the adjustment process. To the extent that the confounding factor measured is not a perfect measure of the idealized confounding factor, residual confounding will remain in the data. Residual confounding becomes an especially important concern if the exposure has a weak or zero effect and the confounding factor has a strong effect.

Prevention of Confounding

Three methods are used to prevent confounding in the design of epidemiologic studies. One, randomization, is applicable only in experiments. The other two methods, restriction and matching, are applicable in both experimental and nonexperimental studies.

RANDOMIZATION

Randomization, or random allocation, is a process in experiments that involves random assignment of the subjects to exposure categories. (Randomization should not be confused with "random sampling," which is a sampling method having nothing to do with experimental design.) Random allocation offers strong advantages over alternative assignment schemes, and consequently it is the method of choice for subject assignment in experiments.

The goal in exposure assignment, of course, is to create study groups that have equal propensities for the outcome—that is, equal incidences of disease in the absence of the assigned exposure. If there are only a few factors that determine incidence and if these are known to the investigator, an ideal plan might call for exposure assignment that would lead to identical distributions of the disease determinants in each group, thus providing an equal propensity for disease in each group. To achieve the identical distributions, however, would involve an assignment scheme in which it would be possible to forecast correctly the assignment of subjects with specified characteristics, if the assignments for previously enrolled subjects were already known. This forecasting ability opens the assignment process to manipulation that can defeat the goals of the study. Therefore, it is preferable to use a scheme in which the assignment of any given individual is unknowable until it is made. Randomization fulfills this criterion.

A drawback to randomization is that it does not lead to identical distributions for disease determinants but only to distributions that tend to be identical, the tendency increasing as the size of the study groups increases. Thus, randomization works very well in large studies but is less effective for smaller studies [Rothman, 1977]. In the extreme case in which only one subject is included in each group (as in the community fluoridation trials with one community in each group), randomization is completely ineffective. As compensation for its unreliability in small studies, randomization has the advantage of tending to make identical the distributions for all factors, not merely those that have been identified as important by the investigator. By providing control of all factors, known and unknown, that influence disease incidence and by providing a mechanism for subject allocation that is resistant to manipulation, randomization is a powerful technique for preventing confounding. Its drawback of being unreliable in small studies can be mitigated by evaluating and controlling any confounding by known or suspected risk factors in the data analysis, to the extent permitted by the small study size.

RESTRICTION

Confounding cannot occur if the potentially confounding variate is prohibited from varying. Restricting the admissibility criteria for subjects is therefore an extremely effective method of preventing confounding. If the potentially confounding variable is measured on a nominal scale, such as race, sex, or religion, restriction is accomplished by admitting into the study as subjects only those who fall into specified categories (usually just a single category) of each variable of interest. If the potentially confounding variable is measured on a continuous scale such as age, restriction is achieved by defining a range of the variable that is narrow enough to correspond to a relatively homogeneous range of disease incidence. Only individuals within the range are admitted into the study as subjects. If the age of subjects in a study varies little, then age cannot be a substantial confounding factor in the study.

Restriction is an excellent technique for preventing confounding, since it is not only extremely effective but also inexpensive. The decision about whether to admit a given individual to the study can be made quickly and without reference to other study subjects. The main disadvantage is simply that restriction of admissibility criteria can shrink the pool of available subjects below the desired level. When potential subjects are plentiful, restriction should be employed extensively, since it improves validity at low cost. When potential subjects are less plentiful, the advantages of restriction must be weighed against the disadvantages of a diminished study group.

One possible concern about restriction is that a homogeneous study group will provide a poor basis for generalization of study results. This concern is illusory, however, because scientific generalization is not a statistical process; it is a process of extending knowledge through a series of tested explanations. An inference about disease etiology derived from a homogeneous study group is a far stronger base for scientific generalization about the study problem than whatever inferences would be possible from a set of observations on a heterogeneous study group. In a study based on a heterogeneous group validity is less secure and the conditions under which the observed relation holds are less specifiable than are those in a study based on a homogeneous study group. The inferential process involves the formulation of abstract concepts from concrete, specific observations; by improving the validity and specificity of epidemiologic observations, restriction of admissibility criteria enhances rather than detracts from scientific inference.

MATCHING

A follow-up study is a generalization of the scientific paradigm, the experiment. To prevent confounding in follow-up studies in which the investigator cannot assign exposures, it seems natural to select subjects in such a way that potentially confounding factors are identically distributed in each of the compared groups. If restriction is not used, identical distributions for the compared groups can still be achieved through matching of characteristics in subject selection. An index series, which would be the exposed group in follow-up studies, is admitted without any restrictions; then the comparison (unexposed) series is selected to have distributions identical to the index series for one or more potentially confounding factors. The comparison subjects can be matched individually to single subjects in the index series, or they can be matched by groups ("frequency matching"). In a follow-up study with matching, none of the potentially confounding variables that have been matched for can be confounding because none will be associated with the exposure in the study population. Despite the apparent simplicity of this argument, matching is one of the most complicated topics in epidemiologic theory. The complications arise because the lucid way in which matching prevents confounding in follow-up studies does not apply to case-control studies.

Matching is rarely used in follow-up studies because it is too costly. To find a comparison subject with just the right set of characteristics with respect to each of the matching factors can involve extensive searching and laborious record-keeping. The typical large size of follow-up studies makes matching an expensive method for controlling confounding in such studies. Matching actually increases the efficiency of a follow-up study when efficiency is judged as the amount of information per subject, but when efficiency is judged as the amount of information per unit cost, matching in follow-up studies is an extremely inefficient method of controlling confounding. Walker [1982] has proposed a method that greatly enhances the cost-efficiency of matched follow-up studies; the method involves collecting data on confounding factors only for the small subset of subjects that will contribute to the estimation of the effect. Nevertheless, it is generally more cost-efficient to control confounding in the analysis of a follow-up study than to try to prevent it by matching.

The expense of matching is a serious drawback even in case-control studies, which tend to be considerably smaller than follow-up studies. Matching the controls to cases for even a modest list of characteristics is a difficult task, one that consumes substantial effort and consequently is expensive compared with alternative methods such as restriction or techniques for controlling confounding in the data analysis. Earlier in this chapter matching was mentioned as a way of enhancing precision and thereby improving study efficiency. The improved precision may come at a considerable cost, however. As with follow-up studies, the efficiency of a case-control study is best judged by relating the information obtained or the precision of measurement not to the number of subjects studied but rather to the cost of obtaining the information. Judging efficiency in this way, the apparently more efficient design achieved by matching may turn out to be less cost-efficient than admitting a large pool of potential controls to the study and controlling for confounding in the analysis by stratification. A more detailed treatment of this topic is given in Chapter 13.

REFERENCES

Antunes, C. M. F., Stolley, P. D., Rosenstein, N. B., et al. Endometrial cancer and estrogen use. Report of a large case-control study. *N. Engl. J. Med.* 1979;300:9–13.

Greenland, S. The effect of misclassification in the presence of covariates. *Am. J. Epidemiol.* 1980;112:564–569.

Greenland, S., and Neutra, R. An analysis of detection bias and proposed corrections in the study of estrogens and endometrial cancer. *J. Chron. Dis.* 1981;34:433–438.

Gutensohn, N., Li, F. P., Johnson, R. E., et al. Hodgkin's disease, tonsillectomy and family size. *N. Engl. J. Med.* 1975;292:22–25.

Horwitz, R. I., and Feinstein, A. R. Alternative analytic methods for case-control studies of estrogens and endometrial cancer. *N. Engl. J. Med.* 1978;299:1089–1094.

Hutchison, G. B., and Rothman, K. J. Correcting a bias? *N. Engl. J. Med.* 1978;299:1129–1130.

Humble, C. G., Samet, J. M., and Skipper, B. E. Comparison of self- and surrogate-reported dietary information. *Am. J. Epidemiol.* 1984;119:86–98.

Kupper, L. L. Effects of the use of unreliable surrogate variables on the validity of epidemiologic research studies. *Am. J. Epidemiol.* 1984;120:634–638.

Mack, T. M., Pike, M. C., Henderson, B. E., et al. Estrogens and endometrial cancer in a retirement community. *N. Engl. J. Med.* 1976;294:1262–1267.

Mendlewicz, J., Fleiss, J. L., Cataldo, M., et al. Accuracy of the family history method in affective illness. Comparison with direct interviews in family studies. *Arch. Gen. Psychiatry* 1975;32:309–314.

Miettinen, O. S. Individual matching with multiple controls in the case of all-or-none response. *Biometrics* 1969;25:339–355.

Morgenstern, H., and Winn, D. M. A method for determining the sampling ratio in epidemiologic studies. *Statistics Med.* 1983;2:387–396.

Paffenbarger, R. S., and Hale, W. E. Work activity and coronary heart mortality. *N. Engl. J. Med.* 1975;292:545–550.

Pickle, L. W., Brown, L. M., Blot, W. J. Information available from surrogate respondents in case-control interview studies. *Am. J. Epidemiol.* 1983;118:99–108.

Robison, L. L., and Daigle, A. Control selection using random digit dialing for cases of childhood cancer. *Am. J. Epidemiol.* 1984;120:164–166.

Rothman, K. J. Epidemiologic methods in clinical trials. *Cancer* 1977;39:1771–1775.

Smith, D. C., Prentice, R., Thompson, D. J., et al. Association of exogenous estrogen and endometrial carcinoma. *N. Engl. J. Med.* 1975;293:1164–1167.

Waksberg, J. Sampling methods for random digit dialing. *J. Am. Stat. Assoc.* 1978;73:40–46.

Walker, A. M. Efficient assessment of confounder effects in matched follow-up studies. *Appl. Stat.* 1982;31:293–297.

Walter, S. D. Determination of significant relative risks and optimal sampling procedures in prospective and retrospective comparative studies of various sizes. *Am. J. Epidemiol.* 1977;105:387–397.

Ward, E. M., Kramer, S., and Meadows, A. T. The efficacy of random digit dialing in selecting matched controls for a case-control study of pediatric cancer. *Am. J. Epidemiol.* 1984;120:582–591.

Ziel, H. K., and Finkle, W. D. Increased risk of endometrial carcinoma among users of conjugated estrogens. *N. Engl. J. Med.* 1975;293:1167–1170.

9. THE ROLE OF STATISTICS IN EPIDEMIOLOGIC ANALYSIS

Many statisticians have contributed to the development of epidemiologic theory, and many prominent epidemiologists have had their primary professional training in statistics. Thus it is not surprising that statistical concepts dominate the thinking of much that is published in epidemiology. Proper understanding and application of statistical concepts is essential for epidemiologic data analysis, but statistical practices and ideas have often been transferred to epidemiology without adequate consideration of how well they apply.

Statistics performs two major roles in epidemiologic analysis: to assess random variation and to control confounding. Although there are other pertinent statistical applications in epidemiology, such as the evaluation of interactions between factors, these two functions represent the fundamental areas in epidemiology that require statistical methods.

ASSESSMENT OF RANDOM VARIABILITY
Statistical Hypothesis Testing

Historically, the scientific assessment of random variability has been done predominantly by means of statistical hypothesis testing, or "significance testing." More than 40 years ago, Berkson [1942] wrote

It is hardly an exaggeration to say that statistics, as it is taught at present in the dominant school, consists almost entirely of tests of significance, though not always presented as such, some comparatively simple and forthright, others elaborate and abstruse.

The ubiquitous use of "P-values" and reference to "statistically significant" findings in the current medical literature demonstrates the dominant role that statistical hypothesis testing still plays in data analysis in the biomedical sciences. Many researchers believe that it would be fruitless to submit for publication any paper that lacks statistical tests of "significance." Their belief is not entirely ill-founded, since journal editors and referees commonly rely on tests of "significance" as indicators of sophisticated and meaningful statistical analysis as well as the primary means of assessing sampling variability in a study. Preoccupation with "significance" tests is embodied in the focus on whether the "P-value" is less than 0.05; results are considered "significant" or "not significant" according to whether or not the "P-value" is less than or greater than 0.05.

The roots of the preoccupation with "significance" testing derive from the research topics that were of interest to statisticians who pioneered in the development of statistical theory earlier in this century. Their research problems were industrial and agricultural and typically involved experiments that formed the basis for a choice between two or more alternative

Nul Hyp. - P values → decision

causes of action. Such experiments were designed to produce results enabling a decision to be made, and the statistical methods employed were intended to facilitate decision making. The concepts that grew out of this heritage and are today applied in clinical and epidemiologic research strongly reflect the background of decision making.

Statistical hypothesis testing focuses on the *null hypothesis,* which is a hypothesis of no association between two variables. If the data provide evidence against the null hypothesis, then this hypothesis can be rejected in favor of some non-null alternative hypothesis. Typically, the alternative hypothesis is vague: If the null hypothesis states that there is no association, then the alternative hypothesis might state simply that there is an association. The alternative hypothesis could be one-sided, stating that there is specifically a positive (or negative) association. In terms of an epidemiologic effect measure, the alternative hypothesis includes a wide range of values, extending from a minute effect to an extremely large effect. The wide range of possible effects consistent with the usual alternative hypothesis implies a wide range of possible outcomes for the data that are consistent with the alternative hypothesis. The null hypothesis, on the other hand, corresponds to a single value of effect and therefore is consistent with a much narrower range of possible outcomes for the data. If we accept the thinking of Popper that we can falsify hypotheses but not confirm them, it is natural to focus on a hypothesis that is as specific as possible because falsification of a specific hypothesis is easier than falsification of a vague one. Statistical hypothesis testing amounts to an attempt to falsify the null hypothesis and by exclusion accept the alternative.

Decision making is ingrained in the process of statistical testing, since rejecting or accepting a hypothesis is itself a decision. The *P-value* is the main statistic used to test hypotheses. It indicates the probability, assuming that the null hypothesis is true, that the observed data will depart from an absence of association to the extent that they actually do, or to a greater extent, by chance alone. *P*-values are calculated from statistical models that are thought to describe the pattern of observations when chance is the sole reason for their variability. The *P*-value is a continuous statistic with a range of zero to 1. Small values of P indicate a low degree of compatibility between the null hypothesis and the observed data by virtue of the low probability that a result as extreme or more extreme than the observed data could have been generated if the null hypothesis were true. Low *P*-values, therefore, shift credibility away from the null hypothesis toward the alternative hypothesis, which serves as a relatively better explanation for the data. Though the *P*-value is a reasonably meaningful continuous measure, it is often used to force a qualitative decision about rejection of the null hypothesis. An arbitrary point, usually 5 percent, is selected as a criterion by which to judge the *P*-value, and this point is used to classify the observation either as "significant" if $P \leq 0.05$, in which case the null hypothesis is rejected, or "not significant" if $P > 0.05$, in which case the null hypothesis is not rejected. It is generally incorrect, for reasons that will be clear later, to think of "accepting" the null hypothesis in favor of the alternative when it cannot be rejected; therefore, "not rejected" is not equivalent to accepted with regard to the null hypothesis.

What if the null hypothesis is indeed true but is rejected anyway? If the P-value criterion for rejection is 5 percent, then the null hypothesis will be rejected about 5 percent of the time when it is true. Such incorrect rejections are described as type I errors, or alpha-errors. If the null hypothesis is false and is not rejected, the result is a type II error, or beta-error. There is a tradeoff between the probability of a type I or a type II error that depends on the cutoff value that is chosen for "statistical significance": Reducing the type I error when there is no effect requires a smaller cutoff for the P-value to be judged as statistically "significant," but a lower cutoff for "significance" increases the probability of a type II error if there is an effect. Increasing the cutoff value for "statistical significance" reduces the type II error when there is an effect but increases the type I error if there is not.

The concept of type I and type II errors is linked to a decision-making process in research that requires data to be interpreted in a way that produces a decision to reject or not to reject the null hypothesis. The extent to which decision making dominates research thinking is reflected in the frequency with which the P-value, a continuous measure, is reported only as an inequality (such as $P < 0.05$ or $P > 0.05$) or else not at all, with the evaluation focusing instead on "statistical significance" or its absence.

When a study forms the sole basis for a choice between two alternatives, a decision-making mode of analysis is justifiable. This situation virtually never occurs for epidemiologic or, for that matter, any biomedical research, however. This is not to claim, of course, that epidemiologic data do not play instrumental roles in public health decision making. Rather, the results of a single study do not often, if ever, constitute the basis for a decision. Decisions based on results from a collection of studies are not facilitated when each study is classified as a "yes" or "no" decision. The degradation of information into a dichotomy is counterproductive, even to decision making, and can be misleading.

In a review of 71 clinical trials that reported no "significant" difference ($P > 0.05$) between the compared treatments, Freiman et al. [1978] found that in the great majority of such trials the data either indicated or at least were consistent with a moderate or even reasonably strong effect of the new treatment. In all of these trials, the original investigators interpreted their data as indicative of no effect because the P-value was not "statistically significant." The misinterpretations arose because the investigators relied solely on "significance" testing for their statistical analysis rather than on a more descriptive and informative analysis. On failing to reject the null hypothesis, the investigators in these 71 trials inappropriately "accepted" the null hypothesis as correct, resulting in a probable type II error for many of these so-called "negative" studies. Type II errors result when the magnitude of an effect, the amount of information in the data, and random variability combine to give results insufficiently inconsistent with the null hypothesis to reject it. This failure to reject the null hypothesis can occur either because the effect is small, the observations are too few, or both. More to the point, however, is that a type II error (or a type I error) arises because the investigator has attempted to dichotomize the results of a study into the categories "significant" or "not significant." Since this degradation of the study is unnecessary, the "error" that may result from an incorrect classification of the study result is also unnecessary.

Why has such an unattractive methodologic crutch become so ingrained? Undoubtedly much of the romance with "significance" testing stems from the apparent objectivity and definitiveness of the pronouncement of "significance." Declarations of "significance" or its absence can supplant the need for any real interpretation of data; the declarations can serve as a mechanical substitute for thought, promulgated by the inertia of training and common practice. The neatness of an apparent clear-cut result may appear more gratifying to investigators, editors, and readers than a finding that cannot be immediately pigeonholed. The rote process of "significance" testing is only superficially like the intellectual process of conjecture and refutation that Popper described as the scientific method. The unbridled homage paid to "statistical significance" in the social sciences has been attributed to the apparent objectivity that the pronouncement of "significance" can convey [Atkins and Jarrett, 1979]:

"Let's look and see what's significant" is not too far from the approach of some researchers, and when the data involve perhaps several hundred variables the practical temptations to use a ready-made decision rule are enormous. . . . [T]he pressure to *decide,* in situations where the very use of probability models admits the uncertainty of the inference, has certain consequences for the presentation of knowledge. The significance test appears to guarantee the objectivity of the researcher's conclusions, and may even be presented as providing crucial support for the whole theory in which the research hypothesis was put forward. As we have seen, tests of significance cannot do either of these things—but it is not in the interests of anyone involved to admit this too openly.

The origin of the nearly universal acceptance of the 5 percent cutoff point for "significant" findings is tied to the abridged form in which the chi-square table was originally published [Freedman et al., 1978]. Before computers or calculators could easily give quick approximations to the chi-square distribution, tables were used routinely. Since there is a different distribution for chi-square corresponding to every possible value for the degrees of freedom, the tables could not give many points for any one distribution. The tables typically included values at 1 percent, 5 percent, and a few other levels, encouraging the practice of checking the chi-square calculated from one's data to see if it exceeded the cutoff levels in the table.

Interval Estimation

If "significance" testing is misleading, how should results be presented? In the spirit of Kelvin's remark that science is measurement, it is best to conceptualize the problem as a measurement problem rather than as a problem in decision making. To conceptualize a study as a measurement exercise demands more precision in presenting results than the simple dichotomy presented by statistical hypothesis testing. Whatever the parameter that is the object of inference in an epidemiologic study—it usually is a measure of effect, either rate ratio or rate difference, but it can also be simply an incidence rate or any other epidemiologic measure—it will be measured on a continuous scale, that is, a scale with an infinite number of possible values. The data from a study can be used to generate an estimate of the parameter. The best estimate, presented as a single value on the continuous scale of measurement, is referred to as a *point estimate*. A point estimate is an indicator of the extent of association, or the magnitude of effect, in the data. Because it is only one point on a scale of infinite possibilities, it is not a reliable estimate. Mathematically, the probability of the point estimate being correct is 1/infinity, or zero. To incorporate into the estimation process an allowance for random variability in the observations, it is preferable to estimate the effect using a range of values for the parameter. The range represents a set of possible values for the parameter that is consistent with the observed data within specified limits. The range is known as a *confidence interval*, and the process of calculating the confidence interval is known as *interval estimation*.

The width of a confidence interval depends on the amount of variability in the data, but it also depends on an arbitrarily selected value that specifies the degree of consistency between the limits of the interval and the data. This arbitrary value is the level of confidence, which is usually expressed as a percentage. If the level of confidence is 90 percent, the confidence interval is constructed with enough width to have a 90 percent probability of containing within it the parameter value—that is, considering the degree of variability in the data, in 90 percent of replications of the process of obtaining the data the interval will include the parameter (in the absence of biases). The level of confidence can be set to any value because it is arbitrary, but values of 95 percent, 90 percent, or occasionally 80 percent are most commonly used.

Conceptually there is a direct relation between the level of confidence and the alpha-level of hypothesis testing. The confidence level is equivalent to the complement of the alpha-level, that is, $1 - \alpha$. To understand this, consider the diagram in Figure 9-1.

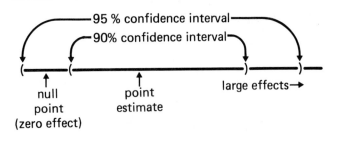

Fig. 9-1. *Two nested confidence intervals with the wider one including the null point.*

Suppose you performed a test of the null hypothesis with $\alpha = 0.10$. The fact that the 90 percent confidence interval does not include the null point indicates that the null hypothesis would be rejected for $\alpha = 0.10$. On the other hand, the fact that the 95 percent confidence interval includes the null point indicates that the null hypothesis would not be rejected for $\alpha = 0.05$. Since a 95 percent interval includes the null point and a 90 percent interval does not, it can be inferred that the P-value is greater than 0.05 and less than 0.10.

The point of the preceding example is not to suggest that confidence intervals can be used as surrogate tests of statistical "significance." Although that is true, to use confidence intervals in this way would defeat all the advantages that confidence intervals have over tests of "significance." The confidence interval does much more than assess the extent to which the null hypothesis is compatible with the data. It provides simultaneously an idea of the magnitude of the effect and the inherent variability in the estimate. The P-value, on the other hand, indicates only the degree of consistency that exists between the data and the null hypothesis and reveals nothing about either the magnitude of the effect or its variability [Bandt and Boen, 1972]. It is not too surprising that a confidence interval conveys more information than a P-value because the confidence interval is defined by two numbers, whereas the P-value is only one number. A reliance on P-values alone can be extremely misleading. The following example illustrates this point.

Consider a study of a new drug, B, which is compared with a standard treatment, A, resulting in the data shown in Table 9-1. A test of the null hypothesis that the two treatments are equally effective gives a result of $P = 0.06$. (The method used to calculate the P-value is described in Chapter 11.) These data might be reported in several ways. The least informative way would be to report that the observed difference is "not significant." Somewhat more information would be given by reporting the actual P-value; to express the P-value as an inequality such as $P > 0.05$ is not much better than reporting the results as "not significant," whereas reporting P

Table 9-1. Hypothetical data from a clinical trial of a new treatment

Outcome	Treatment	
	A	B
Successful	7	14
Unsuccessful	13	6
Total	20	20

= 0.06, at least gives the *P*-value explicitly rather than degrading it into a nominal scale measure. An additional improvement would be to report $P_{(2)} = 0.06$, denoting the use of a two-sided rather than a one-sided alternative hypothesis. Any *P*-value, however, no matter how explicit, fails to convey the descriptive finding that 70 percent of patients were treated successfully with B compared with 35 percent with A, a difference in proportion of 35 percent. A 95 percent confidence interval for the difference in proportion would range from about -1 percent to about $+71$ percent (the positive values favor treatment B). The position of the lower limit of the confidence interval corresponds to the outcome of the "significance" test: The interval includes zero difference, which corresponds to labeling the observed treatment difference as "not significant." Quantitatively, the lower bound of the 95 percent confidence interval extending just slightly beyond zero difference corresponds to a *P*-value that is slightly greater than 0.05. The full confidence interval, however, indicates that these data, although compatible with no real difference between the treatments, are equally compatible with B being markedly more effective; the range of possibilities consistent with the data generally suggests a considerably greater efficacy for treatment B. The complete confidence interval summarizes the findings clearly and unambiguously. The *P*-value, on the other hand, gives no indication of the magnitude of the difference between treatments and, if used merely as a hypothesis test, would result in a type II error, presuming that treatment B is actually better than A, which seems plausible from the data.

Confidence intervals convey information about magnitude and precision of effect simultaneously, keeping these two aspects of measurement closely linked. The use of *P*-values, or "significance" testing, blurs these concepts so that the focus on measurement is lost. Consider a hypothesized cause of disease that is under study; suppose that it is not in fact associated, causally or otherwise, with disease. Study results cannot be reassuring about the safety of the agent if they are reported solely as the results of statistical hypothesis testing. As we have already seen, results that are "not significant" may nevertheless be compatible with substantial effects. Lack of "significance" itself conveys no reassurance.

Standard statistical advice states that when the data indicate a lack of "significance," it is important to consider the power of the study to detect specific alternative hypotheses about the magnitude of the effect as "significant." Power calculations, however, are only indirect indicators of precision, and they require an assumption about the magnitude of the effect. In planning a study, it may be reasonable to make conjectures about the magnitude of an effect. In presenting results, however, it is always preferable to use the information on hand about the effect to estimate it directly rather than to speculate about it. A confidence interval conveys the desired information about reassurance if there is no effect by showing how large an effect is reasonably compatible with the observations, or it may indicate the lack of information necessary for reassurance about an absence of effect. In their reanalysis of the 71 "negative" clinical trials, Freiman et al. [1978] used confidence intervals for the risk difference to reinterpret the findings from these studies. These confidence intervals indicated that many of the treatments under study were indeed beneficial (Fig. 9-2). The inappropriate interpretations of the authors in most of these trials could have been avoided by focusing their attention on the confidence interval rather than on the results of a statistical test.

For a study to be reassuring about the lack of an effect, the limits of an appropriate confidence interval must be near the null value. The question of statistical "significance" is actually irrelevant. Consider the two sets of study results of the same hypothesized cause-effect relation shown in Figure 9-3. Study A was large and gave precise results, that is, a narrow confidence interval, whereas study B was small and led to a large confidence interval. Which study is more reassuring about a potentially harmful effect? Study A indicates that the effect is very likely to be near zero; the upper limit of the confidence interval is near the null point and offers reassurance that the effect under study is not very great. Study B, however, was imprecise, that is, it led to a wide confidence interval, and it does not provide reassurance about the absence of a large effect. Thus, study A is reassuring and study B is not. A statistical test of "significance," though, would not be "significant" for B, but it would be for A, since the null point is within the interval for B but not for A.

In this example, as in the example given in Table 9-1, a reliance on the test of "significance" alone would give precisely the opposite of the correct interpretation of the findings. In Table 9-1, the "significance" test indicated a lack of "significance" when the data indicated a strong effect. In study A in the second example, the "significance" test indicated "significance" although the study is basically "negative" in the sense that it provides evidence against a large effect.

Interval estimation, it has been argued, suffers from a drawback that also applies to "significance" testing—namely, that the procedure is dependent on an arbitrary selection for the confidence level on the one hand or the alpha-level on the other hand. One way to circumvent such arbitrariness

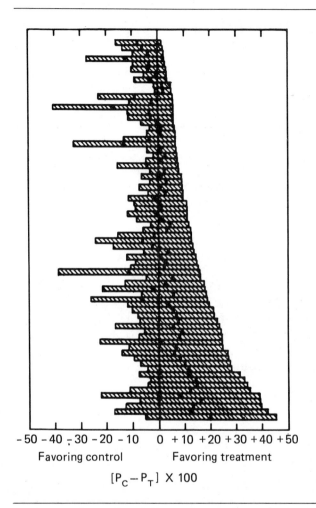

−50 −40 −30 −20 −10   0 +10 +20 +30 +40 +50

Favoring control   Favoring treatment

$[P_C - P_T] \times 100$

Fig. 9-2. Ninety percent confidence limits for the true percentage difference for the 71 trials. The vertical bar at the center of each interval indicates the observed value, $P_c - P_t$, for each trial (copied with the permission of the New England Journal of Medicine *from Freiman et al.* [1978]).

is to consider calculating and reporting a nested series of confidence intervals, for example, the 50 percent, 60 percent, 70 percent, 80 percent, and 90 percent intervals. Intervals with greater confidence are wider and always include within them any intervals of lesser confidence. At the extremes, a 100 percent confidence interval would cover the entire range of the parameter being estimated, and a zero percent confidence interval is simply the point estimate; neither extreme case reveals anything about precision, although the degenerate zero percent confidence interval does

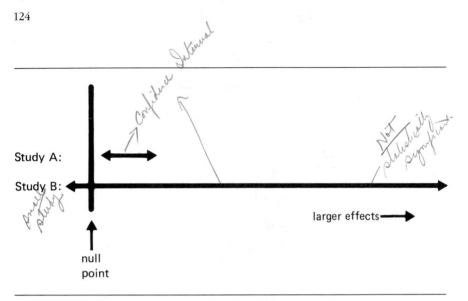

Fig. 9-3. Results from two hypothetical studies.

describe magnitude. As the level of confidence increases from zero to 100 percent, the width of the interval increases but not at a constant rate. From statistical theory, we know that the sampling distribution of the usual estimates of epidemiologic measures is approximately normal. We can therefore infer that a confidence interval does not bracket the parameter value with uniform probability throughout the interval. It is considerably more likely that the parameter is located centrally within an interval than it is that the parameter is located near the limits of the interval. This pattern can be exemplified by the nested confidence intervals shown in Table 9-2, which are based on the data in Table 9-1.

The main implication of the nonuniformity of confidence within the interval is that the precise location of the boundary of an interval is not important for proper interpretation. A series of nested confidence intervals may convey an accurate impression of the precision of estimation, but rarely would different interpretations emerge from consideration of these different confidence intervals because the precise location of the limits of the interval is of little practical consequence. Rather, it is the approximate position of the interval as a whole on its scale of measurement that governs the interpretation. "Significance" testing, on the other hand, is equivalent to funneling all interest into the precise location of one boundary of a confidence interval while the more important information in the data about the likely magnitude of the effect is ignored.

The main thrust of the preceding discussion of the assessment of random variability has been to demonstrate the inadequacy of the most cherished of statistical tools, statistical "significance" testing. This view that estimation is preferable to testing has also been espoused by statisticians [Atkins and Jarrett, 1979]:

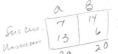

*Table 9-2. Nested confidence intervals for the
difference in proportion for the hypothetical data in table 9-1*

50% Interval:	0.24—0.46
60% Interval:	0.22—0.48
70% Interval:	0.18—0.52
80% Interval:	0.14—0.56
90% Interval:	0.09—0.61

Methods of estimation share many of the problems of significance tests—being
likewise based on probability model assumptions and requiring "arbitrary" limits
of precision. But at least they do not require irrelevant null hypotheses to be set
up nor do they force a decision about "significance" to be made—the estimates
can be presented and evaluated by statistical *and other* criteria, by the researcher
or the reader. In addition the estimates of one investigation can be compared with
others. While it is often the case that different measurements or methods of investigation or theoretical approaches lead to "different" results, this is not a disadvantage; these differences reflect important theoretical differences about the meaning
of the research and the conclusions to be drawn from it. And it is precisely those
differences which are obscured by simply reporting the significance level of the
results.

Indeed, since statistical "significance" testing promotes so much misinterpretation, it would be reasonable to avoid it and the use of *P*-values entirely; routine avoidance of testing might have the desirable effect of ac-
celerating its inevitable demise as a method for inference.

THE ASSESSMENT AND CONTROL OF CONFOUNDING
In an epidemiologic study, if confounding by suspect variables has not
already been prevented by design in the selection of subjects, its assessment and control must be considered in the analysis.

Assessment of Confounding
Because the assessment of confounding often involves a decision about
whether or not to control for a potentially confounding factor in an analysis, there is a natural tendency to use the apparatus of statistical hypothesis testing in the process of assessing confounding: The result is that distributions of "baseline" characteristics between study groups are
compared using *t*-tests, chi-square tests, or other statistical tests. If no statistically "significant" differences are found, the conclusion is drawn that
no confounding exists, whereas statistically "significant" differences are
taken as indicators of potential confounding.

Although hypothesis testing is commonly used to assess confounding, such use is inappropriate. The amount of confounding depends on the combination of two distinct associations: the association between the confounder and the exposure, and the association between the confounder and the disease. If one of these associations is strong and the other is absent, no confounding is present. The result of a statistical test, however, might yield either "significance" or "no significance" depending on which of the two component associations is measured.

The magnitude of confounding, like other biases, does not depend on the size of a study (except in an experiment with randomization); it depends on the magnitude of the associations that give rise to it. *P*-values, on the other hand, depend on both the magnitude of an association and the size of a study. Even as a measure of the magnitude of one of the component associations that determine confounding, then, statistical hypothesis testing is inadequate. A small study might have substantial confounding, yet hypothesis testing might not yield "significant" *P*-values because the numbers generating the associations are small. If the data from the same study were replicated several-fold, the component associations that determine the magnitude of confounding would remain exactly the same; although increasing the size of the study would not affect the magnitude of confounding, it would drive the *P*-value lower, eventually making it "significant." In a sufficiently large study, nearly every association would be statistically "significant," whether the resulting confounding was trivial or important. Thus, the outcome of a "significance" test cannot be interpreted usefully as a measure of confounding.

The entire purpose of a statistical hypothesis test is to evaluate the role of chance as a possible explanation for observed associations. Even in randomized experiments, however, when baseline differences between groups are always explained by chance because a random process produced them, confounding can occur and should be controlled when it does. The compatibility of the baseline differences with chance is irrelevant to the magnitude of confounding.

Proper assessment of confounding involves an appreciation of the degree of bias in a measure of effect that is introduced by the potentially confounding variable. As a practical matter, the assessment of confounding is accomplished by comparing the crude estimate of effect with the estimate obtained after confounding is removed. The extent of confounding can then be inferred from the discrepancy, if any, between the crude estimate and the estimate obtained when confounding is removed.

Control of Confounding

Control of confounding in data analysis is achieved either by *stratification*, which reduces or eliminates confounding by evaluating the effect of an exposure within strata of the confounding variable, or by *multivariate analysis*, which adjusts for confounding through mathematic modeling.

In a stratified analysis, the objective is to compare the exposed and unexposed study groups, or cases and controls, within homogeneous categories or narrow ranges of the confounding variable. Each stratum provides an unconfounded estimate of the effect because the lack of variability of the confounding variable within strata prevents confounding of the within-stratum comparisons. Statistical principles and methods can be applied to combine the results of the stratum-specific comparisons into a single overall estimate. The specific approach used depends on the goal of the analysis and, to some extent, on the data. A detailed discussion of stratified analysis is presented in Chapter 12; the strategy usually adopted calls for combining the stratum-specific estimates of effect into a single overall estimate of effect by taking a weighted average of the stratum-specific effect estimates. The weights used in averaging may be chosen to represent a standard distribution for purposes of comparison, or they may be chosen for statistical efficiency to obtain as precise an estimate of the effect as possible from the stratified analysis.

Multivariate analysis involves the construction of mathematic models to describe simultaneously the effect of exposure and the effect of other factors that may be confounding or modifying the effect of exposure. Statistics plays a role in estimating the parameters of the mathematic model from the data, usually a complicated calculational task that calls for a computer. Statistical considerations should not play a dominant role, however, in constructing the mathematic model. The selection of factors to enter into a model, the mathematic formulation of the model, and the way in which the factors are coded into specific terms for the model are not issues of a statistical nature; rather, they depend on a biologic understanding of the disease process and the mathematic relations of the factors under study.

Multivariate modeling is used in epidemiologic research for two reasons: either for explanatory purposes as a means for scientific inference, or for predictive purposes, to predict disease risks based on the simultaneous consideration of a set of factors. Usually scientific inference about effects is the goal; if the goal is purely prediction without inference, confounding may not be an important issue, since any good set of predictors, causal or noncausal, confounded or not, can accomplish the purpose. (In the long run, however, causal risk factors may prove to be the most reliable for prediction.) In such situations, a major objective may be to reduce a large set of variables to a smaller set that can predict risk efficiently. Statistical algorithms have been developed to reduce a large set of predictors to a smaller set that is nearly as informative. The two most common algorithms, *step-up* and *step-down* procedures, which are named according to whether terms are added to an initial small set or deleted from an initial large set, use statistical hypothesis testing repeatedly to determine the statistical contribution of each term to the overall model.

Although these automatic model-building algorithms are satisfactory for developing prediction models, they are undesirable when scientific inference is the analytic goal. Outside of a situation in which a multivariate model is used for prediction, there is no compelling reason to reduce the model to a small set of terms. It is inadvisable to have so many terms that the number becomes large—say 20 or 30 percent—relative to the number of observations. It is also tedious and expensive to use multivariate models with many dozens of terms. Nevertheless, when inference is the objective, concerns about confounding and the aptness of the model dominate any competing concerns for simplicity in the model. A statistical stepwise algorithm could omit from a model several factors, none of which is individually "statistically significant," but which, when taken together, could account for a substantial amount of confounding. It is always important to keep foremost the goals of the epidemiologic analysis: When attempting to infer the magnitude of the effect of one or more specific factors in a multivariate analysis, it is necessary first to choose an appropriate type of multivariate analysis and then to include in it as complete a set of explanatory factors as possible, eschewing statistical algorithms intended for other purposes.

SUMMARY

Epidemiology, like most modern sciences, relies on statistical principles and applications in data analysis. Statistics, however, serves merely as a tool for epidemiologists to achieve their scientific objectives. Too often statistical procedures have been employed in epidemiologic studies with little regard for epidemiologic objectives. Examples abound: They include the use of survey sampling methods when they are not indicated, the use of analysis of variance or other statistical techniques that do not produce epidemiologic measurements as results, and, most often, the inappropriate reliance on statistical hypothesis testing. The notion of "statistical significance" could be expunged from the lexicon of the epidemiologist with no loss. Used to assess confounding, it is simply incorrect; used to test statistically the association between exposure and disease, it is often misleading and never descriptive of the magnitude of effect or the precision of measurement. In the latter case, the use of confidence intervals rather than P-values or "statistical significance" yields a remarkable improvement in clarity of interpretation for everyone and prevents overt misinterpretation by unwary readers or investigators.

Satisfactory mastery of statistics by the epidemiologist begins with the principle that epidemiologic objectives should set the requirements for study design and data analysis. Statistical methods are adopted or, if necessary, invented to achieve the epidemiologic objectives. Compromises in study design or analysis cannot be defended in pursuit of a statistical goal or to use a statistical method that does not accomplish the study objectives.

REFERENCES

Atkins, L., and Jarrett, D. The significance of 'significance tests.' In J. Irvine, I. Miles, and J. Evans (eds.), *Demystifying Social Statistics*. London: Pluto Press, 1979.

Bandt, C. L., and Boen, J. R. A prevalent misconception about sample size, statistical significance, and clinical importance. *J. Periodont.* 1972;43:181–183.

Berkson, J. Tests of significance considered as evidence. *J. Am. Stat. Assoc.* 1942;37:325–335.

Freedman, D., Pisani, R., and Purves, R. *Statistics*. New York: Norton, 1978.

Freiman, J. A., Chalmers, T. C., Smith, H., et al. The importance of beta, the Type II error and sample size in the design and interpretation of the randomized control trial. Survey of 71 "negative" trials. *N. Engl. J. Med.* 1978;299:690–694.

10. FUNDAMENTALS OF EPIDEMIOLOGIC DATA ANALYSIS

In a well-planned study, the raw observations that constitute the data contain the information that satisfies the objectives of the study. In Chapter 7 it was emphasized that a study is a measurement exercise and that the overall goal for a study is accuracy in measurement. Accordingly, the goal in data analysis is to extract the pertinent measurement information from the raw observations.

Typically, there are several distinct stages in the analysis of data. In the preliminary stage, the investigator should review the recorded data for accuracy, consistency, and completeness; this process is often referred to as *data editing*. Next, the investigator should summarize or transform the data into a concise form for subsequent analysis, usually into contingency tables that tabulate the distribution of the observations according to key factors; this stage of the analysis is referred to as *data reduction*. Finally, the edited and reduced data are used to generate the epidemiologic measures of interest, typically one or more measures of effect (such as relative risk estimates), with appropriate confidence intervals. This last stage of analysis is sometimes considered the analysis proper, but it is more convenient to refer to it as *effect estimation* (or perhaps just *estimation,* if the goal of the analysis is to estimate disease frequency rather than to measure an effect). For some investigators, the last stage of analysis inevitably includes statistical hypothesis testing. The previous chapter explained why hypothesis testing is an undesirable feature of data analysis in most epidemiologic situations. Since the statistical theory behind interval estimation is closely related to statistical hypothesis testing, however, it is useful to consider the issues described in statistical hypothesis testing as a foundation for understanding epidemiologic data analysis.

DATA EDITING

There is no excuse for failing to scrutinize the raw data intensely for errors and to correct such errors whenever possible. Errors are routinely introduced into data in a variety of ways; some errors are detectable in editing and some are not.

The data in an epidemiologic study usually derive from a self-administered or an interviewer-administered questionnaire or from existing records that are transcribed for research. The data from the questionnaire or record-abstraction form may be transcribed from this primary form to a code form for machine entry, usually by keypunching. Coding of responses is often necessary. For example, occupational data obtained from interviews need to be classified into a manageable code, as does drug information, medical history, and many other types of data. Data such as age or year of birth (year of birth is usually preferable to age, since it tends to be reported more accurately and does not change with time), although often grouped into broad categories for reporting purposes, should be recorded in a precise form rather than grouped because the actual values will allow greater flexibility later in the analysis. For example, different groupings may be necessary for comparisons with several other studies. Some nominal scale variables that have only a few possible values can be precoded on the primary forms by checking a designated box corresponding to the appropriate category. For nominal scale variables with many possible categories, however, such as country of birth or occupation, precoded questions are not practical. If all data items can be precoded, it may be feasible to collect the data in a primary form that can be read directly by a machine, by optical scanning, or by some comparable method. Otherwise, it will usually be necessary to translate the information on the primary data form before it is stored in a machine or in machine-readable form.

It is possible and usually desirable to avoid rewriting the data onto a secondary data form during the coding process. Rather than generating additional transcription errors, it is preferable to code the data while simultaneously keying them into a computer storage system. A computer program can be devised to prompt data entry item by item, displaying category codes on a terminal screen to assist in coding. If the data are coded and rewritten by hand, they will often require keypunching anyway, unless they are coded onto optical scanning sheets; consequently, direct data entry during coding reduces both costs and errors. The fewer the number of rewriting operations between the primary record and the machine-stored version, the fewer the errors that are likely to occur. If rewriting is unavoidable, it is useful to assess the extent of coding errors in the rewritten form by coding a proportion of the data forms twice, independently. The information thus obtained can be used to judge the magnitude of bias introduced by misclassification from coding errors.

Basic editing of the data involves checking each variable for illegal or unusual values. For example, gender may be coded 1 for male and 2 for female. Usually a separate value, perhaps 3, is used to designate an unknown value. It is preferable not to assign a code of zero if it can be avoided because missing information or non-numeric codes may be interpreted by some machines or programs as a zero. By not assigning zero as a specific code, not even for unknown information, it may be possible to detect keypunching errors or missing information. The distribution of each variable should be examined in the editing process. Any inadmissible values should be checked against the primary data forms. Unusual values such as unknown gender or unusual age or birth year should also be checked.

In addition to checking for incorrect or unusual values, the distribution of each variable should be examined to see if it appears reasonable. Would you expect about half of the subjects to be males, about 80 percent (a reasonable figure if the subjects have, say, upper respiratory cancer), or about 2 percent (if the subjects are nurses)? Such an evaluation may reveal important problems that might not otherwise come to light. For example, a programming error could shift all the data in each electronic record by one or more characters, thereby producing gibberish that nevertheless might not be detectable in, say, a multivariate analysis (an important drawback of the multivariate approach). The potential for such a disaster heightens the need to check carefully the distribution of each variable during the editing of the data.

The editing checks described so far relate to each variable in the data taken singly. In addition to such basic editing, it is usually desirable to check the consistency of codes for related variables. It is not impossible, but it is improbable that a person 18 years of age will have three children. Males should not have been hospitalized for hysterectomy. People over 2 meters tall are unlikely to weigh less than 50 kilograms. Thorough editing will involve many such consistency checks and is best accomplished by computer programs designed to flag such errors [MacLaughlin, 1980]. Occasionally an apparently inconsistent result may appear on checking to be correct, but many errors will turn up through such editing. It is important, also, to check the consistency of various distributions. If exactly 84 women in a study are coded as premenopausal for a variable, "type of menopause," then it is reassuring that exactly 84 are likewise coded as premenopausal for the variable "age at menopause" (for such a variable, the code "premenopausal" should take a different code number from that assigned to unknown—e.g., 98 for premenopausal and 99 for unknown).

An important advantage of coding and entering data through a computer program is the ability to edit the data automatically during the entry process. Inadmissible or unusual values can be screened as they are entered. Inadmissible values can be rejected and corrected on the spot by programming the machine to print an error message on the screen and give an audible message as well to alert the operator about the error. Unlikely but legal values can be brought to the operator's attention in the same way. A sophisticated data-entry program can also check for consistency between variables and can eliminate some potential inconsistencies by automatically supplying appropriate codes. For example, if a subject is premenopausal, the program can automatically supply the correct code for "age at menopause" and skip the question. (On the other hand, some investigators may prefer the redundancy of the second question to guard against an error in the first.)

Even with sophisticated editing during data entry, it is still important to edit the stored data before analysis, to check on the completeness of the data and the reasonableness of the distribution of each variable. Neither of these features can be evaluated by a data-entry program.

Every experienced investigator knows that even the most meticulous data collection efforts suffer from errors that are detectable during careful editing. If editing is planned as a routine part of handling the data, the existence of such errors is usually not a serious problem. If editing is ignored, momentous problems can result.

DATA REDUCTION

The notion fundamental to data reduction is that certain observations in a set of data are equivalent, and it is easier to deal with equivalent observations after they have been summarized. The summary form usually is a contingency table in which the frequency of subjects (or units of observation) with every specific combination of variable values is tabulated for variables of interest. Such a table is presumed to contain, in summary form, essentially all the relevant information in the data. From the contingency table, the investigator can proceed with effect estimation. In addition, the table displays the distribution of subjects according to key variables and thus conveys directly to the investigator an intimacy with the data that is not easily obtained in any other way.

Data reduction into a contingency table is predicated on an analysis in which there is no concern for confounding or effect modification or there are at most only a small number of variables that might be confounders or effect modifiers. If the analysis must take account of a large number of variables, a multivariate analysis using mathematic modeling will be necessary. For such multivariate analyses, it is not necessary to reduce the data into a contingency table. Nevertheless, to ensure that the investigator acquires some familiarity with the data, it is advisable, even when planning a multivariate analysis, to reduce the data into contingency table format for the variables of central interest. Indeed, proceeding with an abridged analysis based on the contingency table data is a good idea even if the need for the multivariate analysis is certain.

Collapsing the edited data into categories for the contingency table may necessitate some decision making. The process is straightforward for nominal scale variables such as religion or race, which are already categorized. For continuous variables, however, the investigator must decide how many categories to make and where the category boundaries should be. The number of categories will usually depend on the amount of data available. If the data are abundant, it is always preferable to divide a variable into many categories. On the other hand, the purpose of data reduction is to summarize the data concisely and conveniently; creating too many categories would defeat this purpose. For control of confounding, it is rarely necessary to have more than about five categories [Cochran, 1968]. If an exposure variable is categorized to examine effect estimates for various levels of exposure, again it would be unusual to require more than about five categories. Frequently, however, the data are so sparse that it is undesirable to create as many as five categories for a given variable. When the observations are stretched over too many categories, the numbers within categories become statistically unstable and produce large random errors in the effect estimates.

Since most of the confounding from a given factor can be removed by a stratified analysis based on only two categories of a continuous variable [Cochran, 1968], it is desirable with sparse data to keep the number of categories small, perhaps two or three. Even a large body of data can be spread too thin if the contingency table involves too many dimensions, that is, if too many variables are used to classify the subjects. With three variables, apart from exposure and disease, and three categories for each variable, there will be 27 2 × 2 tables (assuming that both exposure and disease are dichotomous). With an additional two variables of three categories each, there will be a total of 243 2 × 2 tables, enough to stretch even a considerable body of data too thin, since a study of 10,000 people would average only about 10 subjects per cell of the multidimensional table. If a stratified analysis is planned and it is necessary to stratify by several variables, it is probable that only a few, perhaps as few as two, categories can be used for each variable. With only two categories per variable, stratification by five variables requires 32 rather than 243 2 × 2 tables, and a study of 10,000 subjects would average 78 subjects per cell rather than 10, thereby gaining precision at the cost of some potential residual confounding within categories.

The investigator must also decide where to draw the boundary between categories. There is no accepted method for doing this. A frequently expressed concern is that boundaries might be "gerrymandered," that is, shifted after a preliminary examination of the effect estimates in such a way that the estimates are altered in a desired direction. This concern imputes a level of dishonesty to the investigator that is presumably uncommon. Furthermore, the shift of a boundary in categorization rarely has a substantial effect on the magnitude of an estimate and then only because of a large random error component. On the other hand, it is frequently useful to inspect the distribution of a variable before deciding at which points to carve categories. There may be "natural" categories if the distribution has more than one mode. The distribution may be sufficiently skewed that preconceived category boundaries would lead to an inefficient separation of subjects, with too few in some categories and too many in others. For these reasons, it is often preferable to define the final categories after reviewing the data, notwithstanding the common advice that it is somehow more "objective" to do so in ignorance of the distribution of observations in hand. Nevertheless, if meaningful category boundaries are inherent in the variable, these can and should be specified a priori. For example, in categorizing subjects according to analgesic consumption, it is desirable to create categories that contrast the various therapeutic indications for analgesic use, the recommended doses for which can be specified in advance. It is often desirable, especially for an exposure variable, to retain extreme categories in the analysis without merging these with neighboring categories, since the extreme categories are often those that permit the most biologically informative contrasts.

A common problem in creating categories is the question of how to deal with the ends of the scale. Open-ended categories can provide an opportunity for considerable residual confounding, especially if there are no theoretical bounds for the variable. For example, age categories such as 65 +, with no upper limit, allow a considerable range of variability within which the desired homogeneity of exposure or outcome may not be achieved. Another example is the separation of the effects of alcohol consumption and tobacco smoking on the risk of oral cancer; within categories of heavy smoking, it is a reasonable possibility that the heaviest smokers drink more alcohol than those who smoke less within that category [Rothman and Keller, 1972]. When residual confounding from open-ended categories is considered likely, strict boundaries should be placed on every category, including those at the extremes of the scale.

A convenient method of assembling the final categories is to categorize the data initially much more finely than is necessary. A fine categorization will facilitate review of the distribution for each variable; more usable categories can then be created by coalescing adjacent categories. The coalescing of adjacent strata for a rank-ordered confounding variable can be justified by the lack of confounding that is introduced by merging the categories; this merging will not introduce confounding if the exposure distribution is the same among the controls or person-time denominators between the strata, or if the proportion of cases or the disease rate is the same among nonexposed subjects between the strata [Miettinen, 1976b]. The advantage of starting with more categories than is ultimately necessary is that the merging of categories can be conveniently accomplished with pencil and paper in seconds or minutes, whereas separating categories into subcategories cannot be done without reading through the entire data file, thus adding another computer run.

EFFECT ESTIMATION (AND HYPOTHESIS TESTING)
Hypothesis Testing

In data analysis, as opposed to the broader area of scientific inference, hypothesis testing generally refers to the evaluation of a null hypothesis. The introduction of the concepts of statistical evaluation early in the twentieth century led to an appreciation of the importance of assessing the role of random error in observations. Hypothesis testing is directed at the question of whether random error might account entirely for an observed association. The statistic used to evaluate this question is the *P-value*.

The *P*-value is usually interpreted as the probability that an association at least as strong as that actually seen in the data might have arisen if the null hypothesis were true, that is, by chance alone. Because a low *P*-value

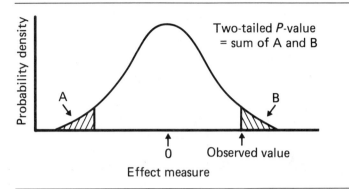

Fig. 10-1. Distribution of effect estimates under the null hypothesis in large studies (continuous distribution).

indicates a low probability, under the null hypothesis, of results as extreme or more extreme than those observed, low P-values are taken as an indication that the data are more compatible with the alternative hypothesis of a nonzero effect than with the null hypothesis. A P-value should not be confused with the probability that the null hypothesis is correct; it is calculated *on the assumption* that the null hypothesis is correct. Extremely low P-values can occur even when the null hypothesis is true; in fact, they are guaranteed to occur a small proportion of the time. The informativeness of the P-value derives solely from the interpretation that small P-values indicate relatively less consistency between the data and the null hypothesis and relatively more consistency with the alternative hypothesis of a nonzero effect.

Imagine that an estimate had a continuous sampling distribution on its scale of measurement, with a value of zero corresponding to the null hypothesis of no effect. Figure 10-1 illustrates the hypothetical probability density of the estimated effect; the bell shape of the curve is ensured for large studies by the central limit theorem in statistics. Values of the estimate equal to or more extreme than that observed correspond in the likelihood of their outcome to the shaded area in the diagram. The definition of *more extreme* can be unidirectional, in which case the P-value is said to be "one-tailed" or "one-sided" and is represented only by the shaded area under one end of the curve, or it can be bidirectional, in which case the "two-tailed" P-value corresponds to the sum of the shaded areas under both ends of the curve.

To calculate the P-value, it is necessary to postulate a statistical model that describes the probability distribution of the data on the assumption of the null hypothesis. If the distribution of effect estimates that are calculable from the data were actually continuous, it would be inconsequential whether the tail area of the curve is defined as the area corresponding

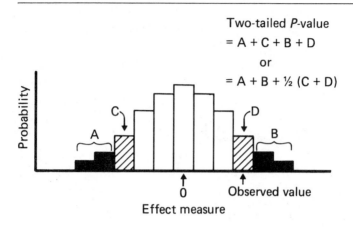

Fig. 10-2. Distribution of effect estimates under the null hypothesis (discrete distribution).

to effect estimates equal to or more extreme than those actually observed, or simply the area corresponding to estimates more extreme than those observed. Typically, however, in epidemiology, the data from which the effect estimates are calculated are discrete frequencies, and the distribution of effect estimates is discrete rather than continuous. The area representing a P-value for a discrete distribution is illustrated in Figure 10-2. Traditionally, the P-value has been defined as the sum of both the lightly shaded areas and the heavily shaded areas in Figure 10-2. The lightly shaded areas correspond to the probability of the actual observations (and the corresponding value in the opposite direction), whereas the darkly shaded areas correspond to the probability of more extreme departures from the null value than those actually observed. Obviously, for discrete distributions it does matter whether the P-value is defined as including the probability of the observed outcome or just the more extreme values.

The problem with the traditional definition of the P-value is that it leads to inconsistencies. For example, what if the observed value of the effect estimate were in the center of the distribution, right on the null value? In the traditional definition, each tail would then include more than half the distribution, and the two-tailed P-value would be greater than 100 percent, which is inconsistent with the view that the P-value represents a probability. An alternative definition of the P-value that overcomes this problem is one in which the probability of the observed value of the effect is partitioned, generally by splitting it into equal parts [Lancaster, 1949; Lancaster, 1961]. Thus, the one-tailed P-value would correspond to the probability of the more extreme values plus one-half the probability of the observed value. This definition of the P-value has been referred to as the "mid-P"

[Lancaster, 1961]. The two-tailed *P*-value is generally obtained by doubling the one-tailed *P*-value, however the *P*-value is defined.

With discrete data, the probability distributions used to calculate the *P*-value can give rise to intricate calculations; *P*-values calculated directly in this way are referred to as *exact P-values*. Usually it is simpler to use an approximation to the discrete distribution, relying on the fact that a normal curve will approximate the shape of the distribution reasonably well; the larger the frequencies involved in the discrete data, the greater the number of values that can be assumed by the effect estimate and the better the normal approximation to the discrete distribution. The advantage of using the normal distribution is that the calculations necessary to obtain the *P*-values are considerably simpler than those needed to get the exact *P*-value.

In an attempt to make the normal approximation better when frequencies are small, Yates [1934] suggested a "correction" procedure that amounts to shifting the observed value of the effect estimate toward the null value by a distance that corresponds to half of the probability of the actual data under the null hypothesis. This adjustment is intended to compensate for the fact that the observed value of the effect actually represents the central value of a range that corresponds to the region on the scale of the effect measure representing each discrete value. Since the probability of the entire range for the observed value is included in the definition of the traditional *P*-value, the Yates "correction" usually improves the approximation to the traditionally defined exact *P*-value. If, however, the mid-*P* definition were used, then the Yates "correction" would actually make the approximation worse, since the observed value already represents the central value of its discrete range. In this text, the Yates "correction" is ignored.

The general form for statistical testing based on a normal distribution around the null value is given by equation 10-1:

$$\chi = \frac{A - E}{\sqrt{V}} \qquad [10\text{-}1]$$

A is the observed value of the effect estimate, E is the expected value for A under the null hypothesis, and V is the variance of A under the null hypothesis. Provided that under the null hypothesis A is normally distributed, then under the null hypothesis χ will also be normally distributed but with a mean of zero and a standard deviation of unity. A normally distributed random variate with a mean of zero and a standard deviation of unity is referred to as a *standard normal deviate;* synonyms are *critical ratio* and *Z-value*. In this text, χ is used as the notation in the formula to emphasize that the square of the standard normal deviate has a chi-square distribution with "one degree of freedom"—indeed, that is how the one degree of freedom chi-square statistic is defined. (Chi-square with n degrees of freedom is simply the sum of n independent chi-squares with one degree of freedom.) The P-value is obtained from the χ value from tables (or computational formulas) of the standard normal distribution. In essence, equation 10-1 converts a normally distributed statistic with a calculated expectation and variance into a standard normal deviate (expectation of zero and standard deviation of unity) for which detailed tables are conveniently available to obtain P-values. It would be possible to square the χ and obtain the P-value from tables of chi-square, but since these usually have considerably less detail than tables of the standard normal distribution, there is no reason to do so.

To this point this discussion has presumed that the observation of interest is the estimate of effect derived from the data. Although this is generally so, in calculating the χ it is usually more convenient to postulate for the random variable A a measure that contains all the essential statistical information about the effect but for which the variance is more easily and accurately calculated. It is convenient to designate A as the number of exposed subjects with disease in the study; with this substitution, the expected number for A under the null hypothesis will not be zero but must be calculated from the data based on the relevant probability model. The models relevant to epidemiologic studies will be described in Chapters 11 and 12.

Estimation of Effects

The single best numerical estimate of an effect from a set of data is referred to as a *point estimate*. Because a point estimate is only one point on a continuous scale with an infinite number of possible values, there is essentially zero probability that it is correct, even if there is no source of bias. Therefore, although point estimates serve as useful indicators of the magnitude of an effect, it is important to supplement the information that they provide with a measure of the random error in the data. Hypothesis testing can accomplish this goal, but the P-value is an undesirable statistic for evaluating random error because it provides no information about magnitude of effect and only indirectly allows assessment of the extent of random error in an estimate. As was emphasized in Chapter 9, the greatest drawback of P-values is that they tend to be used for "significance" testing as an analytic goal, diverting the focus away from the proper goal of estimation of effects. A better approach is the use of confidence intervals, which have none of the drawbacks of P-values.

A confidence interval denotes a range of values surrounding the point estimate that amounts to a "sampling range" for the estimate. The level of confidence, which is arbitrarily selected by the investigator, is the frame of reference by which the sampling range can be interpreted. Most investigators repeatedly use the same level of confidence to ease comparison; 90 and 95 percent are commonly used values.

The connection between confidence intervals and P-values, described

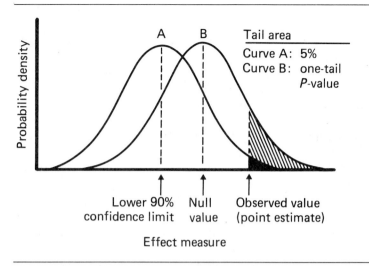

Fig. 10-3. Sampling range of the data in reference to the null value and the lower 90 percent confidence limit.

in Chapter 9, should be expressed in more formal terms. Like a confidence interval, the *P*-value also measures a sampling range, but it specifically measures the sampling range of the data under the null hypothesis. The null point on the effect scale is the reference point for hypothesis testing, and the *P*-value is a measure of the discrepancy of the data with the reference point in probability terms. A confidence interval, in contrast, fixes the probability to an arbitrarily chosen value, which is dependent on the desired level of confidence, and varies the reference point, which becomes the limit to the confidence interval. Thus, in determining the lower boundary of a 90 percent confidence interval, the reference point is adjusted until the upper tail area is exactly 5 percent (Fig. 10-3). For 90 percent confidence limits, the direction of the adjustment of the reference point will be from the null value toward the point estimate if the one-tail *P*-value is less than 5 percent, leading to a lower confidence bound above the null value (for positive effects). If the one-tail *P*-value is greater than 5 percent, the reference point must be adjusted away from the null value in the direction opposite the point estimate to bring the tail area down to 5 percent, resulting in a confidence interval that will bracket the null value. If the one-tail *P*-value is exactly 5 percent, then one boundary of the 90 percent confidence interval will be equal to the null value.

The most accurate way to determine a confidence limit is to use exact calculations analogous to the exact calculations used to calculate *P*-values. The calculations for confidence limits are considerably more difficult, however, for two reasons. First, the adjustment of the reference point in calculating the tail area amounts to the testing of a non-null hypothesis.

The statistical models that describe the non-null situation are highly complicated in comparison with the null-hypothesis models and demand much more involved calculations. Second, these intricate calculations have to be repeated in an iterative process for trial values of the reference point until the tail area conforms with the desired level of confidence. Therefore, calculation of exact confidence limits is practically infeasible without programmable electronic computing equipment.

Fortunately, many simple techniques exist, analogous with formula 10-1, to obtain approximate confidence limits. As with hypothesis testing, the accuracy of all the approximate techniques depends on the number of observations because all the methods depend on the normal distribution of effect estimates guaranteed by the central limit theorem for observations that are sufficiently numerous.

A simplifying assumption that is often made is that the sampling variability of an effect estimate is constant along its scale of measurement, that is, the variance of the effect estimate is a constant, independent of the value of the estimate. This assumption is not necessary for hypothesis testing, since the P-value is calculated on the assumption that the null hypothesis holds, and therefore the concern in hypothesis testing is to estimate the variance only at the null value. With a large set of observations, the sampling range for the effect estimate is narrow enough to make this assumption appropriate; even if the variance changes substantially along the scale of measurement of the effect measure, in a narrow enough range it will be nearly constant. Therefore, the simplifying assumption that the variance is constant is asymptotically correct; that is, the assumption becomes more appropriate as the number of observations used in the estimation process increases.

The usual and simplest approach to calculating approximate confidence limits is to estimate the standard deviation of the normal curve that represents the approximate sampling distribution of the effect estimate. The area under a symmetric segment of a normal curve is a specific function of the standard deviation; in fact, this relation provides the only interpretability for the standard deviation as a measure of variability: If the distribution is not normal, there is no meaningful interpretation of standard deviation, though confidence intervals might nevertheless be obtained by exact calculation. For any normal curve, 68 percent of the area under the curve lies in the region within one standard deviation (SD) of the central point. Thus, measurement values reported with ± SD as a measure of variability amount to a point estimate with an accompanying 68 percent confidence interval, provided that the sampling distribution is indeed normal. When a level of confidence is chosen, usually the value is not 68 percent but commonly 80, 90, or 95 percent. These levels of confidence correspond to regions that are bounded by points 1.282, 1.645, and 1.960 standard deviation units, respectively, from the central value in either direction (Fig. 10-4).

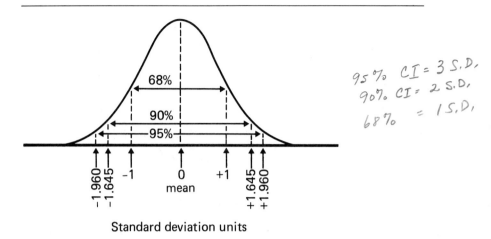

68%

90%

95%

-1.960
-1.645 -1 0 $+1$ $+1.645$
$+1.960$

mean

Standard deviation units

Fig. 10-4. Area under a normal curve.

95% CI = 3 S.D,
90% CI = 2 S.D,
68%   = 1 S.D,

To obtain a confidence interval based on the assumption of a normal sampling distribution it is necessary to estimate both the expected (mean) value of the effect and the standard deviation. The expected value is estimated by the point estimate, and the standard deviation is usually also estimated simply from the observed data. To construct confidence intervals, with rate difference as the effect measure, the resulting formula would be

upper — desired confidence level

$$\hat{RD} \pm Z \cdot \hat{SD}(\hat{RD}) \qquad\qquad [10\text{-}2]$$

lower

in which $\hat{RD}$ indicates the point estimate of rate difference (the caret signifies an estimate), Z is the multiplier for the standard deviation corresponding to the desired level of confidence, and $\hat{SD}(\hat{RD})$ indicates the estimated standard deviation of the point estimate; the minus sign gives the lower limit for the interval, and the plus sign gives the upper limit. The point estimate and the standard deviation are derived from the data, and a value for Z is arbitrarily selected to give the desired confidence level, for example, 1.645 for 90 percent confidence, and so on. Frequently, in a formulation such as that given in equation 10-2, the standard deviation is referred to as the *standard error* (abbreviated SE). In some circumstances there is an important distinction to be made between standard deviation and standard error: The standard error is the standard deviation of the sampling distribution of mean values; if the original observations come from a normal distribution, it is important to distinguish the standard deviation of the latter from the standard deviation of mean values, thus giving rise to the need for a separate term, standard error. In the context of this book, however, we shall generally be interested in the sampling distribution of point estimates, which corresponds to the standard error, although it is also perfectly acceptable to use the term standard deviation, since a standard error is a specific type of standard deviation.

If the effect measure of interest were rate ratio rather than rate difference, it might be reasonable to use formula 10-2 and simply substitute $\hat{RR}$ for $\hat{RD}$. It is preferable, however, to use a different equation because the sampling distribution for $\hat{RR}$ is asymmetric, and consequently the sampling distribution of rate ratio estimates is not normally distributed unless a relatively large number of observations is available. Why is the sampling distribution for $\hat{RR}$ asymmetric? The minimum value for RR is zero, whereas the maximum value is infinity. Random errors can lead to larger discrepancies on the high side of the mean than corresponding discrepancies on the low side of the mean. Notice that for $\hat{RD}$ the sampling distribution is symmetric. Although the sampling distribution for $\hat{RR}$ approaches a normal curve for a sufficiently large number of observations, it is customary to use a scale transformation to introduce symmetry and to set confidence limits on a scale of measurement that gives a better approximation to the normal distribution when the observations are relatively sparse. This is conveniently accomplished by using a logarithmic transformation. For setting confidence limits after logarithmic transformation of rate ratio, the formula is

$$\ln(\hat{RR}) \pm Z \cdot \hat{SD}(\ln(\hat{RR})) \qquad [10\text{-}3]$$

This is analogous to formula 10-2, differing only in that $\ln(\hat{RR})$ has been substituted for $\hat{RD}$. Having set confidence limits on the logarithmically transformed scale, it is necessary to reverse the transformation so that the limits can be interpreted on the original scale. To do so requires taking the antilogarithm of the limits resulting from formula 10-3. The whole process can be summarized by the formula

$$\exp[\ln(\hat{RR}) \pm Z \cdot \hat{SD}(\ln(\hat{RR}))] \qquad [10\text{-}4]$$

Whereas formula 10-2 gives confidence limits that are equidistant from the point estimate, formula 10-4, because of the scale transformation, gives confidence limits that are asymmetric about the point estimate. The limits are symmetric on the logarithmic scale, but on the original scale the point estimate is the geometric mean between the lower and upper limits; that is, the ratio of the upper bound to the point estimate equals the ratio of the point estimate to the lower bound.

Formulas 10-2 and 10-4 are the simplest general formulas for deriving approximate confidence limits for the rate difference and rate ratio measure of effect, respectively. Many specific techniques have been proposed, each striking a different balance between computational ease and accuracy. Some formulas discard the assumption that the standard deviation is uniform along its scale of measurement and use iterative techniques to estimate the value of the standard deviation at the boundary of the interval; the method of Cornfield [1956] for calculating confidence limits for the odds ratio is an example of this approach; Miettinen and Nurminen [1985] have extended Cornfield's approach to the risk ratio and risk difference measures. Iterative calculations usually require programmed computing assistance, so that the theoretical advantages are accompanied by practical disadvantages.

The simplest specific technique for performing interval estimation is the "test-based" method [Miettinen, 1976a], which assumes that the estimate of the standard deviation of the sampling distribution of the effect estimate obtained at the null value is a reasonable estimate of the standard deviation of the distribution elsewhere along the scale. This assumption differs slightly from the usual assumption that the estimated value of the standard deviation at the point estimate will be appropriate at the bounds of the interval; although both approaches assume that the value of the standard deviation estimated at one point along the scale will apply for both lower and upper bounds, the value estimated at the point estimate is more or less centrally placed between the limits of the interval, whereas the null value is not and might even be outside the interval. If the standard deviation changes along the effect-measure scale, the degree of error in the approximate limits is probably less severe if the standard deviation is estimated at a point central to the confidence interval rather than at the null point, which has no connection to the location of the limits. On the other hand, by choosing the null point as the point at which the standard deviation is estimated, the resulting confidence limits will tend to be more accurate when they fall in the vicinity of the null point, and it may be argued that it is worth obtaining greater accuracy in the vicinity of the null value even if it means sacrificing some accuracy for limits calculated to be far from the null value.

Applying the assumption of test-based limits leads to a concise formulation for obtaining confidence limits, based on the test statistics from equation 10-1. Consider the reformulation of equation 10-1 for rate difference:

$$\chi = \frac{\hat{RD} - E}{\hat{SD}(\hat{RD})}$$

where E, the expectation of $\hat{RD}$ under the null hypothesis, is zero, and $\hat{SD}(\hat{RD})$ is calculated on the assumption that the null hypothesis is true. This gives

$$\chi = \frac{\hat{RD}}{\hat{SD}_0(\hat{RD})} \qquad [10\text{-}5]$$

where $\widehat{SD}_0(\widehat{RD})$ indicates that the SD is estimated at the null value. Equation 10-5 can be rewritten as

$$\widehat{SD}_0(\widehat{RD}) = \frac{\widehat{RD}}{\chi}$$

and substituted into formula 10-2, giving, for the lower and upper limits

$$\widehat{RD} \pm Z \frac{\widehat{RD}}{\chi}$$

or

$$\widehat{RD}(1 \pm Z/\chi) \qquad\qquad [10\text{-}6]$$

The χ in formula 10-6 was assumed to be a test statistic evaluating RD per se. Miettinen recommended inserting into formula 10-6 any χ statistic that represents an equally efficient test of the null hypothesis based on the same data. For example, the usual χ based on the distribution of the number of exposed cases could be substituted (see Chap. 11 for the specific application).

The counterpart of equation 10-5 using the rate ratio measure of effect, after logarithmic transformation, is

$$\chi = \frac{\ln(\widehat{RR})}{\widehat{SD}_0(\ln(\widehat{RR}))} \qquad\qquad [10\text{-}7]$$

which can be rewritten as

$$\widehat{SD}_0(\ln(\widehat{RR})) = \frac{\ln(\widehat{RR})}{\chi}$$

and substituted into formula 10-4 to give

$$\exp\left[\ln(\widehat{RR}) \pm Z \frac{\ln(\widehat{RR})}{\chi}\right]$$

which simplifies to

$$\widehat{RR}^{(1 \pm Z/\chi)} \qquad\qquad [10\text{-}8]$$

As with formula 10-6, the attraction of formula 10-8 rests with the substitution for the χ statistic based on $\widehat{RR}$ an alternative and more convenient χ testing the null hypothesis. Indeed, the same χ statistic can be used in formulas 10-6 and 10-8 to generate confidence limits for rate difference and rate ratio. Note that when the χ value equals the Z multiplier, the lower bound should and does correspond exactly to the null value, which is zero for rate difference and unity for rate ratio.

The test-based formulas for approximate confidence limits given in formulas 10-6 and 10-8 are exceedingly easy to apply and produce usable confidence intervals in a wide variety of situations. The only numbers required from the data are an appropriate point estimate of the effect estimate and the χ statistic from hypothesis testing. Indeed, the use of the χ statistic in these test-based formulas is the main justification for any detailed discussion of statistical hypothesis testing in modern epidemiology, since the estimation of a confidence interval is preferable to the use of P-values to evaluate random error, and the P-value adds very little information if a confidence interval is given.

Unfortunately, the principle of test-based limits is invalid as a general method of interval estimation [Halperin, 1977; Gart, 1979]. Simulations have borne out the predictably poor performance of the method for large departures of the odds ratio from the null value [Brown, 1981; Gart, 1982], and Greenland [1984] has provided a counterexample with the SMR that refutes the general validity of the approach. Greenland [1984] states

[T]he problem with test-based limits is not (as has been suggested) lack of variance stabilization in specific applications, but rather that the principle requires us to equate two different large-sample test statistics. Since these statistics are equivalent only in the neighborhood of the null hypothesis, the principle itself is fallacious. ... Unfortunately, the size of the neighborhood for which the principle holds will vary from parameter to parameter.

Despite the theoretical drawbacks, test-based limits can be useful as a "quick-and-dirty" method of interval estimation. The method is known to perform well for odds ratio limits when the odds ratio is between 0.2 and 5.0, and it can also be an acceptable tool in other situations. A comparison of the various methods of confidence interval estimation is illustrated for some simple data in the next chapter.

Adjustment for Multiple Comparisons

Many statisticians have voiced concern about the interpretation of P-values or "significance" tests when multiple comparisons are made. The basis for concern rests on the following argument: Suppose a complex set of completely random numbers were evaluated for 1,000 associations. The premise is that there are no real associations in the data but that 1,000 different measures of association are examined. If "significance" testing is performed, at the 5 percent level of "significance" there would be about 50 "significant" associations in the data, all representing type I or alpha-errors, that is, "statistically significant" associations that occur only by chance.

The point is that chance guarantees a certain proportion of such associations, and when many associations are studied, many false positive associations are possible.

The traditional statistical approach to this "problem" has been to make the "significance" test more stringent, either by changing the criterion to a more stringent value, such as 1 percent instead of 5 percent, or by actually inflating the calculated P-values by some factor that depends on the number of comparisons made. Since epidemiologists, in their usually thorough evaluation of expensively obtained data, typically make multiple comparisons, they have frequently been admonished to be wary of the problem.

It is not clear, however, that the recommended solution is an improvement. In the first place, the above argument, like all hypothesis testing, starts from the premise that the explanation for all the so-called "significant" results is chance, a sort of grand null hypothesis. But why should we assume that chance is a likely explanation for the associations that are observed? Indeed, one might argue that it seldom is (some would say never is) the explanation for findings. If chance is not the explanation for a "significantly" positive association, then the finding does not represent a type I or alpha-error. By making the screening criterion for statistical "significance" more stringent, a penalty is paid: Real non-null associations may go undetected (a type II error) because they fail to meet the more stringent criterion. An elementary consideration of screening principles, which apply here, makes it clear that from a single criterion (the "significance" level) the number of false positives can be reduced only at the expense of an increased frequency of false negatives. Is it worthwhile to reduce false positives at the expense of false negatives? The question cannot be answered generally; it requires a deeper understanding of the consequences of false positive and false negative results in the context of the research setting. One thing, however, is extremely clear: Whatever the arguments might be for reducing the chance of a false positive in favor of a false negative, they have nothing to do with multiple comparisons; they would apply equally well to a single comparison.

The crux of the multiple comparison problem seems to be that in performing many comparisons and reporting only those that are "statistically significant," it is difficult to impute the intended interpretation to the P-value; in the null hypothesis, a well-defined proportion of tests would be "significant," but if the denominator, the number of comparisons, is large and unknown, a reasonable interpretation of the P-values reported is hindered.

If many comparisons were made and each one were reported individually, let us say in a separate publication, it would be absurd to make adjustments to the reported P-values in each report based on the total number of such reports. If such adjustments were indicated, it would also follow that an investigator should keep a cumulative total of comparisons made during a career, and adjust all "significance" tests according to the current total of comparisons made to date. The more senior the investigator, the more the *P*-value would have to be inflated. For that matter, wouldn't such adjustments have to take into account the anticipated number of future comparisons as well as those already made? It should be obvious that these concerns are irrelevant to the research problem; they convert the *P*-value from a statistic conveying information about a specific association in the data to one that depends on the unrelated experiences or psychologic state of the investigator. No one has yet suggested making adjustments for multiple comparisons if the results are reported individually in separate publications. But is it not inconsistent then to consider making such adjustments if the same results are aggregated into one or several publications? Would a review paper of individually reported associations have to adjust the *P*-values? If no adjustments should be made to *P*-values when they are reported individually in separate publications, it follows that the process of lumping the results together in one place should not affect the results themselves, regardless of when and how the lumping is done. Therefore, no adjustments for multiple comparisons should be made even if a large number of comparisons are reported at one time, provided that it is clear how many comparisons have been made and that all "negative" (that is, "nonsignificant") results have been reported along with the "positive" or "significant" results.

A problem does exist when the negative results are not reported; it is then more difficult to interpret properly the *P*-values for the positive findings that are reported. It is still a mistake, however, to believe that interpretation can be improved by adjusting the *P*-value or changing the criterion for "significance." The adjusted values are also impossible to interpret, since they divulge even less about the actual association; changing the criterion for "significance" does not actually solve the problem; as discussed earlier, it merely produces a smaller type I error at the expense of a greater type II error.

As usual, some clarity is gained by considering the use of confidence intervals rather than "significance" tests. The equivalent of multiplying the *P*-value by some adjustment factor to compensate for multiple comparisons would be broadening the confidence interval. But the broader interval has no relation to the amount of information in the data about the effect in question; it depends instead on the number of comparisons that the investigator might have made. The problem with this approach is that it seems to defy the logical presumption that the reported results about an effect should reflect the amount of information about the effect in the data, nothing more and nothing less. If broader confidence intervals were reported to compensate for multiple comparisons, a reader with an interest of the information imparted by the reported findings simply because the original investigator did not also focus solely on that problem. focused solely on the one item would pay an unnecessary penalty in terms

Since no problem calling for any adjustments seems to exist unless the positive results from a large number of comparisons are reported without any information about the total number of comparisons, and since even then it appears that adjustments in the results only make them more difficult to interpret, the best course for the epidemiologist to take when making multiple comparisons is to ignore advice to make such adjustments in reported results. Each finding should be reported as if it alone were the sole focus of a study. If a large number of comparisons makes it infeasible to report all findings, it is important to make it clear how many associations were evaluated. If it cannot be determined how many comparisons were made, then associations not previously reported should be considered merely suggestive. It is worth emphasizing, however, that any new findings should always be considered only suggestive, even if only one comparison is made. Findings that address a previously reported association or lack of association should not become a weaker confirmation or refutation simply because they are accompanied by many other unrelated comparisons, since the previously reported findings on the question amount to a prior hypothesis.

REFERENCES

Brown, C. C. The validity of approximate methods for interval estimation of the odds ratio. *Am. J. Epidemiol.* 1981;113:474–480.

Cochran, W. G. The effectiveness of adjustment by subclassification in removing bias in observational studies. *Biometrics* 1968;24:295–313.

Cornfield, J. A statistical problem arising from retrospective studies. In J. Neyman (ed.) *Proceedings Third Berkeley Symposium,* Vol. 4. Berkeley: University of California Press, 1956, pp. 135–148.

Gart, J. J. Statistical analyses of the relative risk. *Environ. Health Perspect.* 1979;32:157–167.

Gart, J. J., and Thomas, D. G. The performance of three approximate confidence limit methods for the odds ratio. *Am. J. Epidemiol.* 1982;115:453–470.

Greenland, S. A counterexample to the test-based principle of setting confidence limits. *Am. J. Epidemiol.* 1984;120:4–7.

Halperin, M. Re: "Estimability and estimation in case-control studies." Letter to the Editor. *Am. J. Epidemiol.* 1977;105:496–498.

Lancaster, H. O. The combination of probabilities arising from data in discrete distributions. *Biometrika* 1949;36:370–382.

Lancaster, H. O. Significance tests in discrete distributions. *J. Am. Stat. Assoc.* 1961;56:223–234.

MacLaughlin, D. S. A data validation program nucleus. *Comput. Prog. Biomed.* 1980;11:43–47.

Miettinen, O. S. Estimability and estimation in case-referent studies. *Am. J. Epidemiol.* 1976a;103:226–235.

Miettinen, O. S. Stratification by a multivariate confounder score. *Am. J. Epidemiol.* 1976b;104:609–620.

Miettinen, O. S., and Nurminen, M. Comparative analysis of two rates. *Statistics Med.* 1985;4:213–226.

Rothman, K. J., and Keller, A. Z. The effect of joint exposure to alcohol and tobacco on risk of cancer of the mouth and pharynx. *J. Chron. Dis.* 1972;25:711–716.

Yates, F. Contigency tables involving small numbers and the chi-square test. *J. R. Statist. Soc.* Suppl. 1934;1:217–235.

11. ANALYSIS OF CRUDE DATA

The simplest type of epidemiologic analysis, which is based on crude (i.e., unstratified) data, applies when it is not necessary to take into account any factors beyond the exposure and the disease of interest. Although it is not unusual to see data presented solely in crude form, typically the investigator needs first to explore more complicated analyses using stratification or multivariate methods to evaluate the role of other factors. Vigorous restriction by covariates in subject selection (so as to prevent confounding) will often lead to a simple or crude analysis. Clinical trials using random allocation of subjects also can often be analyzed satisfactorily in crude form if the investigators are persuaded that the randomization has successfully prevented confounding. A crude analysis, because of its simplicity, possesses an appealing cogency that is lacking in more complicated analyses.

HYPOTHESIS TESTING WITH CRUDE DATA

The epidemiologist, in conceptualizing types of epidemiologic data, tends to separate follow-up data from case-control data. For statistical hypothesis testing, however, statistical modeling leads to a different kind of separation according to whether the data consist of person-time units or persons as the basic observations. Whereas the units of observation are measured as person-time only in follow-up studies, not all follow-up studies are presented with the data expressed as incidence rates with person-time denominators. If all subjects are followed for a constant period, it may be convenient to express the incidence rates as risk estimates, that is, cumulative incidence data, in which the number of cases is related not to an amount of person-time experience but to the total number of people who were followed. Clinical trials are often presented in this manner. When the denominators of incidence measures are presented as counts of persons rather than as measures of person-time experience, the statistical model that applies for hypothesis testing is the same one that applies to case-control data, in which all observations also are counts of persons.

Hypothesis Testing with Person-Time Data

Crude incidence-rate data consist of the total number of cases and person-time units for both exposed and unexposed categories. We shall use the notation in Table 11-1. The apparent simplicity of this table may mask analytic subtleties that must be considered. Specifically, the person-time experience in the "exposed" column should be defined according to a plausible or tentative model for induction time. Before an individual becomes exposed, all of that individual's person-time experience is, naturally, unexposed person-time (though it is often not included as such in an analysis). If exposure occurs at a point in time and the induction-time model being evaluated calls for a minimum induction time of 5 years, then the 5 years

Table 11-1. Notation for crude incidence-rate data with person-time denominators

	Exposed	Unexposed	Total
Cases	a	b	M_1
Person-time	N_1	N_0	T

after the point of exposure for each individual is likewise unexposed person-time experience rather than exposed, because according to the induction-time model it relates back to a period of time when exposure was absent. Tallying the person-time units into the appropriate exposure categories is a task that must be done subject by subject and may involve complicated rules if the exposure is chronic. Incident cases are tallied into the same category to which the concurrent person-time units are being added—for example, an incident case occurring 4 years after exposure would be tallied in the "unexposed" category if the induction-time model specified a minimum induction time of 5 years.

The statistical model used for hypothesis testing of person-time data is the *binomial distribution* [Shore et al., 1976]. A random event that has only two possible outcomes, X and Y, that occur with fixed probabilities is referred to as a *Bernoulli trial.* Flipping a coin is an example. Let the probability of one of the two outcomes, say X, be p. The probability distribution of the total number of Xs occurring in N independent Bernoulli trials with p constant is referred to as a binomial distribution. Mathematically, the probability is expressed as

$$\Pr(\text{total number of Xs} = x) = \binom{N}{x} p^x (1 - p)^{(N-x)}$$

$$\text{where} \quad \binom{N}{x} \quad \text{is} \quad \frac{N!}{x! \, (N - x)!}$$

The mean of the binomial distribution is Np, and the variance is Np(1 − p).

In applying the binomial model to crude person-time data, each case is considered to be an independent Bernoulli trial, having as its "outcome" the two possibilities of exposed or unexposed. According to the null hypothesis that exposure is unrelated to disease, the probability that a given case will be classified as exposed or unexposed depends only on the proportion of the total person-time experience that is allocated to the exposed category; that is, each case has a probability equal to N_1/T of being classified as exposed under the null hypothesis.

The M_1 cases are thus considered to be M_1 independent Bernoulli trials, and the distribution of exposed cases has a binomial distribution under the null hypothesis, with $p = N_1/T$. The probability of the observed data under the null hypothesis can be written as

$$\text{Pr(number of exposed cases} = a) = \binom{M_1}{a} \left(\frac{N_1}{T}\right)^a \left(\frac{N_0}{T}\right)^b$$

An exact one-tail Fisher P-value can be obtained as

$$\sum_{k=a}^{M_1} \text{Pr(number of exposed cases} = k)$$

The above summation gives the upper tail of the distribution; the lower tail can be obtained by summing k over the range from 0 to a. To obtain the mid-P value instead of the traditional Fisher P-value, only one-half the probability of the observed data should be added to the summation for each tail. When the mid-P values are calculated, the lower and upper tails of the distribution have the desirable property of summing to unity.

With large numbers, these exact calculations are unnecessary because an asymptotic test statistic will give accurate approximations for the P-value. The test statistic is computed from formula 11-1, using the number of exposed cases as the random variate. Based on the formulas for the mean and variance of the number of successes in a binomial distribution, the null expectation for the number of exposed cases is N_1M_1/T, and the variance is $M_1N_1N_0/T^2$, which gives

$$\chi = \frac{a - N_1M_1/T}{\sqrt{\dfrac{M_1N_1N_0}{T^2}}} \qquad\qquad [11\text{-}1]$$

The χ values can then be translated into P-values from tables of the standard normal distribution.

For Example 11-1, the probability of the observed data under the null hypothesis may be calculated as

$$\text{Pr(41 exposed cases)} = \binom{56}{41} \left(\frac{28{,}010}{47{,}027}\right)^{41} \left(\frac{19{,}017}{47{,}027}\right)^{15} = 0.0122$$

An exact upper-tail Fisher P-value may be calculated by repeating the calculation for the more extreme positive outcomes up through 56 exposed cases. For 42 exposed cases, the calculation gives

$$\text{Pr(42 exposed cases)} = \binom{56}{42} \left(\frac{28{,}010}{47{,}027}\right)^{42} \left(\frac{19{,}017}{47{,}027}\right)^{14} = 0.0064$$

Example 11-1. Breast cancer cases and person-years of observation for women with tuberculosis repeatedly exposed to multiple x-ray fluoroscopies, and women with tuberculosis not so exposed [Boice and Monson, 1977]

	Radiation exposure		
	Yes	No	Total
Breast cancer	41	15	56
Person-years	28,010	19,017	47,027

Similarly, Pr(43 exposed cases) = 0.0031, Pr(44 exposed cases) = 0.0013, and Pr(45 exposed cases) = 0.0005. The small magnitude of this last probability indicates that it should not be necessary to calculate the additional terms in the summation, since their contribution would be even smaller and therefore would not affect the sum materially. The one-tail *P*-value thus equals 0.0122 + 0.0064 + 0.0031 + 0.0013 + 0.0005 = 0.024. The one-tail mid-*P* would have ½(0.0122) as the first term, giving 0.017 as the *P*-value (it is actually 0.0174 and would be rounded to 0.018 if the summation were carried a few terms more). Two-tail *P*-values can be obtained simply by doubling the corresponding one-tail *P*-values.

The numbers in the example are large enough to use the normal approximation in formula 11-1, which is a simpler calculation:

$$\chi = \frac{41 - 28,010 \left(\dfrac{56}{47,027} \right)}{\sqrt{\dfrac{(56)\,(28,010)\,(19,017)}{(47,027)^2}}} = \frac{41 - 33.35}{\sqrt{13.49}} = \frac{7.65}{3.67} = 2.08$$

From tables of the standard normal distribution, a χ value of 2.08 corresponds to a one-tail *P*-value of 0.019, which agrees closely with the exact one-tail mid-*P* value.

Hypothesis Testing with Count Data

Follow-up data or prevalence data with denominators consisting of the number of persons at risk can be treated like case-control data for statistical hypothesis testing. For each of these types of data, the basic information can be displayed in a 2 × 2 table in which all four cells of the table are frequencies of subjects classified according to the presence or absence of exposure and disease. The notation we shall use is given in Table 11-2.

Superficially, Table 11-2 resembles Table 11-1 except for the addition of an added row for noncases. The denominators in Table 11-2, however, are frequencies, or counts, of subjects rather than person-time accumulations.

Table 11-2. Notation for crude 2 × 2 table

	Exposed	Unexposed	Total
Cases	a	b	M_1
Noncases	c	d	M_0
Total	N_1	N_0	T

Again, the apparent simplicity of the table may mask some subtleties in determining the classification of subjects.

For case-control data, classification according to exposure depends on an appropriate and meaningful definition of exposure according to a biologic model of induction time that specifies the timing of exposure in relation to disease. In a study of oral cavity cancer, for example, patients with cancer may tend to use mouthwash regularly more frequently than controls, but such use may occur as a consequence of early symptoms of the disease or of its subsequent treatment (radiotherapy in the region of the oropharynx tends to shrink the salivary glands and cause foul breath). A meaningful model for induction time should classify as unexposed only those individuals who were exposed to the agent outside the time window during which exposure might have been etiologically related to the disease.

For follow-up data analyzed with a 2 × 2 table, presumably all subjects were free of disease at the beginning of the follow-up period; the classification of exposure refers to the time of initiation of follow-up, and the classification of disease refers to the time of completion of follow-up. Disease occurrence should not count as such unless it occurs during the time window specified by a meaningful induction-time model. An instance of the illness of interest occurring before or after the hypothesized induction time window should be ignored; if illness occurs before the time window, it may be reasonable to exclude the subject as not being free of disease at the start of the relevant period of follow-up. If the follow-up period has been so long that a substantial proportion of subjects have been lost or have died from causes unrelated to the outcome of interest, it is preferable to use person-time denominators rather than to analyze the data with a 2 × 2 table.

The 2 × 2 table can be considered as representing two independent series of observations: For case-control studies the observations are exposure observations and the two independent series of subjects are the cases and the controls; for follow-up studies the observations are disease observations and the two independent series are the exposed and unexposed groups. The observations made on each of the two independent series can be considered as conforming to the model of a binomial distribution; under the null hypothesis, the probability of a "positive" observation in each of the two independently observed binomial series is the same.

Consider a follow-up study of N_1 exposed subjects and N_0 unexposed subjects. In the exposed series, "a" subjects develop disease, and in the unexposed series, "b" subjects develop disease. The probability that exactly a and b subjects will develop disease among the exposed and unexposed, respectively, is, according to the binomial model,

Pr(a exposed cases and b unexposed cases)

$$= \binom{N_1}{a} (p_1)^a (1 - p_1)^c \cdot \binom{N_0}{b} (p_0)^b (1 - p_0)^d \quad [11\text{-}2]$$

which is the product of the binomial probabilities for each of the two independent groups, exposed and unexposed. The probability of developing disease among the exposed is p_1; among the unexposed, it is p_0. Under the null hypothesis, these two probabilities are equal: $p_1 = p_0 = p$, which gives

Pr(a exposed cases and b unexposed cases)

$$= \binom{N_1}{a} \binom{N_0}{b} \cdot (p)^{M_1} (1 - p)^{M_0} \quad [11\text{-}3]$$

To calculate the value of expression 11-3 for a particular 2 × 2 table, it is necessary to have an estimate of p. Usually p is estimated directly from the data, using the overall disease proportion from the margins of the table, M_1/T. Substituting M_1/T for p gives

Pr(a exposed cases and b unexposed cases)

$$= \binom{N_1}{a} \binom{N_0}{b} \cdot (M_1/T)^{M_1} (M_0/T)^{M_0} \quad [11\text{-}4]$$

From expression 11-4 it is possible to obtain a *P*-value that represents an exact test based on two independent binomial distributions, provided that it is clear how the departures from the null state that are more extreme than those observed are calculated. Let us assume that a positive association is observed between exposure and disease. Assume that a and b are the number of exposed and unexposed cases actually observed. For other possible realizations of the data in which the number of exposed cases exceeds a while the number of unexposed cases is b or less, the overall departure from the null condition is more extreme than that actually observed. Similarly, if the number of exposed cases is a but the number of unexposed cases is less than b, again the departure from the null would be more extreme than that actually observed. The preceding possibilities are easy to classify, but what if the number of exposed cases were a + 1

and the number of unexposed cases were b + 1? What about other combinations such as a + 1 and b + 2? It is difficult to say whether these
possibilities represent situations that depart from the null to a greater extent than the actual observations. To decide definitively if a departure is
more extreme, it would be necessary to evaluate an effect measure for
each hypothetical outcome of the data and compare that measure with the
effect measure calculated from the actual observations. Interestingly, the
decision about which outcomes are more extreme would depend on
which effect measure was used.

To illustrate, consider example 11-2. The "observed" data indicate an
estimated risk difference of 0.05, a risk ratio of 1.11, and an odds ratio of
1.22. Variations 1 and 2 are two other possible outcomes for the data,
presuming that the same number of exposed and unexposed subjects are
studied. Using the risk difference measure to determine departures from
the null, variation 2, but not variation 1, is a more extreme departure from
the null. Using the risk ratio measure, neither variation 1 nor variation 2
is more extreme. For the odds ratio measure, both variations are more
extreme.

The different measures each designate a distinct set of outcomes as
more extreme. This ambiguity makes it problematic to use two independent binomial distributions as a model for hypothesis testing for a 2 × 2
table. Another problem with the use of two binomials is the large number
of possible outcomes. For example, if $N_1 = N_0 = 25$, there are 676 possible outcomes for the data $[(N_1 + 1) \cdot (N_0 + 1)]$. To simplify the calculation, an assumption can be made that addresses both of these problems.
The assumption, for follow-up or prevalence data, is that the total number
of cases actually observed is taken to be a constant [Mantel and Hankey,
1971]. For case-control data, the two binomial distributions refer not to the
exposed and unexposed series but to the case and control series, and the
corresponding assumption is that the total number of exposed subjects is
constant. These assumptions essentially fix all the marginal totals of the 2
× 2 table; therefore, if the a cell increases, the b and c cells must each
decrease an equivalent amount, and the d cell increases by the same
amount. With all the margins held constant, there is only one random
variable to describe: variation in any cell of the 2 × 2 table with fixed
marginal totals is locked together with concomitant variation in each of
the other cells. Usually, then, the focus becomes simply the a cell of the
table, which is taken to be the random variable.

The assumption that all the marginal totals are fixed in a 2 × 2 table
can be justified methodologically as a means of focusing the problem (of
hypothesis testing) directly on the association between exposure and disease. In the jargon of statistics, the "nuisance parameter" is removed by
fixing the marginal totals: Testing the null hypothesis using a model of two
independent binomials requires assessing the values for *two* parameters,
the proportions p_1 and p_0, whereas the analytic problem can be reduced

Example 11-2. Hypothetical data illustrating ambiguity of definition for departures from the null state using the two-binomial model

	"Observed data"		Variation 1		Variation 2	
	Exposed	Unexposed	Exposed	Unexposed	Exposed	Unexposed
Cases	10	45	16	76	13	59
Noncases	10	55	4	24	7	41
Totals	20	100	20	100	20	100
Estimate of						
Risk difference	0.05		0.04		0.06	
Risk ratio	1.11		1.05		1.10	
Odds ratio	1.22		1.26		1.29	

*Example 11-3. History of chlordiazopoxide use in early
pregnancy for mothers of children born with congenital heart
defects and mothers of normal children [Rothman et al., 1979]*

	Chlordiazopoxide use		
	Yes	No	Total
Case mothers	4	386	390
Control mothers	4	1250	1254
Totals	8	1636	1644

to assessing the value of a single measure. That measure is the odds ratio, equal to $p_1(1 - p_0)/[p_0(1 - p_1)]$, which is completely determined by the value of the a cell if the marginal totals are taken as fixed. Testing a departure of the odds ratio from unity is equivalent to testing a departure of p_1 from p_0, since the null condition of $p_1 = p_0$ is equivalent to an odds ratio of unity, but fixing the margins of the 2×2 table greatly simplifies the calculations by reducing the number of parameters in the model from two to one.

The statistical model that describes the variability of the a cell in a 2×2 table with fixed marginal totals is the hypergeometric distribution. The probability of a exposed cases occurring under the assumption that the null hypothesis is correct can be expressed simply as follows [Fisher, 1935]:

$$\text{Pr(a exposed cases)} = \frac{\binom{N_1}{a}\binom{N_0}{b}}{\binom{T}{M_1}} \qquad [11\text{-}5]$$

For the data in example 11-3, the hypergeometric probability for four exposed cases is

$$\text{Pr(4 exposed cases)} = \frac{\binom{8}{4}\binom{1636}{386}}{\binom{1644}{390}} = \frac{390!\ 1254!\ 8!\ 1636!}{1644!\ 4!\ 4!\ 386!\ 1250!}$$

$$= \frac{(390)(389)(388)(387)(1254)(1253)(1252)(1251)(8)(7)(6)(5)}{(1644)(1643)(1642)(1641)(1640)(1639)(1638)(1637)(4)(3)(2)} = 0.0748$$

The probability for an outcome more extreme, five exposed cases, under the hypergeometric model, would be

$$\text{Pr(5 exposed cases)} = \frac{\binom{8}{5}\binom{1636}{385}}{\binom{1644}{390}} = 0.0185$$

The probability for six exposed cases would be 0.0028; for seven exposed cases, 0.0002; and for the most extreme outcome, eight exposed cases, 0.000009. The total one-tail P-value calculated according to Fisher would be $0.0748 + 0.0185 + 0.0028 + 0.0002 + 0.000009 = 0.096$. The one-tail mid-$P$ would be $0.0374 + 0.0185 + 0.0028 + 0.0002 + 0.000009 = 0.059$. The two-tail P-value, either Fisher or mid-P, could be obtained by doubling the one-tail P-value.

For this example, the hypergeometric model requires the calculation of only five probabilities. Had the model of two independent binomial distributions, with 390 cases and 1,254 controls as the two independent series, been used instead, thousands of calculations would be necessary to determine which outcomes were equally or more extreme, and then the probability of each of these outcomes would have to be calculated as well. The simplifying assumption of the hypergeometric distribution, which fixes all the marginal totals, reduces the complexity of the calculations enormously.

The reasonableness of the hypergeometric assumption, even for data such as those given in example 11-3 in which two of the four cell frequencies are small, is evident by comparing the results with the results obtained by using the two-binomial model. Using the two-binomial model and using the magnitude of the odds ratio to determine which outcomes are equally or more extreme departures from the null, the Fisher P-value was found to be 0.094, and the mid-P, 0.071. (This calculation took several hours using a BASIC program on a microcomputer.) The agreement between the two approaches is striking when one considers that only five separate probabilities are included in the hypergeometric calculation, whereas thousands are included in the two-binomial model. With larger cell frequencies, the agreement between the results obtained from the different models improves. Whatever disagreement exists between the results from the two approaches does not indicate any inaccuracy with the hypergeometric approach; since the assumption of fixed marginal totals yields a valid test, even if the margins were not actually fixed by the study design, a test of the null hypothesis based on the hypergeometric model is just as valid as a test based on the two-binomial model. Since the hypergeometric approach is extraordinarily simpler, it is clearly the preferred model.

Unfortunately, even the hypergeometric model can require an onerous number of calculations if all the cell frequencies are sizable. In most applications, therefore, an asymptotic test statistic is used to calculate the P-

value. The asymptotic test statistic can be derived starting from either the two-binomial model or the hypergeometric model. With the hypergeometric model, the random variable would be the a cell, the number of exposed cases. The null expectation for the number of exposed cases is N_1M_1/T, and the hypergeometric variance for the number of exposed cases is $M_1M_0N_1N_0/[T^2(T-1)]$. The χ statistic is

$$\chi = \frac{a - N_1M_1/T}{\sqrt{\dfrac{M_1M_0N_1N_0}{T^2(T-1)}}} \qquad [11\text{-}6]$$

which appears similar to equation 11-1 for person-time data. If an asymptotic test statistic were derived from the two-binomial model rather than from the hypergeometric, one would compare the two observed binomial proportions, a/N_1 and b/N_0. Under the null hypothesis, the expectation of the difference between these proportions is zero. The variance might be estimated in several ways; the usual way is to use a pooled common variance for the two binomial proportions, since under the null hypothesis the binomial probabilities for the two binomial distributions are equal. Thus, M_1/T is taken to be an estimate of the pooled binomial probability, and the variance of the difference in proportions can be expressed as

$$\left(\frac{M_1}{T}\right)\left(\frac{M_0}{T}\right)\left[\frac{1}{N_1} + \frac{1}{N_0}\right]$$

which gives

$$\chi = \frac{\dfrac{a}{N_1} - \dfrac{b}{N_0}}{\sqrt{\left(\dfrac{M_1}{T}\right)\left(\dfrac{M_0}{T}\right)\left[\dfrac{1}{N_1} + \dfrac{1}{N_0}\right]}} \qquad [11\text{-}7]$$

Algebraic manipulation of equation 11-7 gives an expression nearly identical to equation 11-6:

$$\chi = \frac{a - N_1M_1/T}{\sqrt{\dfrac{M_1M_0N_1N_0}{T^3}}} \qquad [11\text{-}8]$$

The only difference between the two formulas is the $T-1$ in the denominator expression in equation 11-6, which is replaced by T in equation 11-8. Since neither formula is applicable unless T is large, for practical purposes these formulas are identical.

If an asymptotic test statistic had been used to calculate the P-value for the data in example 11-3, we would have obtained, using equation 11-6,

$$\chi = \frac{4 - (8)\,(390)/(1644)}{\sqrt{\dfrac{(8)\,(1636)\,(390)\,(1254)}{(1644)^2\,(1643)}}} = 1.75$$

which gives a one-tail P-value of 0.040. As one would expect, the P-value resulting from the asymptotic test is closer to the mid-P exact value than to the Fisher exact value (see Chap. 10), but the approximation is not very good. Notice that under the hypergeometric model there are only nine possible outcomes for the a cell; evidently the number of outcomes is too few for the normal approximation to be valid. A rule of thumb that is often used is that the asymptotic test statistic should be applied only when the smallest null expectation of any cell in the 2 × 2 table, based on the marginal totals, is greater than about 3. If there is any doubt, however, about the adequacy of the asymptotic approximation, it is best to evaluate the P-value exactly.

ESTIMATION OF EFFECTS WITH CRUDE DATA
Estimation with Follow-up Data
POINT ESTIMATION

Point estimation of either difference or ratio measures of effect involves taking the difference or ratio of the observed values of incidence or risk. Thus, the point estimate of incidence rate difference (IRD) would be

$$\widehat{IRD} = \frac{a}{N_1} - \frac{b}{N_0}$$

and the point estimate of incidence rate ratio (IRR) would be

$$\widehat{IRR} = \frac{a/N_1}{b/N_0}$$

Similarly, for risk (cumulative incidence) data, in which denominators are counts rather than measures of person-time, the point estimate of risk difference (RD) would be

$$\widehat{RD} = \frac{a}{N_1} - \frac{b}{N_0}$$

and the point estimate of risk ratio (RR) would be

$$\widehat{RR} = \frac{a/N_1}{b/N_0}$$

If the object of inference is the ratio of incidence rates rather than risk ratio, then the ratio of risks that is directly calculable from risk data using the above formula leads to an underestimate of the effect. The degree of underestimation depends on the level of the risks, being slight for small risks and greater for large risks (see Chap. 4 and Table 6-1). An alternative approach to point estimation with count denominators is to use the odds-ratio formula

$$\widehat{IRR} = \frac{ad}{bc}$$

which overestimates the effect to roughly the same extent that the risk ratio underestimates it (Table 6-1) but has the advantage of being the same estimator used in case-control studies (formula 6-1).

INTERVAL ESTIMATION

Exact Interval Estimation with Follow-up Data. Interval estimation can be exact or approximate. For exact interval estimation, like the calculation of an exact P-value, an appropriate statistical model must be used to describe the probability distribution of the data. The model will generally be an extension of the model used for calculation of an exact P-value. For testing the null hypothesis, an effect of zero is assumed and incorporated into the statistical model; for calculation of exact confidence limits, the statistical model must be able to accommodate nonzero effects.

INCIDENCE RATE (PERSON-TIME) DATA. For incidence rate difference, a difficulty arises in attempting to postulate a statistical model from which an exact confidence interval can be calculated. For hypothesis testing, the binomial model rests on the assumption that M_1, the total number of cases, is a constant. This assumption is analogous to the assumption of fixed marginal totals in the hypergeometric model for 2×2 tables. For interval estimation, the problem with assuming M_1 to be constant is that, with respect to incidence rate difference, the value of M_1 is not simply a "nuisance parameter" that statistically has no bearing on the effect measure; the value of M_1 imposes a limit on the magnitude of the incidence rate difference (a small value of M_1 is compatible only with small values of the rate difference), therefore requiring the sampling variability of M_1 to be taken into account in estimating the incidence rate difference. Thus, the single-binomial model with a fixed M_1 cannot be used to calculate exact confidence limits for incidence rate difference with person-time data. The counterpart for person-time data of the more general two-binomial model for 2 × 2 tables would be a model of two independent Poisson distributions, in which exposed and unexposed cases each occurred independently with frequencies described by a Poisson distribution. The Poisson distribution, however, has no upper limit for the number of events (i.e., cases) that can occur, so it cannot be used for the above calculations without arbitrary truncation. For these reasons, exact interval estimation for incidence rate difference is not easily possible.

It is appropriate, however, to fix M_1 for estimation of incidence rate ratio because the ratio measure depends on the ratio of exposed to unexposed cases, not on the absolute magnitude of the frequencies. Therefore, M_1 can be considered a nuisance parameter that is statistically independent of the rate ratio measure. For estimation, the simple single binomial model used for hypothesis testing must be modified to accommodate a nonzero effect. This can be accomplished by noting that the probability that a case is exposed, given M_1, is related to incidence rate ratio as follows:

$$IRR = \frac{N_0 \cdot Pr(\text{case is exposed})}{N_1 \cdot Pr(\text{case is unexposed})}$$

Exact confidence limits for IRR can be obtained by setting the tail probability of the binomial distribution equal to $\alpha/2$ and $1 - \alpha/2$, where $1 - \alpha$ equals the desired level of confidence. If we denote $\underline{u}$ as the lower confidence bound for the probability that a case is exposed, and $\bar{u}$ as the exact upper confidence bound, then

$$\underline{IRR} = \frac{\underline{u}N_0}{(1 - \underline{u})N_1} \qquad [11\text{-}9]$$

and

$$\overline{IRR} = \frac{\bar{u}N_0}{(1 - \bar{u})N_1} \qquad [11\text{-}10]$$

where $\underline{u}$ and $\bar{u}$ are the solutions to the following equations (for Fisher limits):

$$\alpha/2 = \sum_{k=a}^{M_1} \binom{M_1}{k} \underline{u}^k (1 - \underline{u})^{M_1 - k}$$

and

$$1 - \alpha/2 = \sum_{k=a+1}^{M_1} \binom{M_1}{k} \bar{u}^k (1 - \bar{u})^{M_1 - k}$$

The preceding equations assume that $I\hat{R}R > 1$, and consequently calculate the upper tail of the distribution. If $\hat{IRR} < 1$, then the lower end of the distribution could be used to calculate the tail probabilities:

$$\alpha/2 = \sum_{k=0}^{a} \binom{M_1}{k} \overline{u}^k (1 - \overline{u})^{M_1-k}$$

and

$$1 - \alpha/2 = \sum_{k=0}^{a-1} \binom{M_1}{k} \underline{u}^k (1 - \underline{u})^{M_1-k}$$

If calculations are performed based on the mid-P exact P-value, then the tail probabilities are calculable as

$$\alpha/2 = \frac{1}{2} \binom{M_1}{a} \underline{u}^a (1 - \underline{u})^b + \sum_{k=a+1}^{M_1} \binom{M_1}{k} \underline{u}^k (1 - \underline{u})^{M_1-k}$$

and

$$1 - \alpha/2 = \frac{1}{2} \binom{M_1}{a} \overline{u}^a (1 - \overline{u})^b + \sum_{k=a+1}^{M_1} \binom{M_1}{k} \overline{u}^k (1 - \overline{u})^{M_1-k}$$

These equations must be solved iteratively, by choosing trial values for $\underline{u}$ and $\overline{u}$ and calculating the tail probability repeatedly until it is equal to $\alpha/2$ or $1 - \alpha/2$. Notice the similarity to the calculation of an exact P-value, which involves taking $u = N_1/T$ and calculating the tail probability once. For exact confidence limits, the value of u is adjusted until the tail probability equals the predefined values, $\alpha/2$ or $1 - \alpha/2$.

Consider again the person-time data in example 11-1. Exact Fisher-type 90 percent confidence limits for the IRR would be calculated from equations 11-9 and 11-10 as follows:

$$0.05 = \sum_{k=41}^{56} \binom{56}{k} \underline{u}^k (1 - \underline{u})^{56-k}$$

$$0.95 = \sum_{k=42}^{56} \binom{56}{k} \overline{u}^k (1 - \overline{u})^{56-k}$$

These calculations are best done by computer or by a shortcut method that involves the F-distribution [Rothman and Boice, 1982; Brownlee, 1965]. A trial and error solution of the preceding equations gives $\underline{u} = 0.618$ and $\overline{u} = 0.827$, which gives $\underline{IRR} = 1.10$ and $\overline{IRR} = 3.25$.

If the limits are calculated based on the mid-P exact P-value, then the equations to be solved are

$$0.05 = \frac{1}{2} \binom{56}{41} \underline{u}^{41} (1 - \underline{u})^{15} + \sum_{k=42}^{56} \binom{56}{k} \underline{u}^k (1 - \underline{u})^{56-k}$$

and

$$0.95 = \frac{1}{2} \binom{56}{41} \bar{u}^{41} (1 - \bar{u})^{15} + \sum_{k=42}^{56} \binom{56}{k} \bar{u}^k (1 - \bar{u})^{56-k}$$

The upper and lower 90 percent confidence limits determined by the above mid-P based equations are $\underline{u} = 0.626$ and $\bar{u} = 0.8205$, corresponding to $\underline{IRR} = 1.14$ and $\overline{IRR} = 3.10$.

CUMULATIVE INCIDENCE DATA. If the denominators are counts rather than person-time units, an exact confidence interval for risk difference could theoretically be calculated from the two-binomial model. The calculation, however, would involve iterative determination of the exact tail probability based on two independent binomials and is therefore not readily feasible.

Confidence limits for the risk ratio measure are also subject to the same computational difficulty because the value of the measure is dependent on the total number of cases and requires the use of two independent binomials. If, however, the odds ratio measure is used for estimation, both margins of the 2 × 2 table may be considered fixed, and the calculations can be greatly simplified because the odds ratio measure is independent of the total number of cases. Because the odds ratio is only an approximation of the risk ratio, the calculation of exact limits for the odds ratio does not produce exact confidence limits for the risk ratio. The approximation is good only if the risks are small, in which case the exact confidence interval for the odds ratio can be used as a reasonable surrogate confidence interval for the risk ratio.

The statistical model that describes the variation of the a cell in a 2 × 2 table with fixed margins is the hypergeometric, but for the non-null situation the "noncentral" form of the hypergeometric distribution must be used. The noncentral hypergeometric is more complicated than the null form of the hypergeometric distribution given in formula 11-5 because it accommodates the strength of association between exposure and disease measured by the odds ratio. Given the value of the odds ratio, R, the probability of observing a exposed cases is [Fisher, 1935; Gart, 1971]

$$\text{Pr(a exposed cases)} = \frac{\binom{N_1}{a} \binom{N_0}{b} R^a}{\sum_{k=\max(0,M_1-N_0)}^{\min(N_1,M_1)} \binom{N_1}{k} \binom{N_0}{M_1 - k} R^k}$$

When R = 1, the above formula reduces to expression 11-5. Exact confidence limits for R with a confidence level of 1 − α can be calculated from the formulas

$$\alpha/2 = \frac{\sum\limits_{k=a}^{\min(N_1,M_1)} \binom{N_1}{k}\binom{N_0}{M_1-k}\underline{R}^k}{\sum\limits_{k=\max(0,M_1-N_0)}^{\min(N_1,M_1)} \binom{N_1}{k}\binom{N_0}{M_1-k}\underline{R}^k} \qquad [11\text{-}11]$$

and

$$1-\alpha/2 = \frac{\sum\limits_{k=a+1}^{\min(N_1,M_1)} \binom{N_1}{k}\binom{N_0}{M_1-k}\overline{R}^k}{\sum\limits_{k=\max(0,M_1-N_0)}^{\min(N_1,M_1)} \binom{N_1}{k}\binom{N_0}{M_1-k}\overline{R}^k} \qquad [11\text{-}12]$$

for the Fisher limits and

$$\alpha/2 = \frac{\frac{1}{2}\binom{N_1}{a}\binom{N_0}{b}\underline{R}^a + \sum\limits_{k=a+1}^{\min(N_1,M_1)} \binom{N_1}{k}\binom{N_0}{M_1-k}\underline{R}^k}{\sum\limits_{k=\max(0,M_1-N_0)}^{\min(N_1,M_1)} \binom{N_1}{k}\binom{N_0}{M_1-k}\underline{R}^k} \qquad [11\text{-}13]$$

$$1-\alpha/2 = \frac{\frac{1}{2}\binom{N_1}{a}\binom{N_0}{b}\overline{R}^a + \sum\limits_{k=a+1}^{\min(N_1,M_1)} \binom{N_1}{k}\binom{N_0}{M_1-k}\overline{R}^k}{\sum\limits_{k=\max(0,M_1-N_0)}^{\min(N_1,M_1)} + \binom{N_1}{k}\binom{N_0}{M_1-k}\overline{R}^k} \qquad [11\text{-}14]$$

for mid-P limits. The solution of the foregoing equations can be time-consuming, since each iteration in the process calls for calculating a complicated sum, but it is not nearly as complicated as the calculations that would be required using a statistical model of two independent binomials.

The data in example 11-4 describe partial results from a follow-up study evaluating risk of diarrhea in breast-fed infants in Bangladesh during an

Example 11-4. Diarrhea during a 10-day follow-up period in
30 breast-fed infants colonized with Vibrio cholerae 01, according to
antilipopolysaccharide antibody titers in mother's breast milk [Glass et al., 1983]

	Antibody level	
	High	Low
Diarrhea	7	12
No diarrhea	9	2
Totals	16	14

11-day period following the determination of various antibody titers in the mothers' breast milk. An exact P-value of the null hypothesis of no association gives $P_{(1)} = 0.02$ for the Fisher P-value and $P_{(1)} = 0.01$ for the mid-P value. The estimate of relative risk from these data comparing the group exposed to high titers with the group exposed to low titers is $[7/16]/[12/14] = 0.51$. The odds ratio estimate differs considerably from the relative risk estimate because the risks are so high; the odds ratio estimate is $[7 \times 2]/[12 \times 9] = 0.13$. An exact confidence interval can be calculated for the odds ratio using formulas 11-11 and 11-12 to set the Fisher limits. The 90 percent confidence limits are 0.017 and 0.751, obtained by the trial-and-error solution of equations 11-11 and 11-12. If the mid-P exact limits were desired instead, these could be obtained from equations 11-13 and 11-14 as 0.025 and 0.608. These exact limits for the odds ratio, however, cannot be used as confidence limits for the risk ratio, since the odds ratio is a poor approximation to the risk ratio with these data.

Approximate Interval Estimation with Follow-up Data. Approximate interval estimation from crude follow-up data is straightforward.

INCIDENCE RATE (PERSON-TIME) DATA. Consider first incidence rate data with person-time denominators. Two effect-measures can be estimated, rate difference and rate ratio. Because the rate-difference measure has a symmetric sampling distribution, no scale transformation is needed to obtain accurate approximate confidence limits. The number of exposed and unexposed cases can each be assumed to have a Poisson distribution, from which the variance for each rate can be estimated as a/N_1^2 and b/N_0^2 for exposed and unexposed groups, respectively. The standard deviation of the rate difference, then, is the square root of the sum of the variances of each rate,

$$\text{SD(Incidence rate difference)} \doteq \sqrt{\frac{a}{N_1^2} + \frac{b}{N_0^2}} \qquad [11\text{-}15]$$

From the data in example 11-1, we can estimate the rate difference as

$$\frac{41}{28,010 \text{ yr}} - \frac{15}{19,017 \text{ yr}} = \frac{6.75}{10,000} \text{ yr}^{-1}$$

with a standard deviation for the rate difference of

$$\text{SD} \doteq \sqrt{\frac{41}{(28,010 \text{ yr})^2} + \frac{15}{(19,017 \text{ yr})^2}} = \frac{3.06}{10,000} \text{ yr}^{-1}$$

To obtain an approximate 90 percent confidence interval, the standard deviation is multiplied by 1.645 to get the limits as follows:

$$\frac{6.75}{10,000}\,\text{yr}^{-1} \pm 1.645 \left[\frac{3.06}{10,000}\,\text{yr}^{-1}\right] = \frac{1.7}{10,000}\,\text{yr}^{-1},\ \frac{11.8}{10,000}\,\text{yr}^{-1}$$

Another approach would be to use formula 10-6 for test-based limits,

$$\hat{\text{RD}}\,(1 \pm Z/\chi)$$

Earlier we calculated χ to be 2.08. Using that value in the above formula with $Z = 1.645$ yields an approximate 90 percent confidence interval of $1.4/(10,000\ \text{yr})$, $12.1/(10,000\ \text{yr})$, which compares well with the other approximation.

For the estimation of rate ratio, it is desirable to use a logarithmic transformation to compensate for the asymmetric sampling distribution. By taking confidence limits that are symmetric about the logarithm of the rate ratio and then reversing the transformation by taking antilogarithms, much greater accuracy can be achieved than by taking limits calculated symmetrically around the rate ratio itself. Thus, we calculate

$$\exp\{\ln(\hat{\text{RR}}) \pm Z \cdot \text{SD}[\ln(\hat{\text{RR}})]\} \qquad [11\text{-}16]$$

The standard deviation of the incidence rate ratio can be approximated by

$$\text{SD}[\ln(\hat{\text{RR}})] \doteq \sqrt{\frac{1}{a} + \frac{1}{b}}$$

Again using the data from example 11-1, we can estimate the incidence rate ratio to be

$$\frac{41/28,010\ \text{yr}}{15/19,017\ \text{yr}} = 1.86$$

and $\ln(1.86) = 0.618$. The standard deviation of the log-transformed point estimate is

$$\sqrt{1/41 + 1/15} = \sqrt{0.091} = 0.302$$

A 90 percent confidence interval for the $\ln(\text{RR})$ would then be

$$0.618 \pm 1.645(0.302) = 0.12,\ 1.1$$

which, after taking antilogarithms to reverse the transformation, gives a confidence interval of 1.1 to 3.0. The whole process can be summarized as follows:

$$\exp[\ln(1.86) \pm 1.645 \sqrt{1/41 + 1/15}] = 1.1, 3.0$$

These limits agree well with the exact mid-P 90 percent limits calculated previously as 1.1 and 3.1.

An alternative approach would be to use the test-based formula

$$\widehat{RR}^{(1 \pm Z/x)}$$

in which χ has the value of 2.08 for the data in example 11-1. Using $Z = 1.645$ for 90 percent limits, the test-based approach gives an interval of 1.1 to 3.0, which is also in excellent agreement with the exact mid-P limits.

CUMULATIVE INCIDENCE DATA. To get approximate limits for follow-up data with denominators consisting of persons rather than person-time, slightly different formulas are needed to estimate the standard deviations. For the risk difference, the standard deviation is derived from the sum of two binomial variances and is estimated as

$$\text{SD(Risk difference)} \doteq \sqrt{\frac{a(N_1 - a)}{N_1^3} + \frac{b(N_0 - b)}{N_0^3}} \qquad [11\text{-}17]$$

From the data in example 11-4, the point estimate of rate difference is

$$\frac{7}{16} - \frac{12}{14} = -0.42$$

with an approximate 90 percent confidence interval of

$$-0.42 \pm 1.645 \sqrt{\frac{(7)\,(9)}{(16)^3} + \frac{(12)\,(2)}{(14)^3}}$$

$$= -0.42 \pm 1.645(0.155)$$

$$= -0.68, -0.16$$

Alternatively, the test-based calculation gives

$$-0.42 \left[1 \pm \frac{1.645}{-2.34} \right] = -0.71, -0.12$$

Considering the small numbers involved in these calculations, the agreement between these two approaches seems good.

For the risk ratio, it is again desirable to use a logarithmic transformation, that is, to apply formula 11-16. The standard deviation, however, is estimated as

$$SD[\ln(\hat{RR})] \doteq \sqrt{\frac{c}{aN_1} + \frac{d}{bN_0}}$$

For example 11-4, the risk ratio estimate is $[7/16]/[12/14] = 0.51$, and

$$\ln(\hat{RR}) = -0.673$$

The estimated standard deviation of $\ln(\hat{RR})$ is

$$\sqrt{\frac{9}{7 \cdot 16} + \frac{2}{12 \cdot 14}} = 0.304$$

and the 90 percent confidence interval is

$$\exp[-0.673 \pm 1.645(0.304)] = 0.31, 0.84$$

Alternatively, test-based limits could be calculated as

$$\hat{RR}^{(1 \pm Z/x)} = 0.51^{(1 \pm 1.645/-2.34)} = 0.32, 0.82$$

Once again the two approximate methods for confidence interval estimation are in good agreement.

If the inference from follow-up data with count denominators is to be based on the odds ratio rather than on the risk ratio, then the formula for standard deviation is [Woolf, 1955]

$$SD[\ln(\text{odds ratio})] \doteq \sqrt{\frac{1}{a} + \frac{1}{b} + \frac{1}{c} + \frac{1}{d}}$$

For example 11-4, the odds ratio is $[7 \cdot 2]/[9 \cdot 12] = 0.13$ and the logarithm is $\ln(0.13) = -2.04$. The standard deviation is

$$SD[\ln(\text{odds ratio})] \doteq \sqrt{\frac{1}{7} + \frac{1}{9} + \frac{1}{12} + \frac{1}{2}} = 0.915$$

and the approximate 90 percent confidence interval is

$$\exp[\ln(0.13) \pm 1.645(0.915)] = 0.03, 0.58$$

The test-based confidence limits are calculated as

$$0.13^{(1 \pm 1.645/-2.34)} = 0.03, 0.55$$

Considering the very small numbers involved in the calculations, the above two approximate interval estimates for the odds ratio agree tolerably well not only with one another but also with the exact mid-P confidence interval for the odds ratio, calculated previously to be 0.025 to 0.608.

The Cornfield [1956] approach, which is described in greater detail in Chapter 12, is a theoretically preferable approximate technique since it involves recalculating the standard error using fitted cell frequencies that correspond to the value of the confidence limit. Thus, the procedure is iterative and involves substantially more calculation than the other approximate methods. For the data of example 11-4, the Cornfield approach gives a 90 percent confidence interval of 0.03 to 0.55, agreeing in this instance with the test-based approach.

Case-Control Data

For case-control data, the epidemiologic measure of central interest is the odds ratio, the point estimator for which is

$$\hat{R} = \frac{ad}{bc}$$

Exact confidence interval estimation for the odds ratio is identical for case-control and follow-up data and is based on formulas 11-11 through 11-14. Approximate confidence intervals for the odds ratio from case-control data are determined using the same method used for follow-up data, using the logarithmic transformation with one of the following formulas:

$$\hat{R}^{(1 \pm Z/x)} \qquad \text{or} \qquad \exp\{\ln(\hat{R}) \pm Z \cdot SD[\ln(\hat{R})]\}$$

where

$$SD[\ln(\text{odds ratio})] \doteq \sqrt{\frac{1}{a} + \frac{1}{b} + \frac{1}{c} + \frac{1}{d}}$$

Consider example 11-3. Exact 90 percent confidence limits for the odds ratio, using equations 11-11 and 11-12 for the Fisher limits, are 0.77, 13.6; using equations 11-13 and 11-14 for the mid-P limits, the results are 0.94,

11.1. Approximate 90 percent confidence limits can be determined as follows:

$$\ln(\hat{R}) = \ln(3.24) = 1.175$$

$$SD[\ln(\text{odds ratio})] \doteq \sqrt{\frac{1}{4} + \frac{1}{386} + \frac{1}{4} + \frac{1}{1250}}$$

$$= 0.71$$

$$\exp[\ln(3.24) \pm 1.645(0.71)] = 1.0, 10.4$$

or, using the test-based approach,

$$3.24^{(1 \pm 1.645/1.75)} = 1.1, 9.8$$

As expected, these results agree better with the mid-P exact limits than with the Fisher exact limits. The approximation is not perfect, but neither is it very poor considering that two of the four cells of the 2×2 table have observed frequencies of only four. The Cornfield method gives a 90 percent interval of 1.1 to 9.8, identical to that given by the test-based approach.

REFERENCES

Boice, J. D., and Monson, R. R. Breast cancer in women after repeated fluoroscopic examinations of the chest. *J. Natl. Cancer Inst.* 1977;59:823–832.

Brownlee, K. A. *Statistical Theory and Methodology in Science and Engineering.* New York: Wiley, 1965.

Cornfield, J. A statistical problem arising from retrospective studies. In J. Neyman (ed.), *Proceedings Third Berkeley Symposium,* Vol. 4. Berkeley: University of California Press, 1956, pp. 135–148.

Fisher, R. A. The logic of inductive inference. *J. R. Stat. Soc.,* Series A, 1935;98:39–54.

Gart, J. J. The comparison of proportions: a review of significance tests, confidence intervals and adjustments for stratification. *Rev. Int. Stat. Inst.* 1971;39:148–169.

Glass, R. I., Svennerholm, A. M., Stoll, B. J., et al. Protection against cholera in breast-fed children by antibiotics in breast milk. *N. Engl. J. Med.* 1983;308:1389–1392.

Mantel, N., and Hankey, B. F. Programmed analysis of a 2×2 contigency table. *Am. Stat.* 1971;25:40–44.

Rothman, K. J., and Boice, J. D. *Epidemiologic Analysis with a Programmable Calculator* (2nd ed.). Brookline, MA: Epidemiology Resources Inc., 1982.

Rothman, K. J., Fyler, D. C., Goldblatt, A., et al. Exogenous hormones and other drug exposures of children with congenital heart disease. *Am. J. Epidemiol.* 1979;109:433–439.

Shore, R. E., Pasternack, B. S., and Curnen, M. G. Relating influenza epidemics to childhood leukemia in tumor registries without a defined population base: A critique with suggestions for improved methods. *Am. J. Epidemiol.* 1976;103:527–535.

Woolf, B. On estimating the relation between blood group and disease. *Ann. Hum. Genet.* 1955;19:251–253.

12. STRATIFIED ANALYSIS

Two different analytic concerns motivate the division of data into strata: one is the need to evaluate and remove *confounding;* the other is to evaluate and describe *effect modification*. Because stratification is the preferred means of dealing with both of these analytic issues, the beginning student is apt to become bewildered in the attempt to distinguish between the aims and procedures involved in considering these two aspects of epidemiologic data analysis.

Effect modification refers to a change in the magnitude of an effect measure according to the value of some third variable (after exposure and disease), which is called an *effect modifier*. Effect modification differs from confounding in several ways. The most central difference is that, whereas confounding is a bias that the investigator hopes to prevent or, if necessary, to remove from the data, effect modification is an elaborated description of the effect itself. Effect modification is thus a finding to be reported rather than a bias to be avoided. Epidemiologic analysis is generally aimed at eliminating confounding and discovering and describing effect modification.

It is a useful contrast to think of confounding as a nuisance that may or may not be present depending on the study design. Of course, confounding originates from the interrelation of the confounding factors and study variables in the source population from which the study subjects are selected. Nevertheless, restriction in subject selection, for example, can prevent a variable from becoming a confounding factor in a situation in which it otherwise would be confounding. Effect modification, on the other hand, rather than being a nuisance the presence of which depends on the specifics of the study design, is a natural phenomenon that exists independently of the study. It is a phenomenon that the study is intended to divulge and describe if at all possible. Whereas the existence of confounding with respect to a given factor depends on the design of a study, effect modification has a conceptual constancy that transcends the study design.

Although effect modification is a constant of nature, in its most general sense it cannot correspond to any biologic property because there is one aspect of the concept that is not absolute: Effect modification in its most general context includes modification of an effect without specifying which effect measure is modified. Since there are two effect measures, the difference and ratio measures, that are commonly used in epidemiology as well as others that are used less often, the concept of effect modification without further specification is too ambiguous to be useful as a description of nature.

In Figure 12-1, age can be considered a modifier of the effect of exposure, since the incidence rate difference between exposed and unexposed increases with increasing age. On the other hand, the ratio of incidence among exposed to incidence among unexposed is constant over age. Thus, age modifies the effect of exposure with regard to the difference measure

178

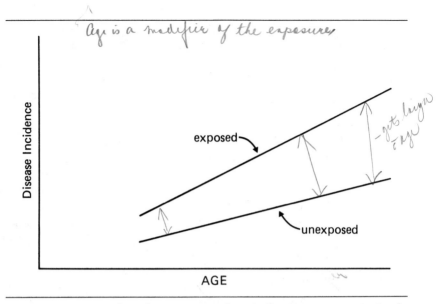

age is a modifier of the exposure

— gets bigger by age

Fig. 12-1. Disease incidence by exposure and age indicating a constant ratio of incidence with age.

of effect but not with regard to the ratio measure. The opposite situation is described in Figure 12-2: The difference in incidence rate between exposed and unexposed is constant over age, but the ratio of incidence among exposed to incidence among unexposed declines with age. These diagrams illustrate why effect modification should be described only in relation to a specific effect measure. If effect modification is absent with regard to either the difference measure or the ratio measure, it will be present with regard to the other measure unless the disease rate among the unexposed is unassociated with the potential effect modifier.

This chapter presents the fundamental analytic strategies for dealing with confounding and effect modification in a stratified analysis. The biologic and public health interpretations of effect modification are considered in Chapter 15.

EVALUATION AND CONTROL OF CONFOUNDING

Confounding is a distortion in an effect measure that results from the effect of another variable that is associated with the exposure under study. In Chapter 7, confounding was defined, and the general characteristics of confounding factors were discussed. To review, a confounding factor must

1. Be a risk factor for the disease among the nonexposed.
2. Be associated with the exposure variable in the population from which the cases derive.

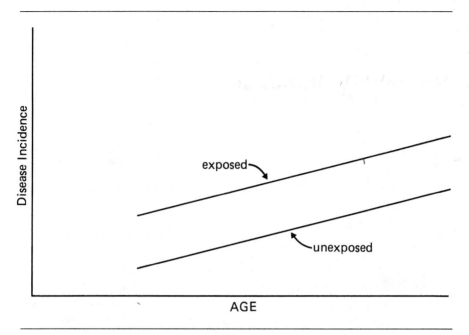

Fig. 12-2. Disease incidence by exposure and age indicating a constant difference of incidence with age.

3. Not be an intermediate step in the causal path between the exposure and the disease.

The case-control data in Example 12-1 demonstrate confounding by age. If the effect of oral contraceptives on the risk of myocardial infarction is estimated from the crude data, the odds ratio estimate is 2.2. If the data are divided, however, into two age categories, the odds ratio estimate in each category is 2.8, which corresponds to a 50 percent greater effect than the estimate of 2.2 ($[2.8 - 1]/[2.2 - 1] = 1.5$).

It is clear that the variable "age" in Example 12-1 meets the criteria for a confounding factor. First, age is a risk factor for myocardial infarction among the nonexposed, that is, nonusers of oral contraceptives. We know in general that age is a strong risk factor for myocardial infarction; more directly, we can see that among the subjects in this particular study who are nonusers the proportion of subjects who are classified as cases is greater in the age category 40 to 44 ($88/183 = 0.48$) than in the age category < 40 ($26/85 = 0.31$). These proportions do not represent any meaningful epidemiologic measure; because these are case-control data, these proportions reflect the overall case-control ratio arbitrarily chosen by the investigators. The proportions might be described as the "prevalence of disease among nonexposed study subjects," which, given the case-control

Example 12-1. Case-control data describing the effect of oral contraceptive use on risk of myocardial infarction, with confounding by age [Mann et al., 1968]

	Age < 40		Age 40–44		Totals	
	User	Nonuser	User	Nonuser	User	Nonuser
Myocardial infarction cases	21	26	18	88	39	114
Controls	17	59	7	95	24	154
Odds ratio estimate	2.8		2.8		2.2	

design, are not meaningful prevalences. Nevertheless, for age to be confounding, these proportions must vary by age.

In addition, for age to be confounding, it must be associated with oral contraceptive use among the source population that gave rise to the cases. Looking among the controls, who are sampled from that source population, we note that the proportion of oral contraceptive users is much greater (17/76 = 0.22) among younger controls than among older controls (7/102 = 0.07), indicating that this condition has been fulfilled.

Since age cannot be construed as a causal link between oral contraceptive use and myocardial infarction, it meets the criteria for a confounding factor in these data. There is a more direct method, however, by which confounding can be assessed. It is possible to evaluate the magnitude of confounding by comparing the estimate of effect derived from the crude data with the estimate derived from the stratified data (provided that the potential confounder is judged not to be a link in the causal path). Ignoring whatever residual age confounding there might be within these two age categories, we can say that the estimate of the incidence rate ratio of oral contraceptive use on the risk of myocardial infarction unconfounded by age is 2.8, since the estimate is 2.8 in each of the two age strata. The estimate based on the crude data, however, is 2.2. If these estimates were identical, the data would indicate no confounding. The magnitude of confounding in the data is estimated by the degree of discrepancy between the crude and unconfounded estimates.

Some investigators have attempted to assess confounding through statistical tests of significance. For example, in a clinical trial, the age distribution in the treatment and comparison groups may be compared by a t test; if the test statistic is "significant," then age would be judged potentially confounding, whereas lack of "significance" would imply that age is not confounding. There is probably no more grievous routine misuse of statistical testing than in this common circumstance. Since confounding is a bias that depends on the magnitude of two component associations, confounder with exposure and confounder with disease, proper assessment of confounding must be based on the magnitude of those associations. Statistical "significance" testing reflects a mixture of both magnitude of association and number of observations and therefore does not correspond to an assessment of magnitude of association alone. A large number of observations will produce statistical "significance" in situations in which the magnitude of one of the component associations of a potentially confounding factor is puny and would preclude any substantial confounding. Conversely, strong associations that produce serious confounding might be judged "not significant" if the number of observations is sparse. Confounding should therefore never be assessed by statistical tests.

Although it is possible to obtain a general appreciation for the presence or absence of confounding in data by examining whether the potentially confounding factor is associated with disease among nonexposed and with exposure among nondiseased, the magnitude of the confounding in the data is difficult to assess in this way because the confounding represents a function of both of these component associations. Furthermore, when several factors are simultaneously confounding, the component associations should ideally be examined conditional on the other confounding factors, thereby complicating the problem. The preferred method of assessing confounding is direct comparison of the crude and unconfounded estimates of effect. (An exception would be the unusual situation in which prior knowledge outweighs the evidence in the data about confounding, as discussed in Chapter 7, or when the potential confounder is judged to be a link in the causal pathway.) This comparison clearly and unambiguously reveals the magnitude of the confounding, which the investigator can then take into account in further analyses or reporting of results. Furthermore, this comparison can be made while controlling for other factors if necessary.

Point Estimation of a Uniform Effect

In Example 12-1, the point estimate of the incidence rate ratio was 2.8 in each of the two age strata, so there is no difficulty in inferring that an overall estimate of effect unconfounded by age should be 2.8. Even if the parameter value of the effect is identical across strata, however, it is reasonable to expect that estimates of the effect will vary among strata because of random error. Typically, then, the investigator must derive an overall estimate of effect from stratified data by taking a weighted average of the stratum-specific effect estimates. If the parameter value of the effect is assumed to be uniform—that is, constant over the range of the confounding variable—then each stratum provides a separate estimate of the same parameter value, the stratum-specific estimates varying only randomly. In weighting the estimates to get an average, it is desirable to assign greater weight to those stratum-specific estimates with smaller random variability and vice versa. Theoretically, the optimum procedure for reducing the variance in the overall weighted average is to assign weights to the stratum-specific values that are inversely proportional to the variance of each stratum-specific estimate:

$$\text{Overall effect estimate} = \frac{\sum_i [w_i \cdot (\text{effect estimate in stratum } i)]}{\sum_i w_i}$$

in which

$$w_i = \frac{1}{(\text{variance of effect estimate in stratum } i)}$$

This method of point estimation, in which the individual strata are weighted to enhance the precision of the overall estimate, is known as *pooling*. (The reader should note that the term *pooled* is sometimes used by statisticians to mean "crude.")

Pooling can be performed by calculating the weights for averaging the stratum-specific effect estimates directly from the estimated variance of the effect calculated from the data in each stratum separately; this method requires enough information within each stratum to get reasonable variance estimates. Another approach, the method of maximum likelihood, involves the solution of a set of equations and produces the pooled estimate without explicitly determining stratum-specific weights. The maximum likelihood approach can be thought of as a weighting process in which the weights are implicit in the equations that yield the point estimate. This description is not literally correct, since, for example, no weighting scheme would work if one of the stratum-specific estimates were infinity, whereas the maximum likelihood approach produces an appropriate finite result in this situation; indeed, the ability to average erratic stratum-specific estimates efficiently when data are relatively sparse is one of the main advantages of the maximum likelihood approach. Another set of pooled estimators, the Mantel-Haenszel estimators, have explicit weights that are built into the formulas; the Mantel-Haenszel estimators are the easiest to calculate, and, considering that their statistical properties are nearly as good as the difficult-to-calculate maximum likelihood estimators, they are often the method of choice.

In the following sections, the above three approaches to pooling are presented: the direct approach, using explicit weights inversely proportional to stratum-specific variance estimates; the maximum likelihood approach; and the Mantel-Haenszel approach. The specific formulas used for determining the pooled estimators depend on the type of data supplied and the effect measure being estimated.

POOLING WITH INVERSE VARIANCES (DIRECT POOLING)
Directly Pooled Point Estimation of a Uniform Effect with Person-Time Data. INCIDENCE RATE DIFFERENCE. Using the notation in Table 12-1, the variance for the estimate of incidence rate difference (IRD) from a single stratum in a stratified analysis is approximately

$$\text{Var}(\widehat{\text{IRD}}_i) \doteq \frac{a_i}{N_{1i}^2} + \frac{b_i}{N_{0i}^2} \qquad [12\text{-}1]$$

(see formula 11-15). Therefore, a pooled estimator for an IRD that is constant over strata can be obtained from

$$\widehat{\text{IRD}} = \frac{\sum\limits_i w_i \, \widehat{\text{IRD}}_i}{\sum\limits_i w_i} \qquad [12\text{-}2]$$

in which

$$w_i = \frac{1}{\text{Var}(\widehat{\text{IRD}}_i)} = \frac{N_{0i}^2 \cdot N_{1i}^2}{a_i N_{0i}^2 + b_i N_{1i}^2} \qquad [12\text{-}3]$$

and

$$\widehat{\text{IRD}}_i = \frac{a_i}{N_{1i}} - \frac{b_i}{N_{0i}}$$

as with crude data.

For an example of pooling used to estimate incidence rate difference, consider the data in Example 12-2. Stratum-specific estimates of incidence rate difference for these data, the corresponding stratum-specific variances, and the weights for pooling are given in Table 12-2, based on formulas 12-1 through 12-3. The pooled estimate of rate difference is obtained by taking the sum of the product of each stratum-specific estimate with the weight and dividing by the sum of the weights. The result is 5.95 $\times$ 10^{-4}yr^{-1}, which is expectedly close to the estimated incidence rate

Table 12-1. Notation for incidence rate data with person-time denominators in stratum i of a stratified analysis

	Exposed	Unexposed	Total
Cases	a_i	b_i	M_{1i}
Person-time	N_{1i}	N_{0i}	T_i

Example 12-2. Age-specific coronary disease deaths among British male doctors by cigarette smoking [Doll and Hill, 1966]

Age	Smokers		Nonsmokers	
	Deaths	Person-years	Deaths	Person-years
35–44	32	52,407	2	18,790
45–54	104	43,248	12	10,673
55–64	206	28,612	28	5,710
65–74	186	12,663	28	2,585
75–84	102	5,317	31	1,462
Total	630	142,247	101	39,220

Table 12-2. Stratum-specific estimates of incidence rate difference, with variances and weights for pooling for the data in example 12-2

Age	Estimate of incidence rate difference ($\times\ 10^4$yr)	Variance ($\times\ 10^8$yr^2)	Weight ($\times\ 10^{-6}$yr^{-2})
35–44	5.04	1.73	57.8
45–54	12.8	16.1	6.21
55–64	23.0	111	0.90
65–74	38.6	535	0.19
75–84	-20.2	1810	0.06

difference for stratum 1, the stratum with the smallest variance and the largest weight. The crude incidence rate difference is

$$\frac{630}{142,247\ \text{yr}} - \frac{101}{39,220\ \text{yr}} = 18.5 \times 10^{-4}\text{yr}^{-1}$$

which differs considerably from the pooled estimate of $5.95 \times 10^{-4}\text{yr}^{-1}$, indicating a substantial amount of age confounding in these data.

INCIDENCE RATE RATIO. For ratio estimators, pooling is performed after a logarithmic transformation of the estimates, which stabilizes the variances. The weights are the inverses of the variances of the logarithmically transformed stratum-specific estimates of incidence rate ratio (IRR). An approximate formula for this variance is

$$\text{Var}[\ln(\widehat{\text{IRR}}_i)] \doteq 1/a_i + 1/b_i \qquad [12\text{-}4]$$

and therefore the weight for pooling is

$$w_i = \frac{a_i b_i}{a_i + b_i}$$

Example 12-3. Mortality by sex and age for patients
with trigeminal neuralgia [Rothman and Monson, 1973]

	Age < 65		Age 65 +		Totals	
	Males	Females	Males	Females	Males	Females
Deaths	14	10	76	121	90	131
Person-years	1516	1701	949	2245	2465	3946

Table 12-3. Stratum-specific estimates of incidence rate ratio, with logarithmic
transformations, variances, and weights for pooling for the data in example 12-3

Age	Estimate of incidence rate ratio	Logarithm of $\widehat{\text{IRR}}$	Variance of $\ln(\widehat{\text{IRR}})$	Weight
< 65	1.57	0.45	0.17	5.83
65 +	1.49	0.40	0.021	46.7

and the pooled estimator, after reversing the logarithmic transformation, is

$$\widehat{\text{IRR}} = \exp\left[\frac{\sum_i w_i \ln(\widehat{\text{IRR}}_i)}{\sum_i w_i}\right] \qquad [12\text{-}5]$$

where

$$\widehat{\text{IRR}}_i = \frac{a_i/N_{1i}}{b_i/N_{0i}}$$

as with crude data.

The application of formula 12-5 is demonstrated using the data of Example 12-3 from a survival study of patients with trigeminal neuralgia. The male-to-female ratio of mortality rates from the crude data is $(90/2465 \text{ yr})/(131/3946 \text{ yr}) = 1.10$. A pooled estimate, controlling for age using the two age categories in Example 12-3, is obtained using the calculations given in Table 12-3. The pooled estimate is obtained by taking the sum of the weight in each stratum multiplied by the logarithm of the stratum-specific point estimate, dividing that sum by the sum of the weights, and then taking the antilogarithm of the result to reverse the transformation, giving 1.50 for the data in Example 12-3. The large discrepancy between this unconfounded estimate and the crude estimate of 1.10 indicates that the crude result was substantially biased by age confounding.

Pooled Estimate compared to crude estimate

Directly Pooled Point Estimation of a Uniform Effect with Cumulative Incidence Data. CUMULATIVE INCIDENCE DIFFERENCE. The notation for stratified 2×2 tables is given in Table 12-4. The approximate variance for the risk difference (RD) in stratum i is

$$\mathrm{Var}(\widehat{\mathrm{RD}}_i) \doteq \frac{a_i(N_{1i} - a_i)}{N_{1i}^3} + \frac{b_i(N_{0i} - b_i)}{N_{0i}^3} \qquad [12\text{-}6]$$

where

$$\widehat{\mathrm{RD}}_i = \frac{a_i}{N_{1i}} - \frac{b_i}{N_{0i}}$$

The weight for pooling stratum-specific estimates of risk difference is the inverse of the variance:

$$w_i = \frac{N_{1i}^3 N_{0i}^3}{N_{0i}^3 a_i(N_{1i} - a_i) + N_{1i}^3 b_i(N_{0i} - b_i)} \qquad [12\text{-}7]$$

A pooled estimator for risk difference is

$$\widehat{\mathrm{RD}} = \frac{\displaystyle\sum_i w_i \widehat{\mathrm{RD}}_i}{\displaystyle\sum_i w_i} \qquad [12\text{-}8]$$

The cumulative incidence data in Example 12-4 indicate a crude risk difference of $30/204 - 21/205 = 0.045$, but this is confounded by age, as is shown in Table 12-5, in which the age-specific risk differences are each seen to be in the vicinity of 0.035.

The unconfounded pooled estimate of cumulative incidence difference is obtained from formulas 12-7 and 12-8; as shown in Table 12-5, the older age category gives an estimate of cumulative incidence difference that has a much greater variance than that from the younger category, and therefore a much greater weight is assigned to the younger age category. The pooled estimate is 0.034, which reflects the greater weight assigned to the younger category.

Table 12-4. Notation for 2 × 2 tables in stratum i of a stratified analysis

	Exposed	Unexposed	Total
Cases	a_i	b_i	M_{1i}
Noncases	c_i	d_i	M_{0i}
Total	N_{1i}	N_{0i}	T_i

Example 12-4. Age-specific comparison of deaths from all causes for tolbutamide and placebo treatment groups, University Group Diabetes Program [1970]

	Age < 55		Age ≥ 55		Totals	
	Tolbutamide	Placebo	Tolbutamide	Placebo	Tolbutamide	Placebo
Dead	8	5	22	16	30	21
Surviving	98	115	76	69	174	184
Totals	106	120	98	85	204	205

Table 12-5. Stratum-specific estimates of cumulative incidence
difference, with variances and weights for pooling for the data in example 12-4

Age	Estimate of cumulative incidence difference	Variance of cumulative incidence difference	Weight
< 55	0.034	0.00099	1009
≥ 55	0.036	0.00357	280

CUMULATIVE INCIDENCE RATIO. The ratio estimator is obtained, as before,
using a logarithmic transformation. The approximate variance of the logarithm of the stratum-specific cumulative incidence ratio (RR) is

$$\mathrm{Var}[\ln(\hat{RR}_i)] \doteq \frac{c_i}{a_i N_{1i}} + \frac{d_i}{b_i N_{0i}} \qquad [12\text{-}9]$$

The weight for pooling is equal to the inverse of this variance:

$$w_i = \frac{a_i b_i N_{1i} N_{0i}}{a_i d_i N_{1i} + b_i c_i N_{0i}} \qquad [12\text{-}10]$$

and the pooled estimator is

$$\hat{RR} = \exp\left[\frac{\sum_i w_i \ln(\hat{RR}_i)}{\sum_i w_i}\right] \qquad [12\text{-}11]$$

where

$$\hat{RR}_i = \frac{a_i/N_{1i}}{b_i/N_{0i}}$$

Let us consider Example 12-4 again, this time for risk ratio estimation.
The crude estimate is $(30/204)/(21/205) = 1.44$. From a visual inspection
it is difficult to assess the extent to which confounding is present, since
the two stratum-specific estimates of cumulative incidence ratio bracket
the crude estimate as shown in Table 12-6. An estimate unconfounded by
age is obtained by applying formula 12-11, using the weights shown in
Table 12-6. The variance for the effect estimate is considerably larger in
the younger age category, just the reverse of the result seen in Table 12-5
for risk difference estimation. Small values of risk lead to stable estimates
of risk difference but unstable estimates of risk ratio. For risk ratio estimation, then, a relatively large weight is assigned to the older age category.

Table 12-6. Stratum-specific estimates of cumulative incidence ratio, with logarithmic transformations, variances, and weights for pooling for the data in example 12-4

Age	Estimate of cumulative incidence ratio	Logarithm of $\widehat{RR}_i$	Variance of $\ln(\widehat{RR}_i)$	Weight
< 55	1.81	0.59	0.31	3.25
≥ 55	1.19	0.18	0.09	11.6

The antilogarithm of the weighted average of the logarithms of the stratum-specific risk ratio estimates gives the pooled estimate, which is 1.31 for the data in Example 12-4. The discrepancy between the crude estimate, 1.44, and the unconfounded estimate, 1.31, indicates the extent of confounding.

Directly Pooled Point Estimation of a Uniform Effect with Case-Control (or Prevalence) Data. The effect parameter of interest with case-control data is the odds ratio, which serves as an estimator of the incidence rate ratio. The odds ratio is also the measure of interest for cross-sectional prevalence data, which should generally be treated as case-control data for the reasons given in Chapter 6. As discussed in Chapter 11, the odds ratio may also be used as an approximate estimator of the risk ratio or prevalence ratio from 2 × 2 tables with cumulative incidence or prevalence data, in which case the same formulas for pooling as given below for case-control data would apply.

For the odds ratio, as for other ratio estimators, a logarithmic transformation is desirable before weighting the stratum-specific estimates. The approximate variance of the stratum-specific estimate of the logarithm of the odds ratio (OR) is [Woolf, 1954]

$$\text{Var}[\ln(\widehat{OR}_i)] \doteq \frac{1}{a_i} + \frac{1}{b_i} + \frac{1}{c_i} + \frac{1}{d_i} \qquad [12\text{-}12]$$

and therefore the weight is

$$w_i = \frac{a_i b_i c_i d_i}{a_i b_i c_i + a_i b_i d_i + a_i c_i d_i + b_i c_i d_i} \qquad [12\text{-}13]$$

$$= \frac{1}{\dfrac{1}{a_i} + \dfrac{1}{b_i} + \dfrac{1}{c_i} + \dfrac{1}{d_i}}$$

Example 12-5. Infants with congenital heart disease and Down syndrome, and healthy controls, according to maternal spermicide use before conception and maternal age at delivery [Rothman, 1982]

	Maternal age < 35			Maternal age 35+			Totals		
	Spermicide use			Spermicide use			Spermicide use		
	+	−	Total	+	−	Total	+	−	Total
Down syndrome	3	9	12	1	3	4	4	12	16
Controls	104	1059	1163	5	86	91	109	1145	1254
Total	107	1068	1175	6	89	95	113	1157	1270

Table 12-7. Stratum-specific estimates of the odds ratio with logarithmic transformations, variances, and weights for pooling for the data in example 12-5

Maternal age	Odds ratio	Logarithm of $\hat{OR}_i$	Variance of $\ln(\hat{OR}_i)$	Weight
< 35	3.4	1.22	0.46	2.20
35+	5.7	1.75	1.54	0.65

and the pooled estimator is

$$\hat{OR} = \exp\left[\frac{\sum_i w_i \ln(\hat{OR}_i)}{\sum_i w_i}\right] \qquad [12\text{-}14]$$

The case-control data in Example 12-5 describe an association between spermicide use near the time of conception and the risk of Down syndrome. The crude estimate of effect is $(4 \cdot 1145)/(12 \cdot 109) = 3.5$. The application of formula 12-14, based on the calculations in Table 12-7, gives a result of $\hat{OR} = 3.8$, which indicates only a modest degree of confounding by maternal age at delivery.

POOLING USING THE METHOD OF MAXIMUM LIKELIHOOD

A full discussion of the maximum likelihood approach to estimation is beyond the scope of this book; the method is described adequately in many statistics texts. Briefly, the approach involves specifying the likelihood equation for the data as a function of the parameter of interest; the maximum likelihood estimate of the parameter is the value of the parameter that makes the observations in hand most probable under the likelihood model. The maximization is usually accomplished by maximizing the logarithm of the likelihood rather than the likelihood itself because the two maxima occur at the same value for the parameter, and the maximum of the logarithm of the likelihood is usually easier to determine. By setting the first derivative of the log-likelihood function equal to zero, an equation or set of equations is derived that yields the maximum likelihood estimate for the parameter.

For most applications, the maximum likelihood estimator requires the iterative solution of a high-order equation or system of high-order equations, clearly a task for a computer rather than pencil and paper. The complicated equations do not involve any direct set of weights by which stratum-specific effect estimates are averaged, but the solution is always within the range of the stratum-specific estimates and behaves as if it were a weighted average in the sense that appropriately large weight is given to the strata with small variances for the effect estimate. In compensation for the difficulty of computation, maximum likelihood estimators have the most desirable statistical properties of all estimators, being highly efficient and minimally biased asymptotically.

A major disadvantage of the directly pooled estimators is that the pooling weight for each stratum is taken as the inverse of the variance of the effect estimate for that stratum, as estimated from the data in that stratum alone. For data with small frequencies, the variance estimates and therefore the weights can be highly inaccurate. Indeed, for data containing one or more zero frequencies, some of the variance estimates given above are infinity, corresponding to a weight of zero. Consider, for example, formula 12-12, which estimates the variance of the logarithm of the odds ratio for a 2 × 2 table. If any of the four cells in the table is zero, this formula gives a value of infinity, and a weight of zero would be assigned to that table. (Furthermore, the logarithm of the odds ratio for that stratum would not be finite with a zero cell.) If the remaining cells in the table are large, there might be a considerable amount of information in the table that would be lost by assigning a weight of zero. Since the odds ratio for the stratum is either zero or infinity, which are the most extreme possibilities, it seems obviously incorrect to ignore such information. One proposed solution to this problem has been to modify formula 12-12 and, by extension, other formulas like it by adding a constant value (usually 0.5 or 1.0) to each observed frequency [Haldane, 1955] or to substitute a small constant for the zero frequencies when they occur. Although this solution mitigates the problem and avoids the difficulty of dividing by zero, it does not completely overcome the inaccuracy of the variance estimates for each stratum-specific estimate of effect when some of the observations are small. The maximum likelihood approach is preferable when some of the observed frequencies are small. Rather than treating each stratum in isolation, as does the directly weighted approach to pooling in the assignment of weights, the maximum likelihood approach automatically "adjusts" the observations in each stratum in a way that integrates the information among all strata.

In the following sections, the equations are presented for maximum likelihood estimation of a uniform effect measure. In each case, the result can be obtained by writing the likelihood equation for the data as a function of a uniform effect measure, the observations, and whatever "nuisance" parameters may be involved, and then setting the derivative of the logarithm of the likelihood equal to zero.

Maximum Likelihood Estimation of a Uniform Effect with Person-Time Data. INCIDENCE RATE DIFFERENCE. The maximum likelihood estimation of incidence rate difference necessitates the solution of a set of equations that number one more than the number of strata. In addition to solving for the incidence rate difference (IRD), it is necessary to solve for the value of the incidence rate among the unexposed group in each stratum, satisfying the following likelihood equations:

$$\sum_i \frac{a_i}{\hat{R}_{0i} + \widehat{IRD}} - \sum_i N_{1i} = 0 \qquad [12\text{-}15]$$

and, for each stratum i,

$$\frac{a_i}{\hat{R}_{0i} + \widehat{IRD}} + \frac{b_i}{\hat{R}_{0i}} - T_i = 0 \qquad [12\text{-}16]$$

where $\widehat{IRD}$ is the pooled estimate of incidence rate difference, $\hat{R}_{0i}$ is the estimate of incidence rate among unexposed in stratum i, and the general notation follows that of Table 12-1. The estimates $\{\hat{R}_{0i}\}$ are estimates of nuisance parameters that must be calculated to solve for the desired estimate, $\widehat{IRD}$. It is convenient to begin the solution to the above equations using the observed rate for unexposed within each stratum as a starting value, but the value for $\hat{R}_{0i}$ that satisfies the equation can differ considerably from the observed value. The overall solution of equations 12-15 and 12-16 is best accomplished by starting with a trial value for $\widehat{IRD}$, solving iteratively for each $\hat{R}_{0i}$, and then evaluating the left side of equation 12-15. Repeated trial values for $\widehat{IRD}$ each require an iterative solution for equation 12-16 in each stratum, making the overall process tedious unless it is done by computer.

For the data in Example 12-2 the maximum likelihood solution for $\widehat{IRD}$ is $5.91 \times 10^{-4} \text{yr}^{-1}$, which is in close agreement with the directly pooled result of $5.95 \times 10^{-4} \text{yr}^{-1}$ obtained previously.

INCIDENCE RATE RATIO. For the maximum likelihood estimation of incidence rate ratio (IRR), no nuisance parameters are involved, and the estimate is obtained by the iterative solution of a single equation:

$$\sum_i a_i - \widehat{IRR} \sum_i \frac{M_{1i}}{\widehat{IRR} + \dfrac{N_{0i}}{N_{1i}}} = 0 \qquad [12\text{-}17]$$

For the data in Example 12-3, the maximum likelihood estimate of IRR is 1.50, which is identical to the result obtained by direct pooling. One would expect good agreement between these two approaches when the observed frequencies are reasonably large, as they are in this example. In addition, the narrow spread between the stratum-specific estimates confines all pooled estimates to the same small range of possible values.

Maximum Likelihood Estimation of a Uniform Effect with Cumulative Incidence Data. CUMULATIVE INCIDENCE DIFFERENCE. The maximum likelihood estimation of cumulative incidence difference (RD) again involves the estimation of a set of nuisance parameters, the risk among the nonexposed group in each stratum. As with person-time data, the number of equations is one more than the number of strata:

$$\sum_i \frac{a_i}{\hat{R}_{0i} + \hat{RD}} - \sum_i \frac{N_{1i} - a_i}{1 - \hat{R}_{0i} - \hat{RD}} = 0 \qquad [12\text{-}18]$$

and, for each stratum i,

$$\frac{a_i}{\hat{R}_{0i} + \hat{RD}} + \frac{b_i}{\hat{R}_{0i}} - \frac{N_{1i} - a_i}{1 - \hat{R}_{0i} - \hat{RD}} - \frac{N_{0i} - b_i}{1 - \hat{R}_{0i}} = 0 \qquad [12\text{-}19]$$

where $\hat{R}_{0i}$ is the maximum likelihood estimate of cumulative incidence among unexposed in stratum i, and the notation follows that in Table 12-4.

Solving the above equations for $\hat{RD}$ using the data from Example 12-4 gives the maximum likelihood estimate of risk difference as 0.034, which is virtually identical to the value derived from direct pooling. The extremely narrow range separating the two stratum-specific point estimates ensures good agreement for any pooled estimators in this example.

CUMULATIVE INCIDENCE RATIO. For maximum likelihood estimation of cumulative incidence ratio (RR), again the risk among unexposed in each stratum is a nuisance parameter that must be estimated, but the maximum likelihood solution for each $\hat{R}_{0i}$ has a closed form solution conditional on $\hat{RR}$. The equations are

$$\sum_i \frac{a_i - (\hat{RR})\hat{R}_{0i}N_{1i}}{1 - (\hat{RR})\hat{R}_{0i}} = 0 \qquad [12\text{-}20]$$

and, for each stratum i,

$$\hat{R}_{0i} = \frac{a_i + N_{0i} + (\hat{RR})(b_i + N_{1i})}{2(\hat{RR})T_i}$$

$$- \left(\left[\frac{a_i + N_{0i} + (\hat{RR})(b_i + N_{1i})}{2(\hat{RR})T_i} \right]^2 - \frac{M_{1i}}{(\hat{RR})T_i} \right)^{1/2} \qquad [12\text{-}21]$$

Solution of these equations for $\hat{RR}$ using the data in Example 12-4 gives the maximum likelihood estimate of 1.31, again identical to the directly pooled estimate.

Maximum Likelihood Estimation of a Uniform Effect with Case-Control (or Prevalence) Data. The maximum likelihood estimation of a uniform odds ratio is the solution, $\hat{OR}$, to the following equations:

$$\sum_i a_i - \sum_i \hat{a}_i = 0 \qquad [12\text{-}22]$$

The quantity $\hat{a}_i$ is the "expected" value for the a cell in each 2×2 table, calculated as a function of the odds ratio. For each 2×2 table $\hat{a}_i$ can be calculated from the formula

$$\hat{a}_i = \frac{\displaystyle\sum_{k=\max(0,M_{1i}-N_{0i})}^{\min(M_{1i},N_{1i})} k \binom{N_{1i}}{k}\binom{N_{0i}}{M_{1i}-k} \hat{OR}^k}{\displaystyle\sum_{k=\max(0,M_{1i}-N_{0i})}^{\min(M_{1i},N_{1i})} \binom{N_{1i}}{k}\binom{N_{0i}}{M_{1i}-k} \hat{OR}^k} \qquad [12\text{-}23]$$

where the notation follows that in Table 12-4. Equation 12-23 can be computationally tedious if the numbers within a stratum are large, but in such circumstances an excellent asymptotic approximation for $\hat{a}_i$ is obtained from the equation

$$\hat{OR} = \frac{\hat{a}_i \hat{d}_i}{\hat{b}_i \hat{c}_i} \qquad [12\text{-}24]$$

in which $\hat{a}_i, \hat{b}_i, \hat{c}_i,$ and $\hat{d}_i$ are the expected cell values that conform to equations 12-22 and 12-24 and to the marginal totals of the 2×2 table [Gart, 1970]. Solving equation 12-24 explicitly for $\hat{a}_i$ in terms of T_i, N_{1i}, M_{1i} and $\hat{OR}$ gives

$$\hat{a}_i = \text{ABS}\left\{ \text{ABS}\left[\frac{1}{2}\left(\frac{T_i}{\hat{OR}-1} + N_{1i} + M_{1i}\right)\right] \right.$$
$$\left. - \sqrt{\left[\frac{1}{2}\left(\frac{T_i}{\hat{OR}-1} + N_{1i} + M_{1i}\right)\right]^2 - \frac{M_{1i}N_{1i}\hat{OR}}{\hat{OR}-1}} \right\} \qquad [12\text{-}25]$$

which is computationally much simpler than equation 12-23. Equation 12-24 represents the maximum likelihood solution for a uniform odds ratio based on 2×2 tables with two independent binomials; this "unconditional" solution (it is conditional on one margin of the 2×2 table but not on both) generally gives nearly identical results to those obtained from the difficult-to-calculate conditional formula 12-23 except when the average number of subjects per stratum is small. In such instances, the unconditional approach can be substantially biased, and it is preferable to use the conditional approach or the Mantel-Haenszel estimator [Breslow, 1981; McKinlay, 1978; Lubin, 1981]. (Directly weighted pooled estimation is also unreliable if the number of subjects per stratum is small.)

Maximum likelihood estimation of the odds ratio in a set of 2×2 tables requires an iterative solution of equation 12-22 coupled with either equation 12-23 or equation 12-25, using trial values for the odds ratio until equation 12-22 is satisfied. For the data in Example 12-5, the conditional maximum likelihood estimate of the odds ratio (i.e., using equation 12-23) is 3.76; the unconditional maximum likelihood estimate (using equation 12-25) is 3.79. Despite the small cell frequencies for the cases and a moderate discrepancy between the stratum-specific estimates of the odds ratio (3.4 for younger mothers and 5.7 for older mothers), the two likelihood approaches give nearly identical results because the total number of subjects per stratum is large. Furthermore, these estimates agree closely with the directly pooled estimate for these data, which is 3.82.

POOLING WITH MANTEL-HAENSZEL ESTIMATORS

Mantel and Haenszel [1959] have proposed a simple formula as an estimator of a uniform odds ratio in a set of 2×2 tables. The estimator is

$$\widehat{OR}_{MH} = \frac{\sum_i a_i d_i / T_i}{\sum_i b_i c_i / T_i} \qquad [12\text{-}26]$$

This formula represents a weighted average, without logarithmic transformation, of the stratum-specific estimates of the odds ratio, with the weight for each stratum equal to $b_i c_i / T_i$:

$$\frac{a_i d_i}{b_i c_i} \cdot \frac{b_i c_i}{T_i} = \frac{a_i d_i}{T_i}$$

These weights are inversely proportional to the variance of the logarithm of the odds ratio under the null condition. Consequently, the Mantel-Haenszel pooled estimator is optimally weighted for stratum-specific odds ratio estimates near 1.0. Theoretical statistical evaluation of the Mantel-Haenszel estimator with respect to bias and precision has shown that it compares favorably with the maximum likelihood estimator (formulas 12-22 through 12-25) under a variety of conditions [Breslow and Liang, 1982]. Whereas the directly pooled estimators require reasonably large frequencies within each stratum, the Mantel-Haenszel estimator, like the conditional maximum likelihood estimators, performs well even if the frequencies within strata are small or if the data contain an occasional zero. Furthermore, it has the advantage of being extremely simple to calculate. For example, the Mantel-Haenszel estimator of a uniform odds ratio for the data in Example 12-5 is calculated as

$$\hat{OR}_{MH} = \frac{(3)\,(1059)/(1175) + (1)\,(86)/(95)}{(104)\,(9)/(1175) + (5)\,(3)/(95)} = 3.8$$

This result is nearly identical to the maximum likelihood estimate (and the directly pooled estimate) but is extraordinarily simpler to produce. The combination of ease of computation and desirable statistical properties make this estimator the preferred choice for most situations in which an estimate of the odds ratio is desired for a set of 2 × 2 tables.

By analogy with the Mantel-Haenszel estimator, it is reasonable to construct estimators for the other ratio measures of effect weighted in a similar way. For incidence rate data, the analogous estimator is [Rothman and Boice, 1982]

$$\hat{IRR}_{MH} = \frac{\sum_i a_i N_{0i}/T_i}{\sum_i b_i N_{1i}/T_i} \qquad [12\text{-}27]$$

This formula is a simple noniterative estimator for a uniform incidence rate ratio that is nearly as efficient as the maximum likelihood estimator [Walker, 1985]. Formula 12-27 may also be used for cumulative incidence to obtain $\hat{RR}_{MH}$ [Nurminen, 1981; Tarone, 1981].

For the data in Example 12-3, formula 12-27 yields

$$\hat{IRR}_{MH} = \frac{(14)\,(1701)/(3217) + (76)\,(2245)/(3194)}{(10)\,(1516)/(3217) + (121)\,(949)/(3194)} = 1.50$$

which is identical for practical purposes with both the maximum likelihood and the directly pooled results.

Formula 12-27 applied to the data in Example 12-4 gives

$$\hat{RR}_{MH} = \frac{(8)\,(120)/(226) + (22)\,(85)/(183)}{(5)\,(106)/(226) + (16)\,(98)/(183)} = 1.33$$

which is reasonably close to both the maximum likelihood and the directly pooled results.

Greenland and Robins [1985] have suggested extending the Mantel-Haenszel approach to difference measures. The statistical properties of the Mantel-Haenszel estimators for difference measures are better than any other approach for very sparse data within strata, but the variance of the

Mantel-Haenszel effect measures is much greater than that of either the directly weighted or maximum likelihood methods when the data are ample. Mantel-Haenszel difference measures are not covered here.

Statistical Hypothesis Testing for Stratified Data

Examples can be found in which a pooled estimate of rate difference shows a negative association whereas a pooled estimate of rate ratio shows a positive association for the same data, apparently indicating that there is not a perfect correspondence between ratio and difference measures with regard to the absence or direction of effect. These discrepancies stem from variation introduced by different weighting schemes. For the purposes of statistical hypothesis testing, there is a theoretical correspondence of different measures at the null point, and consequently only a single hypothesis test need be considered, whatever the parameter used to assess the effect. The tests in common use correspond to the conditional tests for simple data that assume either a fixed number of cases for incidence rate data or fixed marginal totals for 2×2 tables. Strictly speaking, these are tests of a departure from unity of the odds ratio or the incidence rate ratio, but the tests are valid as tests of the null hypothesis whatever the measure of interest.

With stratified data, it is possible that the effect may vary substantially from one stratum to another. Nevertheless, hypothesis testing is generally performed with respect to the overall departure of the data from the null value of no association. That is, even if the parameter value for the effect varies among strata, the hypothesis test represents a test of the departure of some single overall measure of effect from its null value; it is convenient to think of this process as testing the departure of a pooled estimate of effect from the null value. If the stratum-specific values of the odds ratio or incidence rate ratio are identical, the tests described later are extremely powerful; in fact, in the jargon of statistics they are "uniformly most powerful," which means that they are the best possible tests of the null hypothesis in those circumstances. If the values of the odds ratio or incidence rate ratio vary across strata, it is conceivable that specialized tests could be constructed that would be more powerful than the tests of overall departure from the null value described here; the specialized tests would have to be designed to detect a particular pattern of variation of the effect across strata. In general, however, the tests of the departure of the pooled estimate from the null value are still valid, even if they are not theoretically the most powerful tests that might be applied in a given situation. As a practical matter, usually no useful alternative exists.

In certain situations it is conceivable that estimates of an effect could be strongly positive in some strata and strongly negative in others. In such circumstances the pooled estimate of effect may be near the null value as a result of the balancing of the opposing effect estimates in individual strata. A test of the overall departure of the data from the null condition would have little meaning in these circumstances as long as the opposing effect estimates reflect actual divergence of the parameter rather than simply random variability of the effect estimate around the null value.

Statistical hypothesis testing for stratified data represents a straightforward extension of the tests applied to crude data. The exact tests used are based on the probability calculations for a set of strata; the probability of observing a set of outcomes is the product of the probability for each outcome, so the probability of observing the set of observations in stratified data is calculated as the product of the probability of the outcome in each stratum. The latter probability is determined using the same probability model as that used for crude data. Although this extension of exact testing to stratified data is conceptually simple, in practice the large number of combinations of outcomes can make the computations tedious to enumerate and perform except by computer.

The approximate tests for stratified data retain the general form of expression 10-1 and merely extend the formulas for crude data given in Chapter 11 by deriving the components of the test statistics (the observed number of exposed cases, the number expected under the null hypothesis, and the variance) by summing the contributions to each of these three components over the set of strata.

HYPOTHESIS TESTING WITH STRATIFIED PERSON-TIME DATA

Exact Hypothesis Testing with Stratified Person-Time Data. For stratified data, the overall probabilities needed for the calculation of exact P-values are the products of the probabilities obtained within each stratum. The total number of possible outcomes is usually large, especially in comparison with crude data, making exact P-value calculations for stratified data difficult. In practice, they are rarely done. Nevertheless, the principles for obtaining exact P-values with stratified data are straightforward extensions of the principles applicable to crude data, and the computations can be readily programmed into a computer.

The probability formula for the number of exposed cases in a single stratum is identical to the formula used for crude data:

$$\text{Pr(number of exposed cases in stratum } i = a_i) = \binom{M_{1i}}{a_i} \left(\frac{N_{1i}}{T_i}\right)^{a_i} \left(\frac{N_{0i}}{T_i}\right)^{b_i}$$

The probability that a set of N strata will have exactly a_i exposed cases in each stratum i, $i = 1, 2, \ldots N$, is the product of the probability of finding exactly a_i exposed cases in each of the component strata:

$$\text{Pr(the set of observations } \{a_i\}) = \prod_{i=1}^{N} \binom{M_{1i}}{a_i} \left(\frac{N_{1i}}{T_i}\right)^{a_i} \left(\frac{N_{0i}}{T_i}\right)^{b_i} \qquad [12\text{-}28]$$

There is some complexity involved in determining which outcomes of the data are considered equally extreme and more extreme in relation to the actual observations. The problem calls for considering all possible combinations of values for the possible number of exposed cases in each stratum, the number in each stratum being subject to the constraint of the total number of cases, exposed or unexposed, that actually occurred in that stratum.

For example, consider the data presented in Example 12-6. There are a total of 16 cases in the three age strata, of which 9 are exposed. The most extreme outcome, conditional on the number of cases observed in each stratum, would be that all 16 cases were exposed, 2, 12, and 2, respectively, in each of the three age strata. Consider the possible outcomes for which 15 cases are exposed. There are three ways in which 15 of the 16 cases could be exposed: The unexposed case could fall into any of the three age strata. These three possibilities correspond to the distribution of the exposed cases being 1-12-2, 2-11-2, and 2-12-1. A complete enumeration of all the possible outcomes for at least 9 exposed cases is listed in Table 12-8. The 54 combinations constitute the outcomes in the upper tail of the probability distribution for testing the null hypothesis of no association between dose category and thyroid neoplasm. To obtain the exact upper-tail P-value, the probability of each of these 54 possible outcomes must be calculated according to formula 12-28.

For example, the probability of the actual observations 0-7-2 is calculated, according to Formula 12-28, to be

$$\binom{2}{0}\left(\frac{1054}{10{,}996}\right)^{0}\left(\frac{9942}{10{,}996}\right)^{2} \cdot \binom{12}{7}\left(\frac{2665}{18{,}075}\right)^{7}\left(\frac{15{,}410}{18{,}075}\right)^{5}$$

$$\cdot \binom{2}{2}\left(\frac{2217}{3747}\right)^{2}\left(\frac{1530}{3747}\right)^{0} = (0.8175) \times (0.00054036) \times (0.3501) = 0.000155$$

The sum of the probability of all the outcomes in Table 12-8 equals the upper-tail Fisher exact P-value testing the null hypothesis of no association

Example 12-6. Incidence of thyroid neoplasms in females by age, for those exposed to less than 100 rad and those exposed to 300+ rad of radiation [Hempelmann et al., 1975]

	0–14 Years		15–29 Years		30+ Years	
	300+ rad	< 100 rad	300+ rad	< 100 rad	300+ rad	< 100 rad
Cases	0	2	7	5	2	0
Person-years	1054	9942	2665	15,410	2217	1530

Table 12-8. Enumeration of all possible combinations of exposed cases by age category, with at least nine exposed cases, for the data of example 12-6

Total no. exposed cases	Distribution of exposed cases by age category	Total no. exposed cases	Distribution of exposed cases by age category	Total no. exposed cases	Distribution of exposed cases by age category
16	2–12–2	12	0–12–0	10	0–10–0
15	1–12–2	12	0–11–1	10	0–9–1
15	2–12–1	12	0–10–2	10	0–8–2
15	2–11–2	12	1–11–0	10	1–9–0
14	0–12–2	12	1–10–1	10	1–8–1
14	1–12–1	12	1–9–2	10	1–7–2
14	1–11–2	12	2–10–0	10	2–8–0
14	2–12–0	12	2–9–1	10	2–7–1
14	2–11–1	12	2–8–2	10	2–6–2
14	2–10–2	11	0–11–0	9	0–9–0
13	0–12–1	11	0–10–1	9	0–8–1
13	0–11–2	11	0–9–2	9	0–7–2
13	1–12–0	11	1–10–0	9	1–8–0
13	1–11–1	11	1–9–1	9	1–7–1
13	1–10–2	11	1–8–2	9	1–6–2
13	2–11–0	11	2–9–0	9	2–7–0
13	2–10–1	11	2–8–1	9	2–6–1
13	2–9–2	11	2–7–2	9	2–5–2

between level of radiation exposure and incidence of thyroid neoplasm. Algebraically, the tail probability is expressed as

$$\Pr(k \geq a) = \sum_{k=a}^{M_1} \prod_{i=1}^{N} \binom{M_{1i}}{k_i} \left(\frac{N_{1i}}{T_i}\right)^{k_i} \left(\frac{N_{0i}}{T_i}\right)^{M_{1i} - k_i} \qquad [12\text{-}29]$$

where k_i represents the value for the number of exposed cases in stratum i, $k = \Sigma k_i$, $a = \Sigma a_i$, and $M_1 = \Sigma M_{1i}$. The sum of all the probabilities for the combinations listed in Table 12-8 is 0.000600. Interestingly, the sum of the probabilities for the nine combinations that are just as extreme as the actual observation, with exactly nine exposed cases, is 0.000522, nearly as great as the sum for all 54 outcomes listed in Table 12-8. If the nine combinations with 10 exposed cases are included, the sum increases to 0.000592, and by including the possibilities with 11 exposed cases it increases to 0.000599. Clearly it is not necessary to carry out all 54 computations to get an answer accurate enough for any scientific interpretation, since one digit of precision is usually adequate for the *P*-value.

For the lower-tail Fisher exact P-value, which would be calculated when the observed effect is less than the null value, the summation is

$$\Pr(k \leq a) = \sum_{k=0}^{a} \prod_{i=1}^{N} \binom{M_{1i}}{k_i} \left(\frac{N_{1i}}{T_i}\right)^{k_i} \left(\frac{N_{0i}}{T_i}\right)^{M_{1i}-k_i} \qquad [12\text{-}30]$$

where again $k = \Sigma k_i$, and so on.

To obtain the exact mid-P value, only half the probability of all observations as extreme as that observed should be included in the summation:

$$\text{Upper-tail probability} = \frac{1}{2} \sum_{k=a}^{N} \prod_{i=1}^{N} \binom{M_{1i}}{k_i} \left(\frac{N_{1i}}{T_i}\right)^{k_i} \left(\frac{N_{0i}}{T_i}\right)^{M_{1i}-k_i}$$

$$+ \sum_{k=a+1}^{M_1} \prod_{i=1}^{N} \binom{M_{1i}}{k_i} \left(\frac{N_{1i}}{T_i}\right)^{k_i} \left(\frac{N_{0i}}{T_i}\right)^{M_{1i}-k_i} \qquad [12\text{-}31]$$

$$\text{Lower-tail probability} = \frac{1}{2} \sum_{k=a}^{N} \prod_{i=1}^{N} \binom{M_{1i}}{k_i} \left(\frac{N_{1i}}{T_i}\right)^{k_i} \left(\frac{N_{0i}}{T_i}\right)^{M_{1i}-k_i}$$

$$+ \sum_{k=0}^{a-1} \prod_{i=1}^{N} \binom{M_{1i}}{k_i} \left(\frac{N_{1i}}{T_i}\right)^{k_i} \left(\frac{N_{0i}}{T_i}\right)^{M_{1i}-k_i} \qquad [12\text{-}32]$$

For the data in Example 12-6, the exact upper mid-P value would be one-half of 0.000522, which was the probability for the nine possible outcomes with exactly nine exposed cases, plus the probability of all the possible outcomes more extreme than nine exposed cases, which was a total of 0.000078. Therefore, the exact upper mid-P value is 0.00034.

Approximate Hypothesis Testing with Stratified Person-Time Data. For stratified data, asymptotic test statistics are constructed according to the same principles used for crude data. The test variable is still the number of exposed cases, which is the sum of a_i over the strata. The null expectation and the variance for the number of exposed cases is calculated within each stratum, and these results are summed over the strata. Thus, the null expectation for the number of exposed cases is

$$E(A) = \sum_{i=1}^{N} \frac{N_{1i} M_{1i}}{T_i}$$

and the variance, based on the binomial model, is

$$\text{Var}(A) = \sum_{i=1}^{N} \frac{M_{1i} N_{1i} N_{0i}}{T_i^2}$$

which gives as the test statistic

$$\chi = \frac{\displaystyle\sum_{i=1}^{N} a_i - \sum_{i=1}^{N} \frac{N_{1i}M_{1i}}{T_i}}{\sqrt{\displaystyle\sum_{i=1}^{N} \frac{M_{1i}N_{1i}N_{0i}}{T_i^2}}} \qquad [12\text{-}33]$$

Formula 12-33 is identical to formula 11-1 for crude person-time data except that the three components of the test statistic are obtained by summing their stratum-specific contributions over the strata.

For the data in Example 12-6, the test statistic is calculated as follows:

$$A = \text{no. of exposed cases} = 0 + 7 + 2 = 9$$

$$E(A) = 2\left(\frac{1054}{10{,}996}\right) + 12\left(\frac{2665}{18{,}075}\right) + 2\left(\frac{2217}{3747}\right) = 3.14$$

$$Var(A) = 2\left(\frac{1054}{10{,}996}\right)\left(\frac{9942}{10{,}996}\right) + 12\left(\frac{2665}{18{,}075}\right)\left(\frac{15{,}410}{18{,}075}\right)$$

$$+ 2\left(\frac{2217}{3747}\right)\left(\frac{1530}{3747}\right) = 2.16$$

and

$$\chi = \frac{A - E(A)}{\sqrt{Var(A)}} = \frac{9 - 3.14}{\sqrt{2.16}} = 3.98$$

which corresponds to a one-tail P-value of 0.000034 or a two-tail P-value of 0.000069.

The P-value calculated from this approximate test statistic, like the exact P-value, is very small, but the two P-values do not agree closely. The exact mid-P value is about 10 times the magnitude of the approximate P-value. The discrepancy stems from the small numbers involved but is also related to the fact that the normal approximation is poorer in the extremities of the distribution.

Nevertheless, comparison between the exact and the asymptotic test raises the question of the nature of the applicability criteria for the asymptotic test statistic with regard to the number of observations. There is no simple answer to this question, but one important point should be emphasized: The large-number condition need apply only to the summations involved in formula 12-33, not to each individual stratum. For person-time data, then, formula 12-33 would apply even if each stratum had only one case, provided that there were enough such strata to allow the distribution of the total number of exposed subjects in all strata to be well enough approximated by a normal distribution. The large-number condition necessary for formula 12-33 to apply, then, could be reached by having few strata with many observations in each one or many strata with sparse data. With one stratum, formula 12-33 reduces to formula 11-1. A stratum with no cases has no information and contributes nothing to A, E(A), or Var(A).

As a second example of the application of formula 12-33, consider the data in Example 12-3. The large number of cases in each of these two strata make it unnecessary to contemplate any exact test. The P-value can be determined as follows (considering male gender as "exposed"):

$$A = \text{no. of exposed cases} = 14 + 76 = 90$$

$$E(A) = 24 \left(\frac{1516}{3217}\right) + 197 \left(\frac{949}{3194}\right) = 69.8$$

$$\text{Var}(A) = 24\left(\frac{1516}{3217}\right)\left(\frac{1701}{3217}\right) + 197 \left(\frac{949}{3194}\right)\left(\frac{2245}{3194}\right) = 47.1$$

$$\chi = \frac{90 - 69.8}{\sqrt{47.1}} = 2.94$$

$$P_{(1)} = 0.0017$$

HYPOTHESIS TESTING WITH STRATIFIED CUMULATIVE INCIDENCE, PREVALENCE OR CASE-CONTROL DATA (2 × 2 TABLES)

Exact Hypothesis Testing for Stratified 2 × 2 Tables. As with person-time data, exact hypothesis testing for stratified 2 × 2 tables can be accomplished by enumerating all possible outcomes of the number of exposed cases across strata. The joint probability of each combination is calculated as the product of the hypergeometric probabilities of each 2 × 2 table. The exact P-value is determined in the usual way by summing the probabilities in the tail of the distribution. Each 2 × 2 table is considered to have all marginal totals fixed. Using the notation of Table 12-4, we have, for the Fisher P-values,

$$\Pr(k \geq a) = \sum_{k=a}^{\min(N_1, M_1)} \prod_{i=1}^{N} \frac{\binom{N_{1i}}{k_i}\binom{N_{0i}}{M_{1i} - k_i}}{\binom{T_i}{M_{1i}}} \qquad [12\text{-}34]$$

for the upper tail, when the effect estimate is greater than the null value, and

$$\Pr(k \le a) = \sum_{k=\max(0, M_1 - N_0)}^{a} \prod_{i=1}^{N} \frac{\dbinom{N_{1i}}{k_i} \dbinom{N_{0i}}{M_{1i} - k_i}}{\dbinom{T_i}{M_{1i}}} \qquad [12\text{-}35]$$

for the lower tail, when the effect estimate is less than the null value. The summations are for $k = \Sigma k_i$, where k_i is the number of exposed cases in each 2×2 table, and a, N_1, N_0, and M_1 refer to Σa_i, ΣN_{1i}, ΣN_{0i}, and ΣM_{1i}, respectively.

To obtain the exact mid-P value, only half of the probability for the equally extreme outcomes should be added to the tail summation:

Upper-tail probability

$$= \frac{1}{2} \sum_{k=a}^{N} \prod_{i=1}^{N} \frac{\dbinom{N_{1i}}{k_i} \dbinom{N_{0i}}{M_{1i} - k_i}}{\dbinom{T_i}{M_{1i}}} + \sum_{k=a+1}^{\min(N_1, M_1)} \prod_{i=1}^{N} \frac{\dbinom{N_{1i}}{k_i} \dbinom{N_{0i}}{M_{1i} - k_i}}{\dbinom{T_i}{M_{1i}}} \qquad [12\text{-}36]$$

$$\text{Lower-tail probability} = \frac{1}{2} \sum_{k=a}^{N} \prod_{i=1}^{N} \frac{\dbinom{N_{1i}}{k_i} \dbinom{N_{0i}}{M_{1i} - k_i}}{\dbinom{T_i}{M_{1i}}}$$

$$+ \sum_{k=\max(0, M_1 - N_0)}^{a-1} \prod_{i=1}^{N} \frac{\dbinom{N_{1i}}{k_i} \dbinom{N_{0i}}{M_{1i} - k_i}}{\dbinom{T_i}{M_{1i}}} \qquad [12\text{-}37]$$

These formulas can be used to derive an exact P-value for the data in Example 12-5. There were four exposed cases, three in the "young" stratum and one in the "old" stratum. In the young stratum, the number of exposed cases can range from zero to 12 within the constraints imposed by the marginal totals. In the old stratum, the corresponding number can range from zero to 4. Overall, there are $13 \times 5 = 65$ possible outcomes for the two strata. Of these 65 possibilities, 50 are more extreme positive departures from the null condition than the outcome actually observed; a total of five possibilities, including the observed data, are equally extreme with exactly four exposed cases. These 55 equally or more extreme outcomes are enumerated in Table 12-9.

The probability of observing the actual outcome in Example 12-5 is determined as

$$\text{Pr(observed data)} = \frac{\binom{107}{3} \binom{1068}{9} \binom{6}{1} \binom{89}{3}}{\binom{1175}{12} \binom{95}{4}}$$

$$= \frac{(107!) \, (1068!) \, (6!) \, (89!) \, (1163!) \, (12!) \, (91!) \, (4!)}{(1175!) \, (95!) \, (104!) \, (3!) \, (1059!) \, (9!) \, (5!) \, (86!) \, (3!)} = 0.0150$$

The probabilities for all five of the possible outcomes resulting in four exposed cases are, in the order the outcomes are listed in Table 12-9, 0.0118, 0.0150, 0.0039, 0.0002, and 0.0000 (the last one is actually 0.00000149), which totals to 0.0309. The corresponding total for the outcome with five exposed cases is 0.0066, and for six exposed cases, 0.0010. The Fisher P-value for the upper tail of the distribution can therefore be estimated as $0.0309 + 0.0066 + 0.0010 = 0.0385$, assuming that the outcomes with more than six exposed cases do not contribute materially to the summation. The full tail probability is actually 0.0387, based on all 55 possibilities in Table 12-9, so that the truncation after six exposed cases is reasonable. The remaining 10 outcomes with three or fewer exposed cases, which are not listed in Table 12-9, account, in probability terms, for $1 - 0.0387$ or about 96 percent of the distribution; in fact, the outcomes 0-0 and 1-0 together account for about 54 percent of the distribution.

To get the exact mid-P value for the upper tail, only half of the probability of getting four exposed cases should be included, which results in a P-value of 0.0233.

Approximate Hypothesis Testing for Stratified 2 × 2 Tables. The extension of formula 11-6 to stratified 2 × 2 tables is analogous to the extension of formula 11-1 for person-time data. As before, the contribution to each of the three components of the test statistic—the number of exposed cases, the null expectation for the number of exposed cases, and the variance—is derived separately for each stratum and then summed over the strata. Thus, the null expectation for the number of exposed cases is

$$E(A) = \sum_{i=1}^{N} \frac{N_{1i} M_{1i}}{T_i}$$

and the variance, based on the hypergeometric model, is

$$\text{Var}(A) = \sum_{i=1}^{N} \frac{N_{1i} N_{0i} M_{1i} M_{0i}}{T_i^2 (T_i - 1)}$$

Table 12-9. Enumeration of all possible combinations of exposed cases by age category, with at least four exposed cases, for the data in example 12-5

Total no. exposed cases	Distribution of exposed cases by age category	Total no. exposed cases	Distribution of exposed cases by age category	Total no. exposed cases	Distribution of exposed cases by age category
16	12–4	10	10–0	6	6–0
15	12–3	10	9–1	6	5–1
15	11–4	10	8–2	6	4–2
14	12–2	10	7–3	6	3–3
14	11–3	10	6–4	6	2–4
14	10–4	9	9–0	5	5–0
13	12–1	9	8–1	5	4–1
13	11–2	9	7–2	5	3–2
13	10–3	9	6–3	5	2–3
13	9–4	9	5–4	5	1–4
12	12–0	8	8–0	4	4–0
12	11–1	8	7–1	4	3–1
12	10–2	8	6–2	4	2–2
12	9–3	8	5–3	4	1–3
12	8–4	8	4–4	4	0–4
11	11–0	7	7–0		
11	10–1	7	6–1		
11	9–2	7	5–2		
11	8–3	7	4–3		
11	7–4	7	3–4		

which gives as the test statistic

$$\chi = \frac{\sum\limits_{i=1}^{N} a_i - \sum\limits_{i=1}^{N} \frac{N_{1i}M_{1i}}{T_i}}{\sqrt{\sum\limits_{i=1}^{N} \frac{N_{1i}N_{0i}M_{1i}M_{0i}}{T_i^2(T_i - 1)}}} \qquad [12\text{-}38]$$

The above test statistic, first proposed by Mantel and Haenszel in 1959 and known as the Mantel-Haenszel test, is widely used in epidemiologic analyses and other applications in which stratified 2 × 2 tables are used. It is optimal in statistical power when the odds ratio is uniform across strata, but it is generally the most useful and convenient test even if the odds ratio varies across strata. The χ takes a value of zero only when the Mantel-Haenszel pooled estimator of the odds ratio (formula 12-26) equals unity, so that the test statistic may be considered a test of the departure of $\hat{OR}_{MH}$ from unity. The large-number applicability condition does not refer to individual strata but only to the summations in formula 12-38. Individual strata may each have as few as two subjects as long as no marginal total is zero; if a marginal total is zero, the stratum has no information. The test statistic will be applicable if there is a sufficient number of strata, even with sparse data. As we shall see in Chapter 13, the test is the one that applies even to the analysis of matched-pair data.

The null hypothesis of no relation between tolbutamide and death in the University Group Diabetes Program for the age-stratified data in Example 12-4 can be evaluated with the Mantel-Haenszel test. The number of exposed cases, where "exposed" indicates tolbutamide therapy, is $8 + 22 = 30$. The expected number under the null hypothesis is

$$E(A) = \frac{(106)\,(13)}{226} + \frac{(98)\,(38)}{183} = 6.10 + 20.35 = 26.45$$

and the variance of the number of exposed cases is

$$Var(A) = \frac{(106)\,(120)\,(13)\,(213)}{(226)^2\,(225)} + \frac{(98)\,(85)\,(38)\,(145)}{(183)^2\,(182)}$$

$$= 3.06 + 7.53 = 10.60$$

The test statistic is

$$\chi = \frac{30 - 26.45}{\sqrt{10.60}} = 1.09$$

which gives a one-tail P-value of 0.14, or a two-tail P-value of 0.28. Note that since tolbutamide has been considered a preventive of the complications of diabetes, departures from the null value were expected to occur in the direction of preventing death rather than in the opposite direction. Therefore, a one-tail P-value should technically be the lower tail of the distribution, in the direction of prevention, rather than the upper tail. Since the data demonstrate a positive association between tolbutamide and death, the one-tail P-value should be $1 - 0.14$ or 0.86. The two-tail P-value is 0.28 whichever the direction of the prior expectation about departures from the null value.

If the Mantel-Haenszel test is applied to the sparse data in Example 12-5, the test statistic is

$$\chi = \frac{4 - \left[\dfrac{(12)\,(107)}{1175} + \dfrac{(6)\,(4)}{95}\right]}{\sqrt{\dfrac{(107)\,(1068)\,(12)\,(1163)}{(1175)^2\,(1174)} + \dfrac{(6)\,(89)\,(4)\,(91)}{(95)^2\,(94)}}} = 2.41$$

which gives $P_{(1)} = 0.008$, a result that is considerably different from the exact mid-P value of 0.023. The discrepancy is not surprising in view of the small numbers and the striking asymmetry of the distribution, in which more than half of the probability distribution corresponds to the two most extreme outcomes out of the 17 possibilities for the number of exposed cases.

Confidence Intervals for Pooled Estimates of Effect

Confidence intervals for pooled estimates of effect can be calculated exactly from the statistical models adopted to describe the variability of the data, or they can be calculated approximately from asymptotic formulas. The exact calculations are exceedingly complicated and increase quickly in difficulty as the number of observations increases. Nevertheless, ready availability of microcomputers now makes it convenient to calculate exact confidence limits for pooled effect estimates in many applications, since the programming and memory requirements are not great; the calculation time may be long even with a computer, but the cost of computer time for such applications is becoming negligible. In view of the relatively large effort expended on the collection and processing of epidemiologic data, it seems worthwhile to obtain exact confidence limits for sparse data, even if stratified, if the means to do so are at hand. Consequently, exact formulas for confidence limits are presented in the following discussion whenever applicable.

For most situations, on the other hand, it will be preferable to use the straightforward and convenient noniterative approximate formulas for the calculation of confidence limits. The choice of an approximate formula for interval estimation generally depends on the type of point estimator used, since the variance approximation depends on how the point estimate is calculated. Therefore, the description of types of approximate confidence limits is presented according to the types of pooled point estimators described earlier in this chapter.

CONFIDENCE INTERVALS FOR STRATIFIED PERSON-TIME DATA

Incidence Rate Difference. No method exists for obtaining exact confidence limits for incidence rate difference because the total number of cases is not independent of the rate difference. Approximate confidence limits can be obtained in several ways according to the method of point estimation.

DIRECTLY WEIGHTED POINT ESTIMATE. The basic approach relies on the general statistical rule that the variance of a sum of independent random variables is the sum of the variance of each random variable. Since the directly pooled estimator for incidence rate difference is a sum of random variables (the stratum-specific estimates of incidence rate difference) multiplied by a constant (the weight for pooling), an overall variance for the pooled estimator would be

$$\text{Var(pooled } \hat{\text{IRD}}) \doteq \text{Var}\left[\sum_i \frac{w_i}{\sum_i w_i} (\hat{\text{IRD}}_i)\right] \doteq \sum_{i=1}^{N} \frac{w_i^2}{\left(\sum_i w_i\right)^2} \text{Var}(\hat{\text{IRD}}_i)$$

The weight is squared because any constant multiplier of a random variable is squared as a multiplier of variance. Each w_i is taken as the inverse of the variance of $\hat{\text{IRD}}_i$ in pooling, so the overall variance is

$$\text{Var(pooled } \hat{\text{IRD}}) \doteq \sum_{i=1}^{N} \frac{w_i}{\left(\sum_i w_i\right)^2} = \frac{\sum_i w_i}{\left(\sum_i w_i\right)^2} = \frac{1}{\sum_i w_i} \qquad [12\text{-}39]$$

This variance can be used with the pooled estimator and formula 10-2 to compute approximate confidence limits.

Consider the pooled estimate of incidence rate difference for the data in Example 12-2, $5.95 \times 10^{-4}\text{yr}^{-1}$. From equation 12-39, the variance of the estimate is approximately the inverse of the sum of the weights, or

$$1/(65.16 \times 10^6 \text{yr}^2) = 1.535 \times 10^{-8}\text{yr}^{-2}$$

which gives a standard deviation of

$$\sqrt{1.535 \times 10^{-8}\text{yr}^{-2}} = 1.239 \times 10^{-4}\text{yr}^{-1}$$

A 90 percent confidence interval for the pooled estimate is obtainable as

$$5.95 \times 10^{-4}\text{yr}^{-1} \pm 1.645 \,(1.239 \times 10^{-4}\text{yr}^{-1})$$

$$= 3.9 \times 10^{-4}\text{yr}^{-1}, 8.0 \times 10^{-4}\text{yr}^{-1}$$

A second method of obtaining approximate confidence limits for incidence rate difference is to compute test-based limits from the point estimate and the χ from formula 12-33, using formula 10-6. For the data in Example 12-2, the χ is 3.319, giving, for 90 percent confidence limits,

$$\hat{\text{IRD}}(1 \pm Z/\chi) = 5.95 \times 10^{-4}\text{yr}^{-1} \,(1 \pm 1.645/3.319)$$

$$= 3.0 \times 10^{-4}\text{yr}^{-1}, 8.9 \times 10^{-4}\text{yr}^{-1}$$

a wider result than that obtained above. The test-based approach gives wide results because it does not assign an extremely heavy weight to the youngest age stratum as the direct approach does; the small numbers in the youngest stratum result in a small variance for the incidence rate difference estimated from that stratum.

MAXIMUM LIKELIHOOD POINT ESTIMATE. The maximum likelihood estimation of $\hat{IRD}$ requires the simultaneous maximum likelihood estimation of the nuisance parameters R_{0i} for each stratum. These fitted or smoothed estimates of R_{0i} can be used in conjunction with the pooled estimate of IRD to get an improved estimate of the variance for the incidence rate difference in each stratum by substituting $\hat{R}_{0i}$ for b_i/N_{0i} and $\hat{R}_{0i} + \hat{IRD}$ for a_i/N_{1i} in formula 12-1. The improved variance estimate is

$$\text{Var}(\hat{IRD}_i) \doteq \frac{\hat{R}_{0i} + \hat{IRD}}{N_{1i}} + \frac{\hat{R}_{0i}}{N_{0i}} \qquad [12\text{-}40]$$

The overall variance of the pooled maximum likelihood estimate can be obtained by taking

$$w_i = \frac{N_{1i}N_{0i}}{N_{0i}(\hat{R}_{0i} + \hat{IRD}) + N_{1i}(\hat{R}_{0i})} \qquad [12\text{-}41]$$

which is the reciprocal of the variance in formula 12-40; these weights are then used to get the overall variance as in equation 12-39.

For the data in Example 12-2, the weights estimated according to formula 12-41 are, from the youngest to the oldest age categories, $57.6 \times 10^6\text{yr}^2$, $4.9 \times 10^6\text{yr}^2$, $0.7 \times 10^6\text{yr}^2$, $0.7 \times 10^6\text{yr}^2$, and $0.2 \times 10^6\text{yr}^2$. The sum of these weights is $64.1 \times 10^6\text{yr}^2$, and therefore the variance is taken as

$$\text{Var}(\hat{IRD}) = \frac{1}{64.1 \times 10^6\text{yr}^2} = 1.56 \times 10^{-8}\text{yr}^{-2}$$

which is close to the value of $1.53 \times 10^{-8}\text{yr}^{-2}$ obtained from the directly pooled weights. A 90 percent confidence interval for the maximum likelihood estimate of $5.91 \times 10^{-4}\text{yr}^{-1}$ is obtained as

$$5.91 \times 10^{-4}\text{yr}^{-1} \pm 1.645\,(\sqrt{1.56 \times 10^{-8}\text{yr}^{-2}})$$

$$= 3.9 \times 10^{-4}\text{yr}^{-1}, 8.0 \times 10^{-4}\text{yr}^{-1}$$

which is virtually identical to the limits obtained from the weights used in direct pooling.

Incidence Rate Ratio. Confidence limits for the pooled estimate of the ratio of incidence rates from stratified data can be obtained by exact computation or by approximate methods. The exact computation requires iterative calculation of a complicated sum of probabilities and consequently requires a computer.

EXACT CONFIDENCE LIMITS. Obtaining the exact limits necessitates expressing the tail probability for the observations in terms of the incidence rate ratio (IRR). In stratum i, let the probability that a case is exposed be u_i. From formula 11-9 or 11-10 the following relation can be derived:

$$u_i = \frac{N_{0i}(IRR)}{N_{0i}(IRR) + N_{1i}} = \frac{IRR}{IRR + \dfrac{N_{0i}}{N_{1i}}} \qquad [12\text{-}42]$$

Exact Fisher limits for $\underline{IRR}$ and $\overline{IRR}$ can be determined from formula 12-42 and the following modification of formula 12-29:

$$\alpha/2 = \sum_{k=a}^{M_1} \prod_{i=1}^{N} \binom{M_{1i}}{k_i} (\underline{u_i})^{k_i} (1 - \underline{u_i})^{M_{1i} - k_i} \qquad [12\text{-}43]$$

and

$$1 - \alpha/2 = \sum_{k=a+1}^{M_1} \prod_{i=1}^{N} \binom{M_{1i}}{k_i} (\overline{u_i})^{k_i} (1 - \overline{u_i})^{M_{1i} - k_i} \qquad [12\text{-}44]$$

in which k_i represents the number of exposed cases in stratum i, $k = \Sigma k_i$, $a = \Sigma a_i$, and $M_1 = \Sigma M_{1i}$. The value for IRR that satisfies equations 12-42 and 12-43 corresponds to the Fisher exact lower confidence bound; using equation 12-44 instead of 12-43 gives the Fisher exact upper confidence bound. Mid-P exact limits are obtainable by allotting only half the probability for $k = a$ into the tail:

$$\alpha/2 = \frac{1}{2} \sum_{k=a}^{N} \prod_{i=1}^{N} \binom{M_{1i}}{k_i} (\underline{u_i})^{k_i} (1 - \underline{u_i})^{M_{1i} - k_i}$$
$$+ \sum_{k=a+1}^{M_1} \prod_{i=1}^{N} \binom{M_{1i}}{k_i} (\underline{u_i})^{k_i} (1 - \underline{u_i})^{M_{1i} - k_i} \qquad [12\text{-}45]$$

gives the lower bound, and substituting $1 - \alpha/2$ for $\alpha/2$ will give the upper bound.

With the help of a computer, exact 90 percent confidence limits for the incidence rate ratio using the data in example 12-6 can be calculated. The Fisher-type 90 percent interval is 2.43 to 18.0, and the mid-P 90 percent interval is 2.71 to 16.0.

APPROXIMATE CONFIDENCE LIMITS. The formulation of the approximate limits for the three different types of point estimates are as follows:

1. *Directly Weighted Point Estimate.* The variance of the directly pooled incidence rate ratio should be estimated after a logarithmic transforma-

tion, so that the limits can be set on the logarithmic scale. The variance formula resembles 12-39:

$$Var[\ln(\text{pooled } \hat{IRR})] = \frac{1}{\sum_i w_i} \qquad [12\text{-}46]$$

where

$$w_i = \frac{a_i b_i}{a_i + b_i} \qquad [12\text{-}47]$$

For the data in Example 12-3, $w_1 = 140/24 = 5.83$, $w_2 = 9196/197 = 46.7$, and

$$Var[\ln(\text{pooled } \hat{IRR})] = \frac{1}{5.83 + 46.7} = 0.019$$

The directly pooled point estimate is 1.50, giving a 90 percent confidence interval of

$$\exp[\ln(1.50) \pm 1.645 \sqrt{0.019}] = 1.20, 1.88$$

2. *Maximum Likelihood Point Estimate.* The asymptotically efficient maximum likelihood estimator of the incidence rate ratio has a variance estimate of

$$Var(\hat{IRR}) = \frac{\hat{IRR}}{\displaystyle\sum_{i=1}^{N} \frac{M_{1i} N_{0i}/N_{1i}}{\left(\hat{IRR} + \dfrac{N_{0i}}{N_{1i}}\right)^2}} \qquad [12\text{-}48]$$

It is necessary to divide the above by $(\hat{IRR})^2$ to approximate the variance of $\ln(\hat{IRR})$:

$$Var[\ln(\hat{IRR})] = \frac{1}{(\hat{IRR}) \displaystyle\sum_{i=1}^{N} \frac{M_{1i} N_{0i}/N_{1i}}{\left(\hat{IRR} + \dfrac{N_{0i}}{N_{1i}}\right)^2}} \qquad [12\text{-}49]$$

The above formula is identical to formula 12-46 if a_i/b_i is replaced by $(\hat{IRR})N_{1i}/N_{0i}$ in the weight given in formula 12-47.

For the data in Example 12-3, the maximum likelihood estimate of IRR is 1.50, and the variance of $\ln(\hat{IRR})$ is

$$\frac{1}{(1.50)\dfrac{24(1701/1516)}{(1.50 + 1701/1516)^2} + \dfrac{197(2245/949)}{(1.50 + 2245/949)^2}} = 0.019$$

which gives a 90 percent confidence interval of

$$\exp[\ln(1.50) \pm 1.645 \sqrt{0.019}] = 1.20, 1.88$$

This interval estimate is virtually identical to that obtained by the directly weighted approach.

For the data in Example 12-6, the approximate 90 percent confidence interval around the maximum likelihood estimate of IRR, which is 6.55, is 2.77 to 15.5, which agrees quite well with the 90 percent exact mid-P interval of 2.71 to 16.0.

3. *Mantel-Haenszel Point Estimate.* The Mantel-Haenszel estimator for incidence rate ratio (formula 12-27) can be considered a weighted average of stratum-specific estimates of the incidence rate ratio with weights equal to $b_i N_{1i}/T_i$ and the approximate confidence limits calculated on this basis. A more stable formula for the variance, however, can be obtained by considering each a_i and b_i to be an independent Poisson variate [Tarone, 1981], or by considering each a_i to be an independent binomial variate conditional on N_{1i} [Greenland and Robins, 1985]. The latter approach yields

$$\text{Var}[\ln(\widehat{\text{IRR}}_{\text{MH}})] \doteq \frac{\displaystyle\sum_{i=1}^{N} M_{1i} N_{1i} N_{0i}/T_i^2}{\left[\displaystyle\sum_{i=1}^{N} \frac{a_i N_{0i}}{T_i}\right]\left[\displaystyle\sum_{i=1}^{N} \frac{b_i N_{1i}}{T_i}\right]} \qquad [12\text{-}50]$$

For Example 12-3, the above formula gives $\text{Var}[\ln(\widehat{\text{IRR}}_{\text{MH}})] = 0.019$, the same as the result obtained using the directly weighted procedure above. The resulting confidence interval, 1.20–1.88, is likewise identical to the interval for the directly weighted point estimate.

Test-based limits for the data in Example 12-3 can also be obtained for the Mantel-Haenszel point estimate (1.50) and the χ statistic from formula 12-33 (2.94):

$$1.50^{(1 \pm 1.645/2.94)} = 1.19, 1.87$$

These test-based limits are in close agreement with the results obtained from the other approaches. Test-based limits can also be obtained for the directly weighted point estimate.

For the data in Example 12-6, for which $\widehat{\text{IRR}}_{\text{MH}} = 7.30$, the variance

For the data in Example 12-6, for which $IRR_{MH} = 7.30$, the variance calculated from formula 12-50 is 0.344, which gives a 90 percent confidence interval for $\hat{IRR}_{MH}$ of 2.8 to 19. For the same data, the test-based 90 percent confidence limits can be calculated from the χ of 3.98 as

$$7.30^{(1 \pm 1.645/3.98)} = 3.2, 17$$

Considering the small numbers involved, both of these approximate intervals are in reasonably good agreement with the mid-P exact 90 percent confidence interval of 2.7 to 16.

CONFIDENCE INTERVALS FOR STRATIFIED CUMULATIVE INCIDENCE DATA
Risk Difference. Because of the nuisance parameter $\hat{R}_{0i}$ in each stratum, no approach exists for obtaining exact confidence limits for a pooled risk difference or prevalence difference. Approximate confidence limits can be obtained by methods analogous to those described above for incidence rate data.

DIRECTLY WEIGHTED POINT ESTIMATE. The variance of the pooled risk difference can be expressed in terms of the stratum-specific weights in the same way as that used for incidence rate data (formula 12-39):

$$\text{Var(pooled } \hat{RD}) = \frac{1}{\Sigma w_i} \qquad [12\text{-}51]$$

where the weights are those given in formula 12-7:

$$w_i = \frac{N_{1i}^3 N_{0i}^3}{N_{0i}^3 a_i (N_{1i} - a_i) + N_{1i}^3 b_i (N_{0i} - b_i)}$$

The square root of the above variance estimate in formula 12-51 can be used with formula 10-2 to obtain approximate confidence limits. For Example 12-4, the stratum-specific weights are 1,009 and 280 (Table 12-5), so that $\Sigma w_i = 1,289$ and the variance estimate is $1/1,289 = 0.000776$. The square root is 0.028, so that a 90 percent confidence interval estimate, using the weighted point estimate of 0.034, would be

$$0.034 \pm 1.645(0.028) = -0.012, 0.080$$

An alternative is to use test-based confidence limits (formula 10-6), based on the χ from formula 12-38. For the data in Example 12-4, the χ is 1.09 and the test-based confidence interval is

$$0.034(1 \pm 1.645/1.09) = -0.017, 0.086$$

which is slightly wider than the result using the estimates of stratum-specific variance.

MAXIMUM LIKELIHOOD POINT ESTIMATE. Again, the maximum likelihood solutions for the pooled estimate $\hat{RD}$ and the unexposed risk $\hat{R}_{0i}$ in each stratum can be used to improve the variance estimation for the rate difference in each stratum. The improved estimates can be obtained by substituting $\hat{R}_{0i}$ for b_i/N_{0i} and $\hat{R}_{0i} + \hat{RD}$ for a_i/N_{1i}; these substitutions can be made directly into formula 12-7, giving the improved weights

$$w_i = \frac{N_{1i}N_{0i}}{N_{0i}(\hat{R}_{0i} + \hat{RD})(1 - \hat{R}_{0i} - \hat{RD}) + N_{1i}\hat{R}_{0i}(1 - \hat{R}_{0i})} \qquad [12\text{-}52]$$

which can be used in formula 12-51 to get a variance estimate for the maximum likelihood estimate of RD.

For the data in Example 12-4, the weights calculated from formula 12-52 are 1,008 and 280 for strata 1 and 2, respectively, which gives a variance of $1/(1,008 + 280) = 0.000776$. Note that the weights and variance estimate are nearly identical to the results obtained from the noniterative directly weighted procedure because the number of observations within each stratum is large. The resulting 90 percent confidence interval is $-0.012, 0.080$ as it was with the directly weighted approach.

Risk Ratio. Exact confidence limits for risk ratio are not calculable, since the likelihood equation contains the nuisance parameters $\hat{R}_{0i}$ for each stratum i. If risks are small, however, the odds ratio measure may be used to approximate the risk ratio. Since the odds ratio can be estimated without nuisance parameters, the likelihood can be expressed conditionally on all the margins of the 2×2 table, allowing the calculation of exact confidence limits for the pooled odds ratio. This procedure is described below for case-control data.

Approximate confidence limits for pooled estimates of the risk ratio can be obtained for directly weighted, Mantel-Haenszel, or maximum likelihood point estimators.

DIRECTLY WEIGHTED POINT ESTIMATE. As usual, approximate confidence limits for ratio measures should be set on the logarithmic scale. Formulas 12-46 and 12-10 can be used to obtain the variance of the logarithm of the pooled risk ratio estimate. For the data in Example 12-4, the stratum-specific weights, given in Table 12-6, are 3.25 and 11.6. The $\Sigma w_i = 14.85$ and the variance of the logarithmically transformed point estimate is $1/14.85 = 0.0673$. The weighted average of the logarithms of the stratum-specific estimates of the risk ratio is 0.270, which is the antilogarithm of the pooled estimate of the risk ratio, 1.31. Approximate 90 percent confidence limits can be set as follows:

$$0.270 \pm 1.645 (\sqrt{0.0673}) = -0.157, 0.697$$

$$e^{-0.157}, e^{0.697} = 0.86, 2.0$$

MAXIMUM LIKELIHOOD POINT ESTIMATE. Formula 12-10 can be improved by substituting $N_{1i}\hat{R}_{0i}\hat{RR}$ for a_i and $N_{0i}\hat{R}_{0i}$ for b_i, where $\hat{R}_{0i}$ and $\hat{RR}$ are the fitted maximum likelihood estimates. The improved weights are

$$w_i = \frac{(\hat{RR})\hat{R}_{0i}N_{0i}N_{1i}}{(\hat{RR})(1 - \hat{R}_{0i})N_{1i} + (1 - \hat{R}_{0i}\hat{RR})N_{0i}} \qquad [12\text{-}53]$$

which may be used in formula 12-46 to get an estimate for the pooled variance. For Example 12-4, the maximum likelihood point estimate of the risk ratio is 1.31, $\hat{R}_{01} = 0.0504$, $\hat{R}_{02} = 0.1781$, and the improved weights are 3.44 and 11.4. The Σw_i for these improved weights is 14.83, and the variance of the logarithmically transformed point estimate is $1/14.83 = 0.0674$, nearly the same result as that obtained from the stratum-specific variance estimates. The 90 percent confidence interval is obtained on the log scale as

$$\ln(1.31) \pm 1.645 (\sqrt{0.0674}) = -0.156, 0.698$$

and the actual limits are

$$e^{-0.156}, e^{0.698} = 0.86, 2.0$$

MANTEL-HAENSZEL POINT ESTIMATE. The Mantel-Haenszel point estimator of the risk ratio from follow-up data with count denominators takes the same form as the point estimator for the rate ratio with person-time denominators (formula 12-27). The variance for the logarithm of RR_{MH} is approximately [Greenland and Robins, 1985]

$$\text{Var}[\ln(\hat{RR}_{MH})] \doteq \frac{\sum_{i=1}^{N} (M_{1i}N_{1i}N_{0i} - a_i b_i T_i)/T_i^2}{\left[\sum_{i=1}^{N} \frac{a_i N_{0i}}{T_i}\right]\left[\sum_{i=1}^{N} \frac{b_i N_{1i}}{T_i}\right]} \qquad [12\text{-}54]$$

For the data in Example 12-4, the above expression gives $\text{Var}[\ln(\hat{RR}_{MH})] \doteq 0.0671$; coupled with the point estimate of $RR_{MH} = 1.33$, the approximate 90 percent confidence limits are

$$\exp(\ln(1.33) \pm 1.645 \sqrt{0.0671}) = 0.87, 2.0$$

which are nearly identical to the limits calculated for the directly weighted point estimate and the maximum likelihood point estimate.

CONFIDENCE INTERVALS FOR THE ODDS RATIO FROM STRATIFIED CASE-
CONTROL (OR PREVALENCE) DATA

Confidence limits for the pooled estimate of the odds ratio from stratified
2 × 2 tables can be obtained by exact computation or by approximate
methods. The exact computation is exceedingly complex for any but the
most sparse data and requires a computer program [Thomas, 1975].

Exact Confidence Limits. The expression for the probability of the observations in a single set of N 2 × 2 tables, conditional on the marginal totals
for each 2 × 2 table and the odds ratio, is

$$\text{Pr(data)} = \prod_{i=1}^{N} \frac{\binom{N_{1i}}{a_i} \binom{N_{0i}}{b_i} OR^{a_i}}{\sum_{k=\max(0,M_{1i}-N_{0i})}^{\min(M_{1i},N_{1i})} \binom{N_{1i}}{k} \binom{N_{0i}}{M_{1i} - k} OR^{k}} \qquad [12\text{-}55]$$

Tail probabilities for exact confidence limits can be calculated by taking
the sum of the probabilities calculated in expression 12-55 for all possible
values of Σa_i equal to or greater than the actual value observed, and for
all possible combinations of cell frequencies that yield a given value for
Σa_i. To get mid-*P* exact limits, only one-half the probability determined by
expression 12-55 should be added to the summation for every possible
combination in which Σa_i equals the observed value. The exact lower confidence limit is obtained by determining through trial and error the value
of the odds ratio that produces an upper-tail probability of $\alpha/2$ (α equals
the complement of the desired confidence level). The upper confidence
limit is obtainable by summing over all values of Σa_i that are less than or
equal to the observed value and finding the value of the odds ratio that
gives a lower-tail probability of $\alpha/2$.

   For the data in Example 12-5, the observed value for Σa_i is 4; the 55
combinations for which $\Sigma a_i \geq 4$ are listed in Table 12-9. Using expression
12-55 to determine the contributions to the tail probability, 90 percent
exact mid-*P* confidence limits are found to be 1.30, 9.78. The corresponding Fisher limits are 1.09, 10.9.

Approximate Confidence Limits. DIRECTLY WEIGHTED POINT ESTIMATE. Formulas 12-46 and 12-13 can be used to obtain approximate confidence limits for the directly weighted pooled estimate of the odds ratio. As usual
with a ratio measure, the limits are first set on the logarithmic scale and
then translated back to the original scale. For the data in Example 12-5,
using the weights indicated in Table 12-7, the sum of the weights is 2.85,

and the estimated variance of the logarithm of the pooled odds ratio is $1/2.85 = 0.351$. Approximate 90 percent confidence limits are

$$\exp[\ln(3.82) \pm 1.645 \sqrt{0.351}] = 1.44, 10.1$$

which differ somewhat from the exact limits, but the discrepancy is tolerable, especially considering the width of the interval. In view of the small number of cases in the analysis, the approximation seems reasonably good.

MAXIMUM LIKELIHOOD POINT ESTIMATE. With maximum likelihood point estimation, fitted cell entries in the 2×2 tables can be used to derive an estimate of the variance. The values for $\hat{a}_i$, $\hat{b}_i$, $\hat{c}_i$, and $\hat{d}_i$ that satisfy equation 12-23 or equation 12-24 and the marginal totals of each 2×2 table can be substituted in equation 12-13:

$$w_i = \frac{1}{\dfrac{1}{\hat{a}_i} + \dfrac{1}{\hat{b}_i} + \dfrac{1}{\hat{c}_i} + \dfrac{1}{\hat{d}_i}} \qquad [12\text{-}56]$$

The variance of the logarithmically transformed odds ratio point estimate is $1/\Sigma w_i$.

For the data in Example 12-5, the cell frequencies for the unconditional maximum likelihood estimate, satisfying equation 12-24, are given in Table 12-10. From these fitted cell frequencies, $w_1 = 2.31$ and $w_2 = 0.54$, which gives $\Sigma w_i = 2.85$ and a variance of 0.351. Approximate 90 percent confidence limits are

$$\exp[\ln(3.79) \pm 1.645 \sqrt{0.351}] = 1.43, 10.0$$

Using equation 12-23 rather than 12-24 to calculate the fitted frequencies according to the conditional likelihood is considerably more difficult; for these data the a cells for the two strata using equation 12-23 are 3.238 and 0.762, which are nearly identical to the unconditional values in Table 12-10 and produce the same approximate confidence interval. Because the computation necessary to get the conditional fitted cell entries from the iterative solution of equations 12-22 and 12-23 is difficult, it is easier to calculate the exact confidence limits instead.

Another approach, which was proposed initially by Cornfield [1956] for a single 2×2 table, was extended by Gart [1971] for a set of 2×2 tables. The approximate lower limit is the solution to the equation

$$Z_{\alpha/2} = \frac{\Sigma a_i - \Sigma E_i}{\sqrt{\text{Var}(\Sigma a_i)}} \qquad [12\text{-}57]$$

Table 12-10. Fitted maximum likelihood cell entries for the
data in example 12-5; pooled estimate of odds ratio is 3.79

| | Maternal age < 35 | | | Maternal age 35+ | | |
| | Spermicide use | | | Spermicide use | | |
	+	−	Total	+	−	Total
Down syndrome	3.247	8.753	12	0.753	3.247	4
Control	103.753	1059.247	1163	5.247	85.753	91
Total	107	1068	1175	6	89	95

where E_i is the expected value of a_i conditional on the value of the odds ratio at the lower boundary of the confidence interval,

$$R = \frac{E_i(M_{0i} - N_{1i} + E_i)}{(M_{1i} - E_i)(N_{1i} - E_i)}$$

$Z_{\alpha/2}$ is the value of the standard normal statistic that corresponds to the desired level of confidence, and

$$\mathrm{Var}(\Sigma a_i) = \sum_{i=1}^{N} \left[\frac{1}{E_i} + \frac{1}{M_{1i} - E_i} + \frac{1}{N_{1i} - E_i} + \frac{1}{M_{0i} - N_{1i} + E_i} \right]^{-1}$$

To obtain the upper bound to the interval, $Z_{\alpha/2}$ is replaced by $-Z_{\alpha/2}$. Equation 12-57 must be solved iteratively for each limit. In principle this method has the advantage of approximating the variance using the cell frequencies that correspond to the confidence limit value of the odds ratio rather than the point estimate.

For the data in Example 12-5, the fitted cell frequencies for the a cell using equation 12-57 to obtain the lower limit of a 90 percent confidence interval are 1.542 for the young stratum and 0.356 for the older stratum; note that these do not add to $\Sigma a_i = 4$ as in point estimation, though the fitted cell frequencies within each table still conform to the marginal totals of the individual table. The lower confidence limit satisfying equation 12-57 is 1.48. For the upper limit, a separate iterative solution is required to get the fitted frequencies for the a cell of 5.772 and 1.370 for the young and old strata, respectively. The upper confidence limit corresponding to these values is 9.72.

MANTEL-HAENSZEL POINT ESTIMATE. The statistical properties of the Mantel-Haenszel estimator of the odds ratio have been elaborated under two different limiting situations: Either the number of subjects per stratum becomes large, or the number of strata becomes large with few subjects per stratum [Hauck, 1979; Breslow, 1981]. Variance formulas have been proposed for the Mantel-Haenszel odds ratio estimator for each of these limiting situations; Breslow and Liang [1982] proposed weighting the two formulas to derive a combined formula that is generally applicable. More recently, Robins and coauthors [1985] have developed a single variance formula that should be generally applicable for the Mantel-Haenszel odds ratio estimator:

$$\mathrm{Var}[\ln(\hat{OR}_{MH})] \doteq \frac{\sum_{i=1}^{N} P_i R_i}{2\left[\sum_{i=1}^{N} R_i\right]^2} + \frac{\sum_{i=1}^{N} (P_i S_i + Q_i R_i)}{2\sum_{i=1}^{N} R_i \sum_{i=1}^{N} S_i} + \frac{\sum_{i=1}^{N} Q_i S_i}{2\left[\sum_{i=1}^{N} S_i\right]^2} \qquad [12\text{-}58]$$

where

$$P_i = (a_i + d_i)/T_i$$
$$Q_i = (b_i + c_i)/T_i$$
$$R_i = a_i d_i/T_i$$

and

$$S_i = b_i c_i/T_i$$

For the data in Example 12-5, the above formula gives an estimated variance of 0.349, which yields a 90 percent confidence interval of 1.43 to 10.0, a result that is nearly identical to the limits for the directly weighted and maximum likelihood point estimates.

Test-based 90 percent confidence limits for the data in Example 12-5 are obtained as

$$3.78^{(1 \pm 1.645/2.41)} = 1.53, 9.37$$

which are narrower than the limits obtained from formula 12-58. The test-based approach for approximate confidence limits can also be used with the directly weighted point estimate.

EVALUATION AND DESCRIPTION OF EFFECT MODIFICATION

The techniques for deriving a pooled estimate of an effect that is uniform across categories of a third variable should not be applied if it appears unreasonable to assume that the effect is indeed uniform. When an effect is believed to vary across strata—that is, when effect modification is presumed to exist—the focus of data analysis and presentation should shift from the control of confounding to a description of how the effect is modified by the stratification factor. It is important to realize that confounding, when present, is manifest only in the crude measure of effect; when effect modification is present in the data, none of the options for describing the effect involves the crude measure, so the issue of confounding is superseded by the description of effect modification. Determining whether effect modification is present in the data is clearly an important decision that should be addressed in every stratified analysis.

It is important to inject a note of caution about the methodology for assessing effect modification. The evaluation of effect modification often appears to rest on a seemingly mechanical application of statistical tests. The epidemiologic issues of interaction underlying the statistical evaluation of effect modification are subtle and can become muddled in a purely mechanical approach. These issues are discussed in Chapter 15, which supplies an epidemiologic perspective for the statistical methods described in the following section.

In addition to the epidemiologic considerations, there are statistical considerations that warrant a cautious approach to the statistical evaluation of effect modification. The more general statistical tests for effect modification have low power because the alternatives to the null hypothesis that they test are not very specific. As a result, "nonsignificant" P-values are even more difficult to interpret correctly. Furthermore, given the many influences of selection biases, misclassification, confounding, and other biases as well as causal effects, it is seldom that one would expect any effect to be precisely uniform for any scale of measurement. Thus, the null hypothesis of a uniform effect often amounts to no more than a statistical contrivance that at best should be accepted as only an approximation to reality and generally should be regarded with skepticism.

Evaluation of Effect Modification

The first step in evaluating effect modification is to inspect the stratum-specific estimates of effect. While some random variability in stratum-specific estimates is to be expected even when the underlying parameter is uniform, excessive variability or obvious nonrandom patterns of variation may be evident on inspection. The investigator's judgment about effect modification should not be limited to the appearance of the data in hand; when it is available, outside knowledge from previous studies or more general biologic insight should be integrated into the evaluation process.

Typically, however, outside knowledge is scant, and investigators will desire a more formal statistical evaluation of the extent to which the variability of stratum-specific estimates of effect is consistent with purely random behavior. Toward this end, a variety of statistical tests can be applied. Part of the variety derives from the fact that ratio and difference measures require separate evaluations for effect modification, since uniformity of the ratio measure usually implies effect modification of the difference measure and vice versa. The use of statistical tests has been discussed in Chapter 9, especially with regard to assessing "statistical significance," which trivializes the interpretation of otherwise meaningful measures. The use of significance tests is more defensible, however, when an immediate decision rests on the outcome of a single statistical evaluation. Such may be the case if an investigator is attempting to decide whether the extent of variability in a set of stratum-specific estimates of effect is consistent with the random variation of a uniform effect or, alternatively, whether there is effect modification in the data.

Statistical tests of the null hypothesis that the effect is uniform (i.e., exhibits no effect modification) generally are of two types, one based on a directly pooled estimate of uniform effect and the other on a maximum likelihood estimate.

For the directly pooled estimates, the basic principle of the test is to compare each stratum-specific estimate with the pooled estimate, square the difference, and divide by the variance of the stratum-specific effect estimate. The resulting quotient is summed over all strata, yielding a chi-square statistic with degrees of freedom equal to one less than the number of strata:

$$\chi^2_{N-1} = \sum_{i=1}^{N} \frac{(\hat{R}_i - \hat{R})^2}{\text{Var}(\hat{R}_i)} \qquad [12\text{-}59]$$

For difference measures of effect, the above formula can be applied directly, with $\hat{R}_i$ denoting the stratum-specific difference and $\hat{R}$ denoting the directly pooled estimate of effect. The stratum-specific variances in the denominator are the reciprocals of the weights used to obtain the pooled estimate. For ratio measures of effect, it is desirable to use a logarithmic transformation:

$$\chi^2_{N-1} = \sum_{i=1}^{N} \frac{[\ln(\hat{R}_i) - \ln(\hat{R})]^2}{\text{Var}[\ln(\hat{R}_i)]} \qquad [12\text{-}60]$$

in which $\hat{R}_i$ now denotes the stratum-specific ratio estimate of effect and $\hat{R}$ denotes the directly pooled ratio measure.

As an example of the application of the above test for effect modification of the incidence rate difference, consider the stratified effect estimates presented in Table 12-2. The directly pooled estimate of the incidence rate difference is $5.95 \times 10^{-4} \text{yr}^{-1}$. Using the stratum-specific point estimates and their variances in Table 12-2, formula 12-59 gives a χ^2 of 8.38 with four degrees of freedom. From tables of the chi-square distribution, the corresponding two-tail P-value is 0.08, which indicates the degree of consistency of the data in Example 12-2 with the hypothesis that the incidence rate difference is constant across age categories.

For an illustration of formula 12-60 used to evaluate the heterogeneity of a ratio measure of effect, consider the data in Example 12-5 and the calculations derived from them in Table 12-7. The pooled estimate of the odds ratio is 3.8. Formula 12-60 applied to the stratum-specific estimates in Table 12-7 gives a χ^2 with one degree of freedom of 0.14, which corresponds to a two-tail P-value of 0.7, showing that the data are consistent with the hypothesis of a uniform odds ratio.

The chi-square tests given in formulas 12-59 and 12-60, like the directly weighted pooled estimators on which they are based, depend on an assumption of large numbers of observations within strata. With small frequencies, the tests are unreliable. With zero cell frequencies, it may not even be possible to obtain stratum-specific variance or effect estimates. An alternative approach is to use a statistical test based on the maximum likelihood estimation of a uniform effect measure. This approach, termed a likelihood-ratio test, constructs the test statistic from a comparison of the likelihood equations for the data under two hypotheses: One hypothesis is that the effect is uniform, and the other is that the effect acquires a different value in each stratum. Although the likelihood-ratio test is also asymptotic, the requirement for large numbers within each stratum is not as stringent as it is in formulas 12-59 and 12-60; the test can be used even when there are small cell frequencies in the data. With zero cell frequencies the test fails, although it can be modified slightly by substituting a small positive value for zero to get a reasonably accurate result in many cases. The tests require previous calculation of the maximum likelihood estimate of a uniform effect, but otherwise require no iteration and involve only simple computation. The likelihood-ratio approach should give more accurate results in testing for effect modification when the data are relatively sparse.

The formulation of the likelihood-ratio tests for effect modification depends on the effect measure and the type of data under consideration. For incidence rate difference (IRD), the test is

$$\chi^2_{N-1} = -2 \sum_{i=1}^{N} \left[a_i \ln \left(\frac{(\hat{IR}_{0i} + \hat{IRD})N_{1i}}{a_i} \right) + b_i \ln \left(\frac{\hat{IR}_{0i}N_{0i}}{b_i} \right) \right] \qquad [12\text{-}61]$$

Note that the pooled maximum likelihood estimate of IRD is part of the test formula, as is the maximum likelihood estimate of IR_0 in each stratum. The estimates of IR_0 must be obtained in the estimation of IRD, so no additional estimation beyond maximum likelihood point estimation is required to apply formula 12-61.

For the data in Example 12-2, the pooled maximum likelihood estimate of the incidence rate difference is $5.91 \times 10^{-4}\text{yr}^{-1}$; stratum-specific maximum likelihood estimates of the incidence among nonsmokers are, from the youngest to the oldest, $8.406 \times 10^{-5}\text{yr}^{-1}$, $1.640 \times 10^{-3}\text{yr}^{-1}$, $6.303 \times 10^{-3}\text{yr}^{-1}$, $1.352 \times 10^{-2}\text{yr}^{-1}$, and $1.917 \times 10^{-2}\text{yr}^{-1}$. Using these estimates in formula 12-61 gives a χ^2 value of 7.4 with four degrees of freedom, which corresponds to a two-tail P-value of 0.12. This value compares with the result of 0.08 from formula 12-59.

For incidence rate ratio, the likelihood ratio test of uniformity is

$$\chi^2_{N-1} = -2 \sum_{i=1}^{N} \left[a_i \ln\left(\frac{\widehat{IRR} \cdot M_{1i}}{a_i(\widehat{IRR} + N_{0i}/N_{1i})}\right) \right.$$

$$\left. + b_i \ln\left[\left(\frac{M_{1i}}{b_i}\right)\left(1 - \frac{\widehat{IRR}}{\widehat{IRR} + N_{0i}/N_{1i}}\right)\right] \right] \qquad [12\text{-}62]$$

The formula requires the maximum likelihood estimate of IRR, but no nuisance parameters are involved.

For the data in Example 12-2, the maximum likelihood estimate of IRR is 1.42; the chi-square test in formula 12-62 gives a value of 12.1 with four degrees of freedom, which corresponds to a two-tail P-value of 0.016. Thus, these data are even less consistent with a uniform incidence rate ratio than they are with a uniform incidence rate difference. For the incidence rate ratio the stratum-to-stratum pattern of variation is extremely regular, decreasing steadily from the youngest to the oldest age category. The regular pattern of variation casts additional doubt on the validity of the assumption of a uniform incidence rate ratio.

For cumulative incidence difference, the likelihood-ratio test analogous to formula 12-61 is

$$\chi^2_{N-1} = -2 \sum_{i=1}^{N} \left[a_i \ln\left(\frac{(\hat{R}_{0i} + \widehat{RD})N_{1i}}{a_i}\right) + b_i \ln\left(\frac{\hat{R}_{0i}N_{0i}}{b_i}\right) \right.$$

$$\left. + c_i \ln\left(\frac{(1 - \hat{R}_{0i} - \widehat{RD})N_{1i}}{c_i}\right) + d_i \ln\left(\frac{(1 - \hat{R}_{0i})N_{0i}}{d_i}\right) \right] \qquad [12\text{-}63]$$

which again involves not only the maximum likelihood estimate of the risk difference but also the nuisance parameters $\{R_{0i}\}$.

For the data in Example 12-4, the maximum likelihood estimate of the risk difference is 0.0343 under the uniformity assumption. Stratum-specific maximum likelihood estimates of the risk among unexposed persons are 0.0415 and 0.1892 in the young and old strata, respectively. The two stratum-specific estimates of risk difference are 0.0338 and 0.0363, showing extremely little variation. Accordingly, the χ^2 from formula 12-63 is 0.001 with one degree of freedom, corresponding to a P-value of 0.97; this indicates the extraordinarily high consistency between the data and the statistical hypothesis of a uniform risk difference in these two age categories.

For cumulative incidence ratio, the likelihood-ratio test of uniformity is

$$\chi^2_{N-1} = -2 \sum_{i=1}^{N} \left[a_i \ln\left(\frac{\hat{R}_{0i}(RR)N_{1i}}{a_i}\right) + b_i \ln\left(\frac{\hat{R}_{0i}N_{0i}}{b_i}\right) \right.$$

$$\left. + c_i \ln\left(\frac{(1 - \hat{R}_{0i}RR)N_{1i}}{c_i}\right) + d_i \ln\left(\frac{(1 - \hat{R}_{0i})N_{0i}}{d_i}\right) \right] \quad [12\text{-}64]$$

which differs notably from the corresponding test for incidence rate ratio (formula 12-62). The difference derives from the fact that formula 12-62 is developed from a likelihood expression that is conditional on the total number of cases in each stratum, thereby eliminating the nuisance parameters. For cumulative incidence data, however, it is not correct to condition on the total number of cases in a stratum, and therefore an unconditional likelihood expression must be used; one consequence is that the estimates of the nuisance parameters $\{R_{0i}\}$ are part of the test statistic.

The data in Example 12-5 can be evaluated for uniformity of the risk ratio. The maximum likelihood estimate is 1.311, based on the assumption of uniformity. The nuisance parameter estimates (i.e., maximum likelihood estimates of the risk among unexposed for each stratum) are 0.0504 and 0.1781 in the younger and older categories, respectively. The one degree of freedom χ^2 statistic from formula 12-64 is 0.452, which corresponds to a P-value of 0.5. Thus, the data are reasonably consistent with a uniform risk ratio despite the apparent variation in stratum-specific estimates of the risk ratio (1.8 and 1.2).

For case-control (or prevalence) data, the likelihood ratio test of uniformity of the odds ratio is

$$\chi^2_{N-1} = -2 \sum_{i=1}^{N} \left[a_i \ln\left(\frac{\hat{a}_i}{a_i}\right) + b_i \ln\left(\frac{\hat{b}_i}{b_i}\right) + c_i \ln\left(\frac{\hat{c}_i}{c_i}\right) + d_i \ln\left(\frac{\hat{d}_i}{d_i}\right) \right] \quad [12\text{-}65]$$

where the fitted cell frequencies $\hat{a}_i$, $\hat{b}_i$, $\hat{c}_i$, and $\hat{d}_i$ are the values satisfying equation 12-24,

$$\hat{OR}_{ML} = \frac{\hat{a}_i \hat{d}_i}{\hat{b}_i \hat{c}_i}$$

For the data in Example 12-5, the (unconditional) maximum likelihood estimate of the odds ratio is 3.79. The fitted cell frequencies for the a cell are 3.2473 and 0.7527 for the younger and older strata, respectively; the other fitted cell frequencies are obtained from the margins of each 2 × 2 table by subtraction. Formula 12-65 yields a chi-square of 0.13 with one degree of freedom, which corresponds to a two-tail P-value of 0.7. These results are nearly identical to those obtained with formula 12-60.

Another test of uniformity of the odds ratio over a set of 2 × 2 tables was proposed by Zelen [1971]. Zelen's test calls for summing the chi-square calculated for each 2 × 2 table (the square of formula 11-6 or 11-8) and subtracting from the sum the square of the Mantel-Haenszel chi-square (formula 12-38). Zelen's procedure, however, is not generally valid; counterexamples have been cited in which a uniform odds ratio gives a large chi-square for Zelen's test and a zero chi-square results when stratum-specific odds ratios differ considerably [Mantel et al., 1977]. This procedure is not recommended.

None of the tests considered in this section takes into account the pattern of variability of the effect estimates across strata. The chi-square values calculated in the application of these tests are independent of any ordering of the strata: If the strata were reordered, the test result would not differ. In principle, it is possible to construct more powerful tests directed at specific patterns of variation of the effect estimates over the strata as an alternative to uniformity. To do so, it would be necessary to postulate the pattern. For example, the likelihood test of uniformity of the incidence rate ratio for the data given in Example 12-2 produces a P-value of 0.016; the effect estimates decline nearly exponentially, however, so that a more powerful test of uniformity can be constructed using an exponential curve as the alternative pattern of variation. With this more powerful approach, a substantially smaller P-value results [Miettinen and Neff, 1971]. The improved test takes into account the declining pattern of the incidence rate ratio estimates with increasing age.

Description of Effect Modification

When the stratum-specific estimates vary enough to indicate that there is likely to be variation in the underlying effect, it is improper to present either the crude estimate of effect or a pooled estimate. The pooled estimate of effect is a weighted average of the stratum-specific estimates, but the weights are intended to promote precision and therefore reflect the number of observations in individual strata. The pooled estimate is consequently potentially misleading unless it is reasonable to assume that the effect estimates vary only randomly around a uniform effect value. If the effect itself varies over strata, then the value of the pooled estimate calculated on the assumption of uniformity will depend on the distribution of subjects over strata in a way that is peculiar to the individual study and difficult to specify. The crude estimate is a worse alternative, since it does not even represent a weighted average of the stratum-specific estimates.

How, then, should the effect be described when the effect is judged to vary over strata? One simple approach is to present the estimates separately for each stratum: The study can be considered a set of individual substudies that are reported separately. Point estimates and confidence intervals can be reported for each stratum. This approach is often used when effect modification occurs for a dichotomous factor such as sex.

STANDARDIZED EFFECT ESTIMATES

The drawback of reporting the results separately by stratum is that the overall body of data becomes divided, resulting in less precise estimates of effect in individual strata. If the stratification variable has many categories, there will be comparatively little precision for each of the several estimates. Furthermore, a set of many estimates of effect may offer a more detailed description of the effect than would a summary of the overall effect in a single number, but it also provides much less cogency in its detailed description. The entire purpose of data analysis is to reduce inherently complex information into a less complex and therefore more readily interpretable form. With this goal in mind, it is appropriate to consider whether there is not some meaningful way in which a set of stratum-specific estimates might be reduced into a single overall measure. The difficulty with the pooled estimate is the unpredictable or unspecifiable way in which it combines the information over strata. A reasonable way to avoid this difficulty is to combine the information over the strata using a specified system of weights—that is, to standardize the component rates of the effect measure to a standard distribution for the stratification variable. The advantage of standardization is that the weighting of stratum-specific information is easily specified, allowing the averaging of different values of the effect estimate from different strata to occur in a theoretically replicable and epidemiologically meaningful way.

Investigators may occasionally be cautioned to avoid standardization of effect estimates if there is "excessive" variability in the estimates over the strata, since that variability will be obscured in the overall estimate. For example, if effect estimates in two strata point in opposite directions, let us say indicating prevention for males and causation for females, a standardized estimate could indicate prevention, causation, or no effect depending on the choice of standard. This problem exists, however, for any single summary measure. A standardized summary measure at least has the advantage that it weights the divergent estimates in a definable way. It is incorrect to make uniformity of effect a prerequisite for standardization, with uniformity, pooling is preferable to standardization to optimize precision. Standardization is useful principally when the effect does vary over strata. Of course, it is always true that a summary measure can obscure an underlying variability. If the variability is extreme, as it often is when effect estimates point in opposite directions, it may be reasonable to report the stratum-specific details. In other instances, the investigator may properly decide that a summary result will convey enough of the intended message without obfuscating important detail to permit standardization. After all, there is no limit to the process of separating data into levels of detail; even small and apparently homogeneous subgroups represent the aggregate experience of some individuals who experienced the effect of interest and others who did not.

Table 12-11. Incidence rate ratio estimates of
coronary death for smokers relative to nonsmokers
among British male doctors, by age (data of example 12-2)

Age	Point estimate of IRR	Exact (mid-P) 90 percent confidence interval*
35–44	5.74	1.91, 24
45–54	2.14	1.32, 3.63
55–64	1.47	1.06, 2.07
65–74	1.36	0.98, 1.91
75–84	0.90	0.65, 1.28

*Confidence intervals calculated from formulas 11-9 and 11-10.

Consider again the incidence rate data given in Example 12-2. It is apparent that the incidence rate ratio is not uniform over age, declining from an estimated value of 5.7 in the youngest stratum to just below unity in the oldest. A reasonable approach to the presentation of these data might be to show the stratum-specific results rather than any summary figure (Table 12-11). On the other hand, despite the interesting variability apparent in the data, a single summary estimate might be desired and could be defended. In that case, a standardized estimate of incidence rate ratio should be used; one reasonable choice for a standard would be the person-year distribution of smoking British male doctors, which would lead to the SMR:

$$SMR = \frac{630}{[(2/18,790)(52,407) + \ldots]} = \frac{630}{444.41} = 1.42$$

Naturally, a different choice of standard would affect the reported estimate of effect. For example, if each age category were assigned an equal weight, the resulting standardized rate ratio would be

$$SRR = \frac{\dfrac{32}{52,407yr} + \dfrac{104}{43,248yr} + \ldots}{\dfrac{2}{18,790yr} + \dfrac{12}{10,673yr} + \ldots} = 1.16$$

The relatively great difference in the above two effect estimates reflects only the different choice of weights involved in the selection of a standard. The second approach assigns relatively larger weights to the older age categories in which the effect is small.

Standardized estimates, like pooled estimates, are always weighted averages of stratum-specific effect estimates. For difference measures of effect, the weighting is the same as the standard weights, since the standardized rate difference may be expressed as

$$\text{SRD} = \frac{\Sigma w_i R_{1i}}{\Sigma w_i} - \frac{\Sigma w_i R_{0i}}{\Sigma w_i} = \frac{\Sigma w_i (R_{1i} - R_{0i})}{\Sigma w_i} = \frac{\Sigma w_i (\hat{RD}_i)}{\Sigma w_i}$$

where w_i is the standard weight for category i, R_{1i} is the rate among exposed in stratum i, R_{0i} is the rate among unexposed in stratum i, and $\hat{RD}_i$ is the estimate of rate difference in stratum i. For rate ratio measures of effect, however, the standardized rate ratio is a weighted average of stratum-specific values that weights the stratum-specific rate ratios according to the product of the weight from the standard and the rate among the nonexposed:

$$\text{SRR} = \frac{\Sigma w_i R_{1i}/(\Sigma w_i)}{\Sigma w_i R_{0i}/(\Sigma w_i)} = \frac{\Sigma w_i R_{0i} \hat{RR}_i}{\Sigma w_i R_{0i}} = \frac{\Sigma w_i' \hat{RR}_i}{\Sigma w_i'} \qquad [12\text{-}66]$$

where $\hat{RR}_i$ is the estimate of rate ratio in stratum i and $w_i' = w_i R_{0i}$.

The structure of formula 12-66 reveals why the two standardized rate ratios combining the stratum-specific point estimates in Table 12-11 are influenced heavily by the small effect estimates in the older age categories. Since w_i' is a product of the weight for standardization and R_{0i}, the value of R_{0i} will influence the weighting of the stratum-specific estimates. As it happens, R_{0i} increases steeply with age for the data of Example 12-2, thereby magnifying the influence of the older age groups on the overall standardized rate ratio. Even the SMR, standardized as it is to the young age distribution of the smokers themselves, is only a modest 1.42 because of the influence of the R_{0i} in expression 12-66.

Equation 12-66 can be applied, under certain conditions, to case-control data to obtain standardized rate ratio estimates from case-control studies [Miettinen, 1972]. Consider the SMR, which, as always, is standardized to the distribution of the exposed population. If N_{1i} is the numerator and D_{1i} is the denominator of the rate for the exposed source population of subjects in category i, then $a_i = f_{ca(i)} (N_{1i})$ and $c_i = f_{co(i)} (D_{1i})$, where a_i is the number of exposed cases in stratum i of the case-control study, c_i is the number of exposed controls in stratum i, and $f_{ca(i)}$ and $f_{co(i)}$ are the sampling fractions of cases and controls in stratum i of the source population. To standardize to the distribution of the exposed population, w_i should be taken as $D_{1i} = c_i/f_{co(i)}$. R_{1i} may be written as

$$R_{1i} = \frac{a_i/f_{ca(i)}}{c_i/f_{co(i)}}$$

so that $\Sigma w_i R_{1i} = \Sigma a_i / f_{ca(i)}$. Similarly,

$$R_{0i} = \frac{b_i / f_{ca(i)}}{d_i / f_{co(i)}}$$

and

$$\Sigma w_i R_{0i} = \sum_{i=1}^{N} \frac{b_i c_i}{d_i f_{ca(i)}}$$

If the sampling fraction for cases is constant over the strata, which will be true if the cases have been selected independently of the stratification factor, then

$$SMR = \frac{\displaystyle\sum_{i=1}^{N} a_i}{\displaystyle\sum_{i=1}^{N} \frac{b_i c_i}{d_i}} \qquad [12\text{-}67]$$

Expression 12-67 has the usual form for an SMR, namely, the ratio of the observed number of exposed cases to an "expected" or null number. The expected number is not identical to the expected number used for statistical hypothesis testing, since hypothesis testing is premised on the correctness of the null hypothesis, which cannot be assumed for estimation. The expected number in expression 12-67 indicates how many exposed cases would have been observed if the exposure had no effect, but it involves no marginal totals that include the a cell, since the a cell is the one cell in each 2 × 2 table that differs from its null value when the exposure has an effect.

It is possible to choose other standards for the standardization of rate ratio estimates in case-control studies. For example, if w_i is taken as the size of the denominator for the unexposed population in category i, equal to $D_{0i} = d_i / f_{co(i)}$, then

$$SRR = \frac{\displaystyle\sum_{i=1}^{N} \frac{a_i d_i}{c_i}}{\displaystyle\sum_{i=1}^{N} b_i} \qquad [12\text{-}68]$$

assuming once again that the sampling fraction for cases is constant over the strata.

Confidence intervals for standardized effect measures can be calculated, but they must reflect the pattern of the weights assigned by the standard. For standardized rate differences, an approximate variance formula is

$$\text{Var(SRD)} \doteq \frac{1}{(\Sigma w_i)^2} \sum_{i=1}^{N} w_i^2 \text{Var(RD}_i) \qquad [12\text{-}69]$$

where w_i is the weight from the standard for category i and $\text{Var}(\hat{RD}_i)$ is obtained from formula 12-1 or 12-6, depending on the type of data. The square root of Var(SRD) can be used for the standard deviation in formula 10-2 to obtain approximate confidence limits. For rate ratio measures, the usual logarithmic transformation should be used. With follow-up data, an approximate variance formula for the logarithm of a standardized rate ratio is

$$\text{Var[ln(SRR)]} \doteq \frac{\Sigma w_i^2 \text{Var}(R_{1i})}{(\Sigma w_i R_{1i})^2} + \frac{\Sigma w_i^2 \text{Var}(R_{0i})}{(\Sigma w_i R_{0i})^2} \qquad [12\text{-}70]$$

where $\text{Var}(R_{1i})$ and $\text{Var}(R_{0i})$ can be estimated from the first and second terms, respectively, of formula 12-1 or 12-6, depending on the type of data; the square root of Var[ln(SRR)] can be used in expression 10-4 to find approximate confidence limits.

To exemplify the application of formula 12-70, let us determine the approximate 90 percent confidence limits for the SMR calculated from Example 12-2. The weights from the standard, which for an SMR is always the exposed group, and the terms of the necessary sums for the variance of the logarithm of the SMR are given in Table 12-12. The variance is

$$\text{Var[ln(SMR)]} \doteq \frac{630}{630^2} + \frac{1997.56}{444.41^2} = 0.00159 + 0.01025 = 0.01184$$

The standard deviation is therefore $\sqrt{0.01184} = 0.1088$, and a 90 percent confidence interval around the SMR of $630/444.41 = 1.42$ is

$$\exp[\ln(1.42) \pm 1.645(0.1088)] = 1.19, 1.70$$

Table 12-12. Intermediate calculations for the variance
of the logarithm of the SMR for the data of example 12-2

Age category	w_i	$w_i R_{1i}$	$w_i R_{0i}$	$w_i^2 \text{Var}(R_{1i})$	$w_i^2 \text{Var}(R_{0i})$
35–44	52,407	32	5.58	32	15.56
45–54	43,248	104	48.63	104	197.03
55–64	28,612	206	140.30	206	703.04
65–74	12,663	186	137.16	186	671.91
75–84	5,317	102	112.74	102	410.02
Total	142,247	630	444.41	630	1997.56

The analogous calculations for a standard in which a weight of 1.0 is assigned to each category, which gives a standardized rate ratio of 1.16, would result in a variance of 0.0161, corresponding to a standard deviation of 0.1269. The 90 percent confidence interval for the SRR with uniform weights is

$$\exp[\ln(1.16) \pm 1.645(0.1269)] = 0.94, 1.43$$

No general formulation can be made for the variance of the logarithm of a standardized rate ratio calculated from case-control data, since for case-control data the variance formula itself depends on the choice of a standard. For the SMR (calculated from formula 12-67), which uses the distribution of exposed subjects in the source population as the standard, the variance is approximated by

$$\mathrm{Var}[\ln(\mathrm{SMR})] \doteq \frac{1}{\sum_i a_i} + \frac{\sum\limits_{i=1}^{N} \left(\dfrac{b_i c_i}{d_i}\right)^2 \left(\dfrac{1}{b_i} + \dfrac{1}{c_i} + \dfrac{1}{d_i}\right)}{\left(\sum\limits_{i=1}^{N} \dfrac{b_i c_i}{d_i}\right)^2}$$

Using the data from Example 12-5, the SMR is calculable as 3.78, and the Var[ln(SMR)] $\doteq$ 0.350, which gives a 90 percent confidence interval of

$$\exp[\ln(3.78) \pm 1.645(\sqrt{0.350})] = 1.43, 10.0$$

This point estimate and confidence interval happen to agree well in this instance with the (unconditional) maximum likelihood point estimate and the exact mid-P 90 percent confidence interval, which were previously calculated to be 3.79 and 1.30 to 9.78, respectively; while such agreement is reasonably common, it is not guaranteed because different principles are involved in weighting the stratum-specific results for the two approaches.

Using the distribution of the nonexposed subjects in the source population as the standard (i.e., formula 12-68), the variance is estimated as

$$\mathrm{Var}[\ln(\mathrm{SRR})] \doteq \frac{1}{\sum_i b_i} + \frac{\sum\limits_{i=1}^{N} \left(\dfrac{a_i d_i}{c_i}\right)^2 \left(\dfrac{1}{a_i} + \dfrac{1}{c_i} + \dfrac{1}{d_i}\right)}{\left(\sum\limits_{i=1}^{N} \dfrac{a_i d_i}{c_i}\right)^2} \qquad [12\text{-}71]$$

For the data in Example 12-5, the SRR from formula 12-68 is 3.98 and the Var[ln(SRR)] $\doteq$ 0.381, giving a 90 percent confidence interval of

$$\exp[\ln(3.98) \pm 1.645(\sqrt{0.381})] = 1.44, 11.0$$

EFFECT FUNCTIONS

When the effect-modifying factor is measured on a continuous scale such as age it is possible to fit a mathematical equation describing the variation in the effect measure as a function of the effect modifier. For example, if the rate ratio seems to vary linearly with age, it is possible to express the rate ratio as a straight line function of age:

$$RR = a_0 + a_1(age)$$

where a_0 is the "intercept" value and a_1 is a coefficient that describes the change in the rate ratio for a unit increment of age. The coefficients a_0 and a_1 can be estimated by a simple weighted regression procedure.

A linear function is not necessarily a good description of the mathematical relation between the effect measure and the effect modifier; it may be worthwhile to consider transformations that improve the description. The stratum-specific estimates of the incidence rate ratio for the data in Example 12-2 (Table 12-11) illustrate a progressive decline in IRR with age. The stratum-specific estimates are plotted in Figure 12-3. It is evident that a straight line will not provide as good a fit as one might hope. In Figure 12-4, the logarithm of each age-specific estimate of IRR is plotted; for the five age categories from youngest to oldest, these values are 1.7469, 0.7603, 0.3841, 0.3046, and -0.1001, respectively. These values conform better to a linear pattern. For the data of Example 12-2, then, it seems reasonable to describe the effect of smoking, as measured by the incidence rate ratio, as a function of age using a logarithmic transformation of the IRR:

$$\ln(IRR) = a_0 + a_1(age)$$

The coefficients for this equation can be determined easily by a linear regression procedure. It is important to use a weighted regression that assigns to each age-specific observation a weight that reflects the precision of that estimate; a weight proportional to the reciprocal of the variance of $\ln(\hat{IRR}_i)$ accomplishes this purpose. The age-specific weights for the weighted regression are calculated as the reciprocals of the variances determined by formula 12-4; the weights are 1.88, 10.76, 24.65, 24.34, and 23.77 from youngest to oldest, respectively. Note the small weight accorded to the youngest age category, for which only two events were observed among the nonsmokers; the small number of events in the denom-

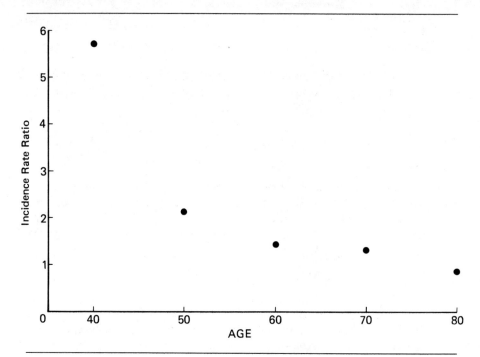

Fig. 12-3. Estimates of incidence rate ratio for coronary death for smoking British doctors, compared with nonsmoking doctors, by age (data of example 12-2).

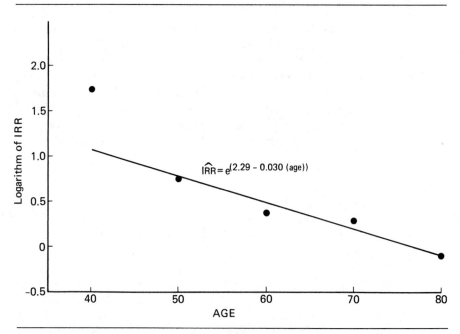

Fig. 12-4. Logarithm of estimates of incidence rate ratio for coronary death for smoking British doctors, compared with nonsmoking doctors, by age (data of example 12-2), and fitted weighted regression line.

inator rate of the rate ratio leads to a large variance for the rate ratio. The youngest category consequently does not contribute much to the fitting of the weighted regression line. A least-squares weighted regression analysis [Kleinbaum and Kupper, 1978] using the above weights gives $a_0 = 2.29$ and $a_1 = -0.030$. To express the IRR as a function of age using these results, we can reverse the logarithmic transformation:

$$\widehat{IRR} = e^{(2.29 - 0.030(\text{age}))}$$

The above fitted equation describes the incidence rate ratio as a function of age and can be used to estimate the IRR at any given age. For example, at age 65 the estimate of IRR is $\exp(2.29 - 0.030(65)) = 1.43$. At age 40 the estimated value of IRR is 3.0; the predicted and observed values are relatively discrepant at age 40 because the entire set of age categories was used to generate the coefficients, but little weight was contributed by the unstable estimate of IRR in the youngest age category. For age 80, however, the estimated IRR of 0.91 from the regression equation is nearly identical to the observed value of 0.90 because of the greater weights assigned to the older age categories. The overall pattern indicates roughly exponential decline in IRR with age, until the effect disappears entirely between ages 75–80 (the apparent reversal in the direction of the effect at the oldest ages is not striking enough to warrant a biologic interpretation).

REFERENCES

Breslow, N. Odds ratio estimators when the data are sparse. *Biometrika* 1981;68:73–84.

Breslow, N. E., and Liang, K. Y. The variance of the Mantel-Haenszel estimator. *Biometrics* 1982;38:943–952.

Cornfield, J. A statistical problem arising from retrospective studies. *Proc. Third Berkeley Sympos.* 1956;4:135–148.

Doll, R., and Hill, A. B. Mortality of British doctors in relation to smoking; observations on coronary thrombosis. In W. Haenszel (ed.), *Epidemiological Approaches to the Study of Cancer and Other Chronic Diseases. Natl. Cancer Inst. Mono.* 1966;19:205–268.

Gart, J. J. Point and interval estimation of the common odds ratio in the combination of 2 × 2 tables with fixed marginals. *Biometrika* 1970;57:471–475.

Gart, J. J. The comparison of proportions: A review of significance tests, confidence intervals and adjustments for stratification. *Rev. Int. Stat. Inst.* 1971;39:148–169.

Greenland, S., and Robins, J. M. Estimation of a common effect parameter from sparse follow-up data. *Biometrics* 1985;41:55–68.

Haldane, J. B. S. The estimation and significance of the logarithm of a ratio of frequencies. *Ann. Hum. Genet.* 1955;20:309–311.

Hauck, W. W. The large sample variance of the Mantel-Haenszel estimator of a common odds ratio. *Biometrics* 1979;35:817–819.

Hempelmann, L. H., Hall, W. J., Phillips, M., et al. Neoplasms in persons treated with x-rays in infancy—fourth survey in 20 years. *J. Natl. Cancer Inst.* 1975;55:519–530.

Kleinbaum, D. G., and Kupper, L. L. *Applied Regression Analysis and Other Multivariate Methods.* North Scituate, MA: Duxbury Press, 1978. P. 243.

Lubin, J. H. An empirical evaluation of the use of conditional and unconditional likelihoods for case-control data. *Biometrika* 1981;68:567–571.

Mann, J. I., Inman, W. H. W., and Thorogood, M. Oral contraceptive use in older women and fatal myocardial infarction. *Br. Med. J.* 1968;2:193–199.

Mantel, N., and Haenszel, W. Statistical aspects of the analysis of data from retrospective studies of disease. *J. Natl. Cancer Inst.* 1959;22:719–748.

Mantel, N., Brown, C., and Byar, D. P. Tests for homogeneity of effect in an epidemiologic investigation. *Am. J. Epidemiol.* 1977;106:125–129.

McKinlay, S. M. The effect of nonzero second-order interaction on combined estimators of the odds ratio. *Biometrika* 1978;65:191–202.

Miettinen, O. S. Standardization of risk ratios. *Am. J. Epidemiol.* 1972;96:383–388.

Miettinen, O. S., and Neff, R. K. Computer processing of epidemiologic data. *Hart Bull.* 1971;2:98–103.

Nurminen, N. Asymptotic efficiency of general noniterative estimators of common relative risk. *Biometrika* 1981;68:525–530.

Robins, J. M., Breslow, N., and Greenland, S. Estimators of the Mantel-Haenszel variance consistent in both sparse data and large strata limiting models. *Biometrics* 1985; in press.

Rothman, K. J. Spermicide use and Down's syndrome. *Am. J. Public Health* 1982;72:399–401.

Rothman, K. J., and Monson, R. R. Survival in trigeminal neuralgia. *J. Chron. Dis.* 1973;26:303–309.

Rothman, K. J., and Boice, J. D. *Epidemiologic Analysis with a Programmable Calculator.* Brookline, MA: Epidemiology Resources, 1982. (First edition published by U.S. Government Printing Office, Washington D.C., NIH Publication No. 79-1649, June, 1979.)

Tarone, R. E. On summary estimators of relative risk. *J. Chron. Dis.* 1981;34:463–468.

Thomas, D. G. Exact and asymptotic methods for the combination of 2 × 2 tables. *Computers and Biomedical Research* 1975;8:423–446.

University Group Diabetes Program. A study of the effects of hypoglycemic agents on vascular complications in patients with adult onset diabetes. *Diabetes* 1970;19(Suppl. 2):747–830.

Walker, A. M. Small sample properties of some estimators of a common hazard ratio. *Appl. Stat.* 1985;34:42–48.

Woolf, B. On estimating the relation between blood group and disease. *Ann. Hum. Genet.* 1954;19:251–253.

Zelen, M. The analysis of several 2 × 2 contingency tables. *Biometrika* 1971;58:129–137.

13. MATCHING

Matching refers to the selection of a comparison series—unexposed subjects in a follow-up study or controls in a case-control study—that is identical, or nearly so, to the index series with respect to one or more potentially confounding factors. The mechanics of the matching may be performed subject by subject, which is described as *individual matching,* or for groups of subjects, which is described as *frequency matching.* The general principles that apply to matched data are identical for individually matched or frequency matched data.

PRINCIPLES OF MATCHING

The topic of matching in epidemiology is beguiling: What at first seems clear is seductively deceptive. Whereas the clarity of an analysis in which confounding has been securely prevented by perfect matching of the compared series seems indubitable and impossible to misinterpret, the intuitive foundation for this cogency attained by matching is a surprisingly shaky structure that does not always support the conclusions that are apt to be drawn. The difficulty is that our intuition about matching springs from knowledge of experiments or follow-up studies, whereas matching is most often applied in case-control studies, which differ enough from follow-up studies to make the implications of matching different and counterintuitive.

Whereas the traditional view, stemming from an understanding based on follow-up studies, has been that matching enhances validity, in case-control studies the effectiveness of matching as a methodologic tool derives from its effect on study efficiency, not on validity. Indeed, for case-control studies it would be more accurate to state that matching introduces confounding rather than that it prevents confounding.

The different implications of matching for follow-up and case-control studies are easy to demonstrate. Consider a source population of 2,000,000 individuals, distributed by exposure and sex as indicated in Table 13-1. Both the exposure and male gender are risk factors for the disease: For the exposure the relative risk is 10, and for males relative to females it is 5. There is also substantial confounding, since 90 percent of the exposed individuals are male and only 10 percent of the unexposed are male. The crude relative risk in the source population, comparing exposed with unexposed, is 32.9, considerably different from the unconfounded value of 10.

Now consider what happens if a follow-up study is planned by drawing the exposed cohort from the exposed source population and matching the unexposed cohort to the exposed cohort for sex. Suppose 10 percent of the exposed source population were included in the follow-up study; if these subjects were selected independently of gender, we would have approximately 90,000 males and 10,000 females in the exposed cohort. A

Table 13-1. *Hypothetical source population of 2,000,000 people, in which exposure increases risk 10-fold, and males have five times the risk of females, and exposure is strongly associated with male gender*

	Males (1,000,000)		Females (1,000,000)	
	Exposed (900,000)	Unexposed (100,000)	Exposed (100,000)	Unexposed (900,000)
One-year risk	0.005	0.0005	0.001	0.0001
No. cases in one year	4500	50	100	90

$$\text{Crude relative risk} = \frac{(4500 + 100)/1,000,000}{(50 + 90)/1,000,000} = 32.9$$

comparison group of unexposed subjects would be drawn from the 1,000,000 unexposed individuals in the source population. If the comparison group were drawn, like the exposed group, independently of gender, the follow-up study would have the same confounding as exists in the source population (apart from sampling variability), since the follow-up study would then be a simple 10 percent sample of the source population. It would be possible, however, to assemble the unexposed cohort so that the proportion of males in it was identical to that in the exposed cohort. The purpose of matching the unexposed cohort to the exposed group by sex is to prevent confounding by sex. Of the 100,000 unexposed males in the source population, 90,000 would be in a matched comparison group, corresponding to the 90,000 exposed males in the study. Of the 900,000 unexposed females, 10,000 would be selected to match the 10,000 exposed females.

The "expected" results from the matched cohort study described here are indicated in Table 13-2. The expected relative risk in the study population is 10 for males and 10 for females and is also 10 in the crude data for the study. The matching has apparently accomplished its purpose: There is no confounding by sex, since sex is unrelated to exposure in the study population because of matching.

The situation differs considerably, however, if a case-control study is conducted instead. Consider a case-control study based on the total of 4740 cases that occur in the source population during one year. Of these cases, 4550 are male. Suppose, then, that 4740 controls were selected from the source population, matched to the cases by gender, so that 4550 of the controls are male. Of the 4550 male controls, we expect about 90 percent, or 4095, to be exposed, since 90 percent of the males in the source population are exposed. Of the 190 female controls, we expect about 10 percent, or 19, to be exposed, corresponding to the 10 percent of females exposed in the source population. For the control series as a whole, the expected number of exposed subjects is 4095 + 19 = 4114 of a total of

Table 13-2. Expectation of the results of a matched
one-year follow-up study of 100,000 exposed and 100,000
unexposed subjects drawn from the source population described in table 13-1

	Males		Females		Total	
	Exposed	Unexposed	Exposed	Unexposed	Exposed	Unexposed
Cases	450	45	10	1	460	46
Total	90,000	90,000	10,000	10,000	100,000	100,000
	$\hat{RR} = 10$		$\hat{RR} = 10$		Crude $\hat{RR} = 10$	

4740. For the cases, $4500 + 100 = 4600$ of the 4740 would be exposed.
The crude estimate of effect, based on the odds ratio from the crude data,
is

$$\text{Crude relative risk} \doteq \frac{(4600)\,(626)}{(4114)\,(140)} = 5.0$$

which is a substantial underestimate of the unconfounded effect of the
exposure. Interestingly, the case-control data give the correct result, $\hat{RR} =$
10, if the data are stratified into male and female strata (Table 13-3). The
discrepancy between the crude results and the stratum-specific results in
Table 13-3 is a manifestation of confounding by sex (note that the sex-
specific effect estimates are identical to one another and distinctly different
from the crude estimate). This confounding is not a reflection of the original confounding by sex in the source population but rather a confounding
that was introduced into the study by the matching process. In case-control
studies, matching on factors associated with exposure builds confounding
into the data, whether or not there was confounding in the source population. If there is confounding initially in the source population, as there
was in the example, the process of matching will substitute a new confounding structure in place of the initial one. The confounding introduced
by matching is generally in the direction of a bias toward the null value of
effect, whatever the nature of the confounding in the source population.
In the example, the strong positive confounding (positive indicating a bias
in the same direction as the effect) in the source population was replaced
by strong negative confounding (negative indicating a bias in the direction
opposite to that of the effect) in the case-control data.

Why does matching in a case-control study introduce confounding? The
purpose of the control series in a case-control study is to provide an estimate of the person-time distribution for the exposed population relative
to the unexposed population in the source population of cases. If controls
are selected to match the cases for a factor that is correlated with the
exposure, then the crude exposure proportion in controls is distorted in

Table 13-3. Expectation of the results of a case-control study of 4740 cases and 4740 matched controls drawn from the source population described in table 13-1

	Males			Females			Total		
	Exposed	Unexposed	Total	Exposed	Unexposed	Total	Exposed	Unexposed	Total
Cases	4500	50	4550	100	90	190	4600	140	4740
Controls	4095	455	4550	19	171	190	4114	626	4740
		$\widehat{RR} = 10$			$\widehat{RR} = 10$			$\widehat{RR} = 5$	

the direction of similarity to that of the cases. If the matching factor were perfectly correlated with the exposure, the exposure distribution of controls would be identical to that of cases, and the crude relative risk estimate would be 1.0, since controls are chosen to be identical to cases with respect to the matching factor. Interestingly, the bias of the effect estimate toward the null value does not depend on the direction of the correlation between the exposure and the matching factor; as long as there is a non-zero correlation, positive or negative, the crude exposure distribution among controls will be distorted in the direction of similarity to that of cases. A perfect negative correlation between the matching factor and the exposure will still lead to identical exposure distributions for cases and controls and a crude relative risk estimate of 1.0 because each control is matched to the identical value of the matching factor of the case, guaranteeing identity for the exposure variable as well.

If the matching factor happens to be uncorrelated with the exposure, then matching does not influence the exposure distribution of the controls, and therefore no bias is introduced by matching. Because matching is ostensibly motivated by the need to control confounding by the matching factor(s), one would generally expect some correlation to exist between the matching factor(s) and the exposure. If the correlation is zero, the matching factor was not confounding in the first place, since a confounding factor must be associated with both the exposure and the disease.

It seems that matching, although intended to control confounding, does not attain that objective in case-control studies. Apparently, it merely accomplishes the substitution of a new confounding structure for the old one. In fact, matching can even introduce confounding where none previously existed: If the matching factor is unrelated to disease in the source population, ordinarily it would not be a confounder; however, if it is correlated with the exposure, it will become a confounder after matching for it in a case-control study. This situation is illustrated in Table 13-4, in which the exposure has an effect corresponding to a relative risk of 5.6, and there is no confounding in the source population; however, if the cases are used as the basis for a case-control study, and a control series is matched to the cases by gender, the expected value for the crude estimate of effect from the case-control study is 2.1 rather than the correct value of 5.6. In the source population sex is uncorrelated with disease among the unexposed, the prevalence of disease being 2 in 1000 for both unexposed males and unexposed females. Sex is strongly correlated with exposure, however. In the case-control study, sex is confounding because it was a matching factor that was correlated with exposure. Despite the absence of correlation between sex and disease among unexposed in the source population, a correlation between sex and disease among unexposed is introduced into the case-control data by matching. The result is a crude estimate of effect, 2.1, that seriously underestimates the correct value of 5.6.

Table 13-4. *Prevalence state of a source population with no confounding by sex and a case-control study drawn from the source population illustrating confounding introduced by matching for sex*

Source population

	Males			Females			Totals	
	Exposed	Unexposed	Total	Exposed	Unexposed	Total	Exposed	Unexposed
Disease	999	20	1019	111	180	291	1110	200
No disease	89,001	9980	1019	9889	89,820	291	98,890	99,800
Totals	90,000	10,000	2038	10,000	90,000	482	100,000	100,000
	$\hat{RR} = 5.6$			$\hat{RR} = 5.6$			Crude $\hat{RR} = 5.6$	

Case-control study drawn from the source population and matched on sex

	Males			Females			Totals		
	Exposed	Unexposed	Total	Exposed	Unexposed	Total	Exposed	Unexposed	Total
Cases	999	20	1019	111	180	291	1110	200	1310
Controls	916	103	1019	29	262	291	945	365	1310
Totals	1915	123	2038	140	342	482	2055	565	2620
	$\hat{RR} = 5.6$			$\hat{RR} = 5.6$			Crude $\hat{RR} = 2.1$		

The confounding introduced by matching in a case-control study is by no means irremediable. Notice that in Tables 13-3 and 13-4 the stratum-specific estimates of effect are valid; the confounding can be removed by a stratified analysis to arrive at a pooled estimate of effect after stratifying by the matching factor(s). Table 13-4 illustrates the need for an analysis to remove confounding by the matching factors, since matching may cause confounding even when none was originally present. In Table 13-4, the selection criterion used in matching controls makes the control series unrepresentative of the source population with regard to exposure; this would lead to a selection bias but for the fact that it can be controlled in the analysis and can be therefore viewed as confounding.

   In a follow-up study that compares risks, no additional action is required in the analysis to control confounding by the matching factors; the process of matching has already eliminated any confounding by the matching factors. In contrast, matching in a case-control study requires further control of confounding by the matching factors in the analysis even if the matching factors were not confounding in the source population, provided that the matching factors are correlated with the exposure. What accounts for this discrepancy? In a follow-up study, matching is undertaken without regard to disease status, which is unknown at the start of follow-up, therefore preventing bias. In a case-control study, on the other hand, matching involves the specification of both the exposure and the disease status and leads to conditional associations between the matching factor(s) and both exposure and disease, thereby resulting in bias. In a case-control study, if the matching factors are not correlated with the exposure, no confounding is introduced by matching; in this situation there could not have been confounding in the source population to begin with, so the matching was unnecessary.

   It is reasonable to ask why one would consider matching at all in case-control studies, since it does not accomplish its intended objective of preventing confounding. The utility of matching in case-control studies derives not from its ability to prevent confounding but from the enhanced efficiency that it affords for the control of confounding. In Table 13-3, the male and female strata each have an equal number of cases and controls because of the matched design. If 4740 controls were selected without matching, half would be male and half would be female. There would thus be a great excess of female controls, since 2370 is an unnecessarily large number of controls for 190 cases; the total amount of information does not increase substantially after five or six controls per case (see Fig. 8-1), and therefore the information collected on so many females is partially wasted. On the other hand, there would be only 2370 male controls for the 4550 male cases. It is generally inefficient to have strata in which the ratio of controls to cases varies substantially on either side of unity. The extreme form of such inefficiency occurs when there are many individual strata with one or more cases and no control subjects (control/case ratio

= 0) and other strata with one or more controls and no cases (control/case ratio = infinity). Such strata provide no information in a stratified analysis. If matching is used in the selection of controls, however, there will be fewer uninformative strata in a stratified analysis than there would have been in such an analysis without matching: A fixed number of matched controls for each case will provide an extremely efficient stratified analysis. The improved efficiency will be manifest in narrower confidence limits about the point estimate than would otherwise be obtainable. Matching in case-control studies can thus be considered a means of providing a more efficient stratified analysis rather than a direct means of preventing confounding. Stratification (or an equivalent multivariate approach) will be necessary to control confounding with or without matching, but matching makes the stratification more efficient.

The efficiency that matching provides in the analysis of case-control data comes at a substantial cost. One part of the cost is a research limitation: If a factor has been matched in a case-control study, it is no longer possible to estimate the effect of that factor, since its distribution is forced to be identical for cases and controls. Consequently, matching factors cannot be the objects of inquiry in a case-control study (except as effect modifiers—see pages 279–282, Evaluation of Effect Modification with Matched Data). Another cost is the added analytic complexity required to control confounding by factors that have not been matched. It is possible to control simultaneously for both matched and unmatched factors but usually only through specialized analyses, usually multivariate models. Conducting these analyses poses no serious difficulties in view of the growing availability of computers, but the investigator is forced to depend on computers and computer programs to analyze data that might otherwise have been analyzed in a more straightforward way.

A further cost involved with individual matching is the literal expense entailed in the process of choosing control subjects with the same distribution of matching factors found in the case series. If several factors are being matched, many potential control subjects must typically be scanned to find one that has the same characteristics as the case. Whereas this arduous process may lead to a statistically efficient analysis, it improves efficiency only at considerable expense.

If the efficiency of a study is judged from the point of view of the amount of information per subject studied (size efficiency), matching can be viewed as a means of improving study efficiency. Alternatively, if efficiency is judged as the amount of information per unit of cost involved in obtaining that information (cost efficiency), matching may paradoxically have the opposite effect of decreasing study efficiency, since the effort expended in finding matched subjects could be spent simply in gathering information for a greater number of unmatched subjects. With or without matching, confounding would have to be controlled in the data analysis. With matching, a stratified analysis would be more size efficient, but without it the resources for data collection can increase the number of subjects, thereby improving cost efficiency. Since cost efficiency is a more fundamental concern to an investigator than size efficiency, the apparent efficiency gains from matching may be illusory.

Thus the beneficial effect of matching on study efficiency, which is the primary reason for employing matching, appears to be ephemeral. Indeed, the decision to match subjects can result in less overall information, as measured by the width of the confidence interval for the effect measure, than would have been obtained without matching if the expense of matching reduces the total number of study subjects. A wider appreciation for the costs that matching imposes and the often meager advantages it offers would presumably persuade epidemiologists to avoid the technique in many settings in which matching is routinely used. Since the intended goal is to control confounding, and this goal is attainable only by proper analysis regardless of whether matching is employed, the routine use of matching is seldom justified.

Nevertheless, there are some situations in which matching is desirable or even necessary. If the process of obtaining the information from the study subjects is expensive, it is desirable to optimize the amount of information obtained per subject. For example, if exposure information in a case-control study involves an expensive laboratory test run on blood samples, the investigator would want the information from each subject to contribute as much as possible. As long as the expense of ascertaining matched controls is small compared with the expense of obtaining the exposure information from each subject, it is preferable to plan for a stratified analysis in which the stratification does not lead to loss of information, that is, it is desirable to match controls during subject selection so that there will be a uniform ratio of controls to cases in the stratified analysis. If no confounding is anticipated, of course, there is no need to match; for example, restriction of both series might prevent confounding without the need for stratification or matching. If confounding is likely, however, matching will ensure that control of confounding in the analysis will not lose information that has been expensively obtained. The essential difference that makes matching attractive in this situation is the high price of expanding the study size; when additional subjects are expensive to obtain, it is worthwhile to pay the cost of matching to take full advantage of the information that is collected. In such a situation, matching serves both size efficiency and cost efficiency.

Sometimes the control of confounding in the analysis is not possible unless matching has prepared the way to do so. Imagine a potential confounding factor that is measured on a nominal scale with many categories; examples would be variables such as neighborhood, sibship, and occupation. Controlling sibship would be impossible unless sibling controls had been selected for the cases, that is, matching on sibship is required to control for it. These variables are distinguished from other nominal scale variables such as sex by their multitude of categories, ensuring that one or very few subjects will fall into each category. Without matching, most strata in a stratified analysis would have only one subject, either a case or a control, and no information about effect unless control subjects had been matched to the cases for the value of the factor in question. Continuous variables such as age also have a multitude of values, but the values are easily combined by grouping, avoiding the fundamental problem. If the categories of a nominal scale variable could be combined in a reasonable way, the need for matching could be avoided. Methods to achieve this have been proposed [for example, see Miettinen, 1976], but they require a multivariate analysis as a preliminary step to the stratified analysis. Matching for nominal scale variables with many categories ensures that, after stratification by the potentially confounding factor, each case will have one or more matched controls for comparison.

A fundamental problem with stratified analysis is the inability to control confounding by several factors simultaneously. Control of each additional factor involves spreading the existing strata over a new dimension; the total number of strata required becomes exponentially large as the number of stratification variables increases. For studies with many confounding factors, the number of strata in a stratified analysis that controls all factors simultaneously may be so large that the situation mimics that in which there is a nominal scale confounder with a multitude of categories: There may be one or very few subjects per stratum and hardly any comparative information about the effect in any strata. If a large number of confounding factors is anticipated, matching may be desirable to ensure an informative stratified analysis. On the other hand, it is not absolutely necessary to match unless there are nominal scale variables with many categories, since a multivariate analysis can cope with confounding by many factors simultaneously even in situations in which stratification fails. Even multivariate analysis, however, is inadequate to control confounding by nominal scale variables with a large number of possible values unless matching has provided the necessary comparative information within categories.

We can summarize the utility of matching in case-control studies as follows: Matching is a useful means for improving study efficiency, in terms of the amount of information per subject studied, if the amount of information obtainable from the more efficient analysis exceeds the amount of information obtainable simply by studying more subjects without matching. Matching is indicated for potentially confounding factors that are measured on a nominal scale with many categories or when the number of potentially confounding variables is so great that stratification would spread the subjects too thinly over the strata. Multivariate analysis is a reasonable alternative in the latter situation; it would be feasible even without matching. Even multivariate analysis, however, is infeasible to control confounding by a nominal scale factor with many categories, unless matching is employed.

Overmatching

A term often used in reference to matched studies is *overmatching*. The interpretation of this term has changed with a sharper understanding of the principles that underlie matched studies. Originally, the term overmatching was used to refer to a loss of validity in a case-control study stemming from a control group that was so closely matched to the case group that the exposure distributions differed very little. This original interpretation for overmatching was based on a faulty analysis that failed to correct for confounding. On proper analysis, no validity problem whatsoever is introduced by matching. Note that in a follow-up study with matching even the crude analysis is valid, so that overmatching was never seen as a problem for follow-up studies. We have seen that indeed a validity problem does exist from matching in a case-control study if the crude data are used for inference. This problem disappears, however, if stratification by the matching factors is employed in the analysis.

The modern interpretation of overmatching relates to study efficiency rather than validity. Consider an individually matched case-control study with one control matched to each case. Each stratum in the analysis will consist of one case and one control unless some strata can be combined. A stratum cannot contribute information to a case-control analysis if any marginal total in the 2 × 2 table is equal to zero. If a case and a single matched control are either both exposed or both unexposed, one margin of the 2 × 2 table will be zero and that pair of subjects will not contribute any information to the analysis. If several controls are matched to a single case and all the controls have the same exposure value as the case, all exposed or all unexposed, the resulting zero margin likewise signals that the matched set of controls and case will not contribute to the analysis. Since matching is intended to select controls identical to the index case with respect to correlates of exposure, typically the information from many subjects is "lost" in a matched analysis. Obviously the loss of information detracts from study efficiency, reducing both information per subject studied and information per dollar spent. Matching has the net effect of increasing study efficiency only because stratified analysis in the absence of matching is ordinarily even less efficient than stratified analysis with matching. Recall, however, that matching in a case-control study can introduce confounding even if none exists in the source population, if the matching factor is correlated with the exposure but not with the disease. In such an instance, matching decreases study efficiency by locking the investigator into an analysis stratified by the matching factor, which will inevitably lose information on the matched sets with completely concordant exposure histories, whereas without matching a much more efficient crude analysis could have been used. Since the matching was not necessary in the first place and has the effect of impairing study efficiency relative to the type of analysis that could have been performed without matching, matching in this situation can properly be described as overmatching.

Overmatching is thus understood to be matching that causes a loss of information in the analysis because the resulting stratified analysis would have been unnecessary without matching. The extent to which information is lost by matching depends on the degree of correlation between the matching factor and the exposure. A strong correlate of exposure that has no relation to disease is the worst factor to match for, since it will lead to relatively few informative strata in the analysis with no offsetting gain. Consider, for example, a study of the relation between coffee drinking and cancer of the bladder; suppose matching for consumption of powdered cream-substitutes were considered along with matching for a set of other factors. Since this factor is a strong correlate of coffee consumption, many of the individual strata in the matched analysis will be completely concordant for coffee drinking and will not contribute to the analysis; that is, for many of the cases, controls matched to that case will be classified identically to the case with regard to coffee drinking simply because of matching for consumption of powdered cream-substitutes. If powdered cream-substitutes have no relation to bladder cancer, nothing is accomplished by the matching. Though no validity problem exists, the matching is counterproductive and can consequently be considered overmatching.

Matching on a risk factor that is not correlated with the exposure under study will not lead to an increased correlation of exposure histories for cases and controls. Such matching could nevertheless be considered overmatching because it adversely affects cost efficiency although it does not affect size efficiency. (Similarly, matching for any factor that is merely a consequence of disease can also be considered overmatching.) On the other hand, overmatching from a factor that is associated with exposure but not with the disease, such as indicators of opportunity for exposure [Poole, 1986], will reduce both cost efficiency and size efficiency, that is, an investigator will spend more to obtain information from the same number of subjects as he could have obtained without matching on the factor and will obtain less information per subject after having spent more. These losses in efficiency are suffered to control a factor that was not confounding anyway.

If a factor is a weak risk factor and a strong correlate of the exposure, it will be a weak confounder; matching for such a factor will involve a relatively large loss of information compared with a crude analysis because of the strong correlation with exposure. A crude analysis is no longer a proper alternative, however, if the factor is a genuine confounding factor. A reasonable alternative to matching of a confounding factor is a stratified analysis without matching. Matching theoretically improves efficiency by stabilizing the control-case ratio in the analysis, but it reduces efficiency by causing the loss of information in some strata in which the exposure information is concordant. If the elementary strata corresponding to each matched set have a reasonably large number of controls, complete concordance is unlikely; on the other hand, such concordance is very likely for matched pairs. If elementary strata can be combined in the analysis, a possibility when there are only a few matching factors with a modest number of categories, it is much less likely that there will be zero margins for the 2 × 2 tables in the analysis. The likelihood is further reduced if the matching factors are not strongly correlated with the exposure, although it should be remembered that the confounding that prompts matching depends on the magnitude of the association between the potential confounding factor and the exposure: With no association, there is no confounding. If it is thought that a study design would lead to many elementary strata with zero margins, then the value of matching in stabilizing the case-control ratio to improve study efficiency must be weighed against the loss of information from concordant exposure histories. It may be considered a form of overmatching to match on a weak confounding factor that is a strong correlate of exposure, since the matching itself is expensive and can lead to a less efficient analysis than the alternative of stratification without matching. The primary way to improve study efficiency when considering matching for a strong correlate of exposure is to increase the ratio of controls to cases, thereby decreasing the likelihood of a zero margin in the 2 × 2 table corresponding to each matched set.

Matching on Indicators of Information Quality

Another reason that matching is sometimes employed is to achieve comparability in the quality of information collected. A typical situation in which such matching might be undertaken is a case-control study in which some or all of the cases have already died, and surrogates must be interviewed for exposure and confounder information. In principle, controls for dead cases should be living, since they constitute a sample from the source population that gave rise to the cases. In practice, since surrogate interview data is usually presumed to differ in quality from interview data obtained directly from the subject, many investigators prefer to match dead controls to dead cases. It is not clear, however, that matching on information quality is justifiable. Whereas using dead controls can be justified in "proportional mortality" studies essentially as a convenience (see Chapter 6), there is no certainty that matching on information quality reduces overall bias. Many of the assumptions about the quality of surrogate data, for example, are unproved [Gordis, 1982]. Furthermore, comparability of information quality still allows bias from nondifferential misclassification, which is more severe in matched than in unmatched studies [Greenland, 1982], and can be more severe than the bias due to differential misclassification arising from noncomparability [Greenland and Robins, 1985b].

To summarize, the intricacies of matching in case-control studies and the relation of matching to confounding and study efficiency are much more complicated than one might at first suppose. Matching has often been employed when simpler and cheaper alternatives would have been preferable. Matching is clearly indicated only in sharply defined circumstances. In many study situations, the decision rests on cost and efficiency considerations that border on the imponderable.

MATCHED CASE-CONTROL ANALYSIS

The most important point in the analysis of matched case-control data is that matching introduces a bias in the crude estimate of effect toward the null value if the matching factor is correlated either positively or negatively with exposure, conditional on disease status. This bias may be viewed as a type of confounding, since it is present in the crude data, but it can be completely removed by stratifying by the matching factors. Therefore, the main task in a matched case-control analysis is to stratify by the matching factors.

Since stratification has already been discussed, there would be no need to elaborate further on matched case-control analysis but for one special feature of these analyses: Often the matching factor or factors have so many possible categories that the stratified analysis consists of one stratum for every case in the study. This feature introduces no new analytic concepts into the stratified analysis beyond those discussed in Chapter 12, but it does often lead to analyses with dozens or hundreds of strata. The formulas of Chapter 12 become tedious to apply by hand if the number of strata is large, but the formulas can be simplified for matched data so that their application with pencil and paper is not arduous even with thousands of strata.

If stratification could be accomplished without creating a large number of strata, a study with matching could be analyzed using an ordinary stratified approach. For example, if subjects are matched only for age and sex, there is no need to conduct a specialized "matched analysis" that amounts to creating individual strata for each matched set of subjects. It is sufficient to consider age and sex as confounding factors that need to be controlled in the analysis and to create only the few strata for age and sex that would have been necessary had no matching been undertaken in subject selection. Additional confounding factors can be easily controlled in such an analysis, even if they are not matching factors, by further stratification or multivariate analysis. Frequency matching is always handled using a "non-matched" analysis, that is, using the usual analytic techniques to control confounding. There is no special principle underlying the methods of a matched analysis. The need for a matched analysis is purely a practical one, stemming from the need to define strata in such a way that a large number of strata is inevitable, as is the case with an analysis in which a nominal scale variable with many categories is one of the matching variables. When such a variable is confounding, individual matching is needed to permit the control of confounding. In other situations, however, frequency matching or no matching at all is a better design option, since it is usually more cost efficient. Even if individual matching is employed, unless the number of categories in the analysis is inevitably large relative to the number of cases, there is no compulsion to use the methods of individually matched analysis as long as the matching factors are all controlled in the analysis.

Point Estimation of the Relative Risk (Odds Ratio) from Matched Case-Control Data

As usual for case-control data, the odds ratio, being an estimate of the incidence rate ratio or relative risk, is the measure of interest. Either the maximum likelihood or the Mantel-Haenszel approach may be used for estimation. The Mantel-Haenszel approach is simpler, but the maximum likelihood approach is not as complicated for matched data as it is for the usual stratified analysis.

Maximum likelihood estimation of the odds ratio in a stratified analysis can be "conditional" on both margins of the 2 × 2 tables or "unconditional," which means conditional on only one margin of the 2 × 2 table. The two approaches give nearly identical results except when the average number of subjects per stratum is small, in which case the unconditional approach can be substantially biased and should not be used [Breslow, 1981; Lubin, 1981]. Matched analyses are the extreme form of stratified analysis in the sense of having the fewest possible subjects per stratum. One case and one control per stratum is the minimum requirement, but studies in which all the strata are matched pairs can nevertheless be extremely informative. For matched analyses, the applicable likelihood methods are those based on the conditional likelihood.

POINT ESTIMATION OF RELATIVE RISK FROM MATCHED CASE-CONTROL PAIRS
When a single control is matched individually to each case, the elementary strata in the analysis are 2 × 2 tables with only two subjects. For a dichotomous exposure, only four possible exposure patterns exist for the two subjects: both exposed, both unexposed, case exposed and control unexposed, and case unexposed and control exposed. These four exposure patterns are shown in Table 13-5. Note that when the exposure history is identical for the case and the control, there is a marginal total equal to zero in the 2 × 2 table. The first and last of the 2 × 2 tables in Table 13-5, A and D, have a zero marginal total and consequently do not contribute to either estimation or statistical hypothesis testing.

The conditional maximum likelihood estimate of the odds ratio is simply the frequency of matched sets of type B divided by the frequency of sets of type C, that is, the ratio of the number of discordant pairs in which the case is exposed to the number of discordant pairs in which the control is exposed. This estimator can be derived easily as follows: If the odds

Table 13-5. *Possible patterns of exposure for a case and a single matched control*

	A			B			C			D		
	E	U	T	E	U	T	E	U	T	E	U	T
Case	1	0	1	1	0	1	0	1	1	0	1	1
Control	1	0	1	0	1	1	1	0	1	0	1	1
Totals	2	0	2	1	1	2	1	1	2	0	2	2

E = exposed; U = unexposed; T = total.

ratio is designated as OR, then from the noncentral hypergeometric distribution (see Chap. 11) the probability of a 2 × 2 table of type B is OR/(OR + 1) and the probability of a table of type C is 1/(OR + 1). Let the frequency of discordant pairs in which the case is exposed be f_{10} and the frequency of discordant pairs in which the control is exposed be f_{01}. Since a discordant pair must contribute either to f_{10} or to f_{01}, we can treat the distribution of discordant pairs of type B as binomial; the likelihood of observing exactly f_{10} type B pairs, given that there are $f_{10} + f_{01}$ discordant pairs is then

$$Pr = \binom{f_{10} + f_{01}}{f_{10}} \left(\frac{OR}{OR + 1}\right)^{f_{10}} \left(\frac{1}{OR + 1}\right)^{f_{01}} \qquad [13\text{-}1]$$

The maximum likelihood estimator of the OR is derived by maximizing the above expression with respect to the OR. The maximization is equivalent to maximizing the logarithm of expression 13-1,

$$\ln(Pr) = \ln\binom{f_{10} + f_{01}}{f_{10}} + f_{10} \ln\left(\frac{OR}{OR + 1}\right) + f_{01} \ln\left(\frac{1}{OR + 1}\right)$$

Taking the derivative and setting it equal to zero gives

$$\frac{d(\ln(Pr))}{d(OR)} = 0 = f_{10} - (\hat{OR})f_{01}$$

$$\hat{OR} = \frac{f_{10}}{f_{01}} \qquad [13\text{-}2]$$

which is the conditional maximum likelihood estimator.

Alternatively, the Mantel-Haenszel estimator of the odds ratio can be used (formula 12-26). For each table of type B, $a_i d_i / T_i = \frac{1}{2}$ and $b_i c_i / T_i = 0$. For each table of type C, $a_i d_i / T_i = 0$ and $b_i c_i / T_i = \frac{1}{2}$. Therefore the Mantel-Haenszel estimator for matched-pair data is

$$\widehat{OR}_{MH} = \frac{\Sigma a_i d_i / T_i}{\Sigma b_i c_i / T_i} = \frac{\frac{1}{2} f_{10}}{\frac{1}{2} f_{01}} = \frac{f_{10}}{f_{01}}$$

the same expression as the maximum likelihood estimator.

POINT ESTIMATION OF RELATIVE RISK WITH R CONTROLS MATCHED TO EACH CASE

For the more general situation of R controls matched to each case, there is a larger number of possible exposure patterns, the exact number depending on the value of R. Considering all R controls as equivalent, there are R + 1 different outcomes possible for each matched set of controls, corresponding to the number of controls in the matched set that are exposed and ranging from zero exposed at one extreme to R exposed at the other extreme. Since the case can be either exposed or unexposed, the total number of possible exposure patterns is 2 (R + 1). A convenient way to summarize the data is simply to tally the frequency of matched sets with each exposure pattern, using the notation of Table 13-6.

The frequency f_{00} is the number of matched sets with no exposed subjects: these elementary strata have a zero marginal total and do not contribute to the analysis. Similarly, f_{1R} refers to the sets with no unexposed subjects; these sets also have a zero marginal total and do not contribute to the analysis. The remaining 2R types of sets are all informative sets, representing elementary 2×2 tables with nonzero marginal totals. Note that as R increases, the probability that a given set will be informative also increases, since the likelihood that all the controls will have the same exposure as the case becomes smaller. If there is a 90 percent probability that a matched control has an exposure history concordant with that of the case, the probability that the matched set for that case will contribute to the analysis ranges from 10 percent for R = 1 to $1 - (0.9)^5 = 41$ percent for R = 5. If a matched control has an 80 percent probability of having a concordant exposure, the probability that a set is informative ranges from 20 percent for R = 1 to 67 percent for R = 5.

Let us denote the total number of exposed subjects in a matched set as m. The value of m ranges from zero to R + 1, but the informative sets are

Table 13-6. Data summary for R controls matched to each case, indicating the frequency (f_{ij}) of matched sets with every possible exposure pattern

	No. exposed controls					
	0	1	2	3	...	R
Exposed cases	f_{10}	f_{11}	f_{12}	f_{13}	...	f_{1R}
Unexposed cases	f_{00}	f_{01}	f_{02}	f_{03}	...	f_{0R}

those for which $1 \leq m \leq R$, keeping all marginal totals nonzero. For a given value of m, there are two possible patterns of exposure for the matched set, corresponding to the case being exposed and $m - 1$ controls being exposed, or the case not being exposed and m controls being exposed. From the noncentral hypergeometric distribution, the probability that the case is exposed, given m exposed subjects, is

$$\text{Pr(case is exposed, given m)} = \frac{m(OR)}{R + 1 - m + m(OR)}$$

$$= \frac{OR}{\dfrac{R + 1 - m}{m} + OR} \qquad [13\text{-}3]$$

and the probability that the case is unexposed is the complement,

$$\text{Pr(case is unexposed, given m)} = \frac{(R + 1 - m)/m}{\dfrac{R + 1 - m}{m} + OR} \qquad [13\text{-}4]$$

It is again convenient to consider the observations as following a binomial distribution, but with R-to-1 matching there is a separate binomial distribution for each value of m. Thus, for $m = 1$, there is a total of $f_{10} + f_{01}$ sets, and, given that exactly one subject in a set is exposed, the probability of exposure is $OR/(OR + R)$, from equation 13-3. The probability of observing exactly f_{10} and f_{01} sets with the case exposed and unexposed, respectively, given a total of $f_{10} + f_{01}$ sets with one exposed subject, is

$$\text{Pr} = \binom{f_{10} + f_{01}}{f_{10}} \left(\frac{OR}{OR + R}\right)^{f_{10}} \left(\frac{R}{OR + R}\right)^{f_{01}}$$

The overall likelihood for the data is the product of the binomial probabilities corresponding to each value of m from 1 to R:

$$\text{Pr} = \prod_{m=1}^{R} \binom{f_{1,m-1} + f_{0,m}}{f_{1,m-1}} \left(\frac{OR}{(R + 1 - m)/m + OR}\right)^{f_{1,m-1}}$$
$$\cdot \left(\frac{(R + 1 - m)/m}{(R + 1 - m)/m + OR}\right)^{f_{0,m}} \qquad [13\text{-}5]$$

The logarithm of the above likelihood expression is

$$\ln(\text{Pr}) = \sum_{m=1}^{R} \left[\ln\binom{f_{1,m-1} + f_{0,m}}{f_{1,m-1}} + f_{1,m-1} \ln\left(\frac{OR}{(R + 1 - m)/m + OR}\right) \right.$$

$$+ f_{0,m} \ln\left(\frac{(R + 1 - m)/m}{(R + 1 - m)/m + OR}\right)\Bigg]$$

Taking the derivative of the above expression with regard to the OR and setting it equal to zero yields the equation for the conditional maximum likelihood solution for the OR [Miettinen, 1970]:

$$\frac{\sum_{m=1}^{R} f_{1,m-1}}{\hat{OR}} - \sum_{m=1}^{R} \frac{f_{1,m-1} + f_{0,m}}{(R + 1 - m)/m + \hat{OR}} = 0 \qquad [13\text{-}6]$$

Equation 13-6 reduces to equation 13-2 for $R = 1$. For $R = 2$, it can be solved explicitly for $\hat{OR}$ [Miettinen, 1970], but for values of R greater than 2 an iterative solution is necessary. Even so, equation 13-6 represents a rather simple computational exercise compared with the onerous computations needed to obtain a conditional maximum likelihood estimate of the odds ratio for unmatched stratified data.

The data in Example 13-1 represent the individual exposure values for each subject in a matched case-control study with 18 cases and four controls matched to each case. The cases were women with ectopic pregnancy; controls were women without ectopic pregnancy drawn from the same source population and matched individually to the cases for number of pregnancies, age, and husband's level of education. All subjects had had at least one previous pregnancy. A positive history indicates that the woman had at least one induced abortion.

If only the first control had been matched to each case, the investigators would have observed nine concordant pairs (four concordant pairs with positive exposure histories and five with negative exposure histories) and nine discordant pairs. In eight of the discordant pairs the case is exposed, compared with only one in which the control is exposed, giving a relative risk estimate of $8/1 = 8$. Considering all controls that were studied, there are $2(4 + 1) = 10$ types of exposure patterns for the matched sets. The distribution of exposure patterns for the data in Example 13-1 is shown in Table 13-7.

Six of the matched sets have completely concordant exposure histories and so are noncontributory to the analysis. The data from the remaining sets can be used to estimate the odds ratio, or relative risk, of ectopic pregnancy after induced abortion by substituting into equation 13-6:

$$\frac{11}{\hat{OR}} - \frac{4}{\hat{OR} + 4} - \frac{5}{\hat{OR} + 3/2} - \frac{3}{\hat{OR} + 2/3} = 0$$

A trial and error solution gives $\hat{OR} = 23$.

Example 13-1. Previous history of induced abortion among women with ectopic pregnancy and matched controls. Data of Trichopoulous et al. [Miettinen, 1969]

Case	Control 1	2	3	4
−	−	−	−	−
+	−	+	−	−
+	−	−	−	−
−	−	−	−	−
−	+	−	−	−
+	−	−	−	−
+	−	−	−	−
−	−	−	−	−
+	+	−	−	+
+	−	+	−	−
+	−	+	+	−
−	−	−	−	−
+	+	+	+	+
+	−	−	+	−
+	−	−	+	−
+	+	−	−	−
−	−	−	−	−
+	+	−	−	+

+ = previous induced abortion; − = no previous induced abortion.

Table 13-7. Pattern of exposure for the 18 matched sets in example 13-1

	No. exposed controls				
	0	1	2	3	4
Exposed cases	3	5	3	0	1
Unexposed cases	5	1	0	0	0

An alternative to the maximum likelihood approach to estimation is the Mantel-Haenszel approach. When the matching ratio exceeds one control per case, the two approaches are not identical. With R-to-1 matching, formula 12-26 can be rewritten as follows:

$$\hat{OR}_{MH} = \frac{\sum\limits_{m=1}^{R} (R + 1 - m)f_{1,m-1}}{\sum\limits_{m=1}^{R} mf_{0,m}} \qquad [13\text{-}7]$$

Applying formula 13-7 to the data in Table 13-7 gives

$$\widehat{OR}_{MH} = \frac{4(3) + 3(5) + 2(3)}{1(1)} = \frac{33}{1} = 33$$

which differs noticeably from the conditional maximum likelihood estimate of 23. The large difference between the two estimates is attributable to the fact that there are only 12 informative sets, and 11 of these are supportive of a positive association, representing an extreme result with somewhat scanty data. Consequently, it is not surprising that two different estimators give somewhat discrepant results. Breslow [1981] has shown that statistically the Mantel-Haenszel estimator is consistent for matched data, is as efficient as the conditional maximum likelihood approach when the OR = 1, and is nearly as efficient over a wide range of conditions.

POINT ESTIMATION OF RELATIVE RISK WITH A VARYING NUMBER OF CONTROLS MATCHED TO EACH CASE

With a varying number of controls matched to each case, the data can be summarized by a set of displays like the one in Table 13-6, each one corresponding to a different value of R. The likelihood for the data is the product of the likelihood expressions corresponding to each value of R, and the equation that yields the maximum likelihood estimate of the OR is a simple extension of equation 13-6:

$$\sum_{R} \left[\frac{\sum_{m=1}^{R} f_{1,m-1}}{\widehat{OR}} - \sum_{m=1}^{R} \frac{f_{1,m-1} + f_{0,m}}{(R + 1 - m)/m + \widehat{OR}} \right] = 0 \qquad [13-8]$$

The data in Example 13-2 are derived from a study of myocardial infarction and history of coffee consumption [Jick et al., 1973]. The authors attempted to match two controls to each case, but for 27 cases only one

Example 13-2. Distribution of cases of myocardial infarction and matched controls according to amount of coffee drinking; subjects drinking one to five cups of coffee per day were excluded [Jick et al., 1973]

| | No. controls drinking 6+ cups/day | | | | |
| | Matched pairs | | Matched triplets | | |
	0	1	0	1	2
Cases					
6+ cups/day	8	8	16	23	4
0 cups/day	8	3	20	22	3

matched control was available. The resulting data consist of 27 matched pairs and 88 matched triplets. The use of these data and equation 13-8 to determine the maximum likelihood estimate of the odds ratio produces the following likelihood equation:

$$\left[\frac{8}{\hat{OR}} - \frac{11}{\hat{OR} + 1}\right] + \left[\frac{39}{\hat{OR}} - \frac{38}{\hat{OR} + 2} - \frac{26}{\hat{OR} + 1/2}\right] = 0$$

Solving the above equation by trial and error gives $\hat{OR} = 2.0$.

The generalization of formula 13-7 for the Mantel-Haenszel estimator of the odds ratio with matched case-control data having a varying number of controls, R, matched to each case can be derived easily from formula 12-26:

$$\hat{OR}_{MH} = \frac{\sum_{R} \sum_{m=1}^{R} \frac{(R + 1 - m)f_{1,m-1}}{R + 1}}{\sum_{R} \sum_{m=1}^{R} \frac{mf_{0,m}}{R + 1}}$$

[13-9]

Applying the above formula to the data of Example 13-2 gives the Mantel-Haenszel estimate as

$$\hat{OR}_{MH} = \frac{8/2 + [2(16) + 23]/3}{3/2 + [22 + 2(3)]/3} = 2.1$$

which is nearly identical to the maximum likelihood estimate and is considerably easier to obtain.

Statistical Hypothesis Testing with Matched Case-Control Data

Since the analysis of matched case-control data is equivalent to an analysis stratifying the data according to the matching factors, hypothesis testing for matched data is accomplished simply by applying the general approach for stratified data to the strata defined by the matching. As with point estimation, some of the formulas can be simplified for matching because the 2×2 tables can have only a limited number of configurations; since a matched analysis typically involves many strata, the simplifications may prove important. Even the two tableaus for displaying the data in Example 13-2 illustrate this point because they summarize data on 115 strata, corresponding to the 115 matched sets.

HYPOTHESIS TESTING FOR MATCHED CASE-CONTROL PAIRS

For matched pairs, an exact P-value can be calculated from equation 13-1 by setting OR = 1 and calculating the tail probability. This calculation is simply the tail probability of a binomial distribution with a probability of 0.5 for each binomial trial. The tail probability for the Fisher P-value is

$$\text{Fisher } P = \sum_{k=f_{10}}^{f_{10}+f_{01}} \binom{f_{10} + f_{01}}{k} \left(\frac{1}{2}\right)^{f_{10} + f_{01}} \quad [13\text{-}10]$$

for $f_{10} \geq f_{01}$. If $f_{01} > f_{10}$, then the lower tail should be calculated by summing over the range $0 \leq k \leq f_{10}$.

To get the exact mid-P value, only half the probability of the observed data should be included. For the upper tail, this modification gives

$$\text{Mid-}P = \frac{1}{2} \binom{f_{10} + f_{01}}{f_{10}} \left(\frac{1}{2}\right)^{f_{10} + f_{01}} + \sum_{k=f_{10}+1}^{f_{10}+f_{01}} \binom{f_{10} + f_{01}}{k} \left(\frac{1}{2}\right)^{f_{10} + f_{01}} \quad [13\text{-}11]$$

If $f_{01} > f_{10}$, then the lower tail should be calculated by summing over the range $0 \leq k \leq f_{10} - 1$.

Consider the data in Example 13-2 relating just to matched pairs. The 16 pairs for which the exposure history was concordant do not contribute to the evaluation and should be ignored. Of the remaining 11 pairs, 8 are discordant with the case exposed. The exact Fisher one-tail P-value is, from formula 13-10,

$$\binom{11}{8} \left(\frac{1}{2}\right)^{11} + \binom{11}{9} \left(\frac{1}{2}\right)^{11} + \binom{11}{10} \left(\frac{1}{2}\right)^{11} + \binom{11}{11} \left(\frac{1}{2}\right)^{11}$$

$$= 0.0806 + 0.0269 + 0.0054 + 0.0005 = 0.11$$

The mid-P value is the same summation except for the first term, which would be $\frac{1}{2}(0.0806)$, giving a one-tail P-value of 0.07.

An approximate P-value can be calculated using the Mantel-Haenszel test statistic (formula 12-38). For matched pairs, the Mantel-Haenszel test simplifies to

$$\chi = \frac{f_{10} - f_{01}}{\sqrt{f_{10} + f_{01}}} \quad [13\text{-}12]$$

which is a form of the test first described by McNemar [1947] and often referred to as the McNemar test.

For the matched pair data in Example 13-2, this test formula gives

$$\chi = \frac{8 - 3}{\sqrt{11}} = 1.51$$

which corresponds to a one-tail P-value of 0.07, agreeing well with the exact mid-P value even for these apparently small numbers.

HYPOTHESIS TESTING FOR R CONTROLS MATCHED TO EACH CASE

Exact hypothesis testing for R controls matched to each case is considerably more complicated than hypothesis testing for matched pairs. The data can be considered a set of R binomial distributions with the likelihood function expressed in formula 13-5. For hypothesis testing, the value of the odds ratio in expression 13-5 is set equal to unity. The upper tail probability is determined by evaluating formula 13-5 for every possible distribution of the data for which the number of exposed cases is equal to or greater than the number observed (the exposed cases for whom all matched controls are also exposed can be ignored). The exact Fisher P-value is therefore

Fisher upper-tail probability

$$= \sum_{k=a}^{M_1} \prod_{m=1}^{R} \binom{f_{1,m-1} + f_{0,m}}{k_m} \left(\frac{m}{R+1}\right)^{k_m} \left(\frac{R+1-m}{R+1}\right)^{f_{1,m-1}+f_{0,m}-k_m} \qquad [13\text{-}13]$$

where a is the total number of exposed cases in sets with at least one unexposed control, M_1 is the total number of sets that are not completely concordant, k_m is the permutation of the possible number of exposed cases with $m - 1$ exposed controls, i.e., the total number of exposed cases that could have been observed among matched sets that actually had m exposed subjects, and k is the sum of k_m:

$$a = \sum_{m=1}^{R} f_{1,m-1}$$

$$M_1 = \sum_{m=1}^{R} f_{1,m-1} + f_{0,m}$$

$$k = \sum_{m=1}^{R} k_m$$

The tail summation includes all the combinations of the data that could give rise to all the values of k in the range from a to M_1. For the lower tail probability, the range of summation for k is from 0 to a.

To obtain the exact mid-P value, it is necessary to include only half the probability for $k = a$, as follows:

Mid-P upper tail probability

$$= \frac{1}{2} \sum_{k=a}^{R} \prod_{m=1}^{R} \binom{f_{1,m-1} + f_{0,m}}{k_m} \left(\frac{m}{R+1}\right)^{k_m} \left(\frac{R+1-m}{R+1}\right)^{f_{1,m-1}+f_{0,m}-k_m}$$

$$+ \sum_{k=a+1}^{M_1} \prod_{m=1}^{R} \binom{f_{1,m-1} + f_{0,m}}{k_m} \left(\frac{m}{R+1}\right)^{k_m} \left(\frac{R+1-m}{R+1}\right)^{f_{1,m-1}+f_{0,m}-k_m} \qquad [13\text{-}14]$$

For the lower tail mid-P value, the second summation in equation 13-14 should be for $0 \leqslant k \leqslant a - 1$ rather than $a + 1 \leqslant k \leqslant M_1$.

Consider the data in Example 13-1 (Table 13-7). Disregarding the exposed case that had four exposed matched controls, there are 11 exposed cases, so $a = 11$. The total number of informative sets, M_1, is $3 + 5 + 3 + 0 + 1 + 0 + 0 + 0 = 12$. There is only one set of values for $\{k_m\}$ for which every informative set has an exposed case; since there are four, five, three, and zero sets, respectively, for $m = 1, 2, 3$, and 4, the values of k_m would be 4, 5, 3, and 0, respectively, to obtain the most extreme outcome, with all the cases exposed. There are three different patterns that could yield $\Sigma k_m = 11$. These are, starting with the observed pattern, 3, 5, 3, 0; 4, 4, 3, 0; and 4, 5, 2, 0. Thus the upper tail has four possible outcomes in it, including the observed data; there are two equally extreme outcomes, and one more extreme outcome.

Let us calculate the probability of each of these four outcomes. Consider first the most extreme outcome, 4, 5, 3, 0. The probability is, using expression 13-13,

$$\binom{4}{4}\left(\frac{1}{5}\right)^4\left(\frac{4}{5}\right)^0 \cdot \binom{5}{5}\left(\frac{2}{5}\right)^5\left(\frac{3}{5}\right)^0 \cdot \binom{3}{3}\left(\frac{3}{5}\right)^3\left(\frac{2}{5}\right)^0$$

$$= \left(\frac{1}{5}\right)^4\left(\frac{2}{5}\right)^5\left(\frac{3}{5}\right)^3 = 0.00000354$$

For the observed data, the probability is

$$\binom{4}{3}\left(\frac{1}{5}\right)^3\left(\frac{4}{5}\right)^1 \cdot \binom{5}{5}\left(\frac{2}{5}\right)^5\left(\frac{3}{5}\right)^0 \cdot \binom{3}{3}\left(\frac{3}{5}\right)^3\left(\frac{2}{5}\right)^0$$

$$= 4 \cdot 4 \left(\frac{1}{5}\right)^4\left(\frac{2}{5}\right)^5\left(\frac{3}{5}\right)^3 = 0.00005662$$

For the remaining two possible outcomes, the probabilities are

$$\binom{4}{4}\left(\frac{1}{5}\right)^4\left(\frac{4}{5}\right)^0 \cdot \binom{5}{4}\left(\frac{2}{5}\right)^4\left(\frac{3}{5}\right)^1 \cdot \binom{3}{3}\left(\frac{3}{5}\right)^3\left(\frac{2}{5}\right)^0$$

$$= 5 \left(\frac{1}{5}\right)^4\left(\frac{2}{5}\right)^4\left(\frac{3}{5}\right)^4 = 0.00002654$$

and

$$\binom{4}{4}\left(\frac{1}{5}\right)^4\left(\frac{4}{5}\right)^0 \cdot \binom{5}{5}\left(\frac{2}{5}\right)^5\left(\frac{3}{5}\right)^0 \cdot \binom{3}{2}\left(\frac{3}{5}\right)^2\left(\frac{2}{5}\right)^1$$

$$= 3 \left(\frac{1}{5}\right)^4\left(\frac{2}{5}\right)^6\left(\frac{3}{5}\right)^2 = 0.00000708$$

The sum of the probabilities for the four possible outcomes is 0.000094, which is the upper Fisher exact P-value. The upper mid-P would include just half the probability for the outcomes for which $\Sigma k_m = 11$, namely,

$$\frac{1}{2} (0.00005662 + 0.00002654 + 0.00000708) + 0.00000354 = 0.000049$$

which is barely more than half of the Fisher exact P-value, since the observed outcome is the second most extreme possible outcome in the upper tail.

Approximate hypothesis testing for R controls matched to each case can once again be performed with the Mantel-Haenszel test (formula 12-38). With one case and R controls in each stratum, the test can be rewritten in terms of the distribution of matched sets as

$$\chi = \frac{\displaystyle\sum_{m=1}^{R} \left[f_{1,m-1} - \frac{m}{R+1} (f_{1,m-1} + f_{0,m}) \right]}{\sqrt{\displaystyle\sum_{m=1}^{R} (f_{1,m-1} + f_{0,m}) \frac{m(R+1-m)}{(R+1)^2}}} \qquad [13\text{-}15]$$

For the data in Table 13-7, the above formula yields

$$\chi = \frac{11 - \dfrac{23}{5}}{\sqrt{\dfrac{16}{25} + \dfrac{30}{25} + \dfrac{18}{25}}} = 4.0$$

which corresponds to a one-tail P-value of 0.00003. This value agrees reasonably well with the exact upper mid-P value considering the small numbers involved and the extremeness of the observed outcome.

HYPOTHESIS TESTING WITH A VARYING NUMBER OF CONTROLS MATCHED TO EACH CASE

Formulas 13-13 and 13-14 can be easily extended to accommodate a varying ratio of controls to cases by taking the product of the binomial probabilities over all values for R:

Fisher upper-tail probability

$$= \sum_{k=a}^{M_1} \prod_{R} \prod_{m=1}^{R} \binom{f_{1,m-1} + f_{0,m}}{k_m} \left(\frac{m}{R+1} \right)^{k_m} \left(\frac{R+1-m}{R+1} \right)^{f_{1,m-1} + f_{0,m} - k_m} \qquad [13\text{-}16]$$

Mid-P upper-tail probability

$$= \frac{1}{2} \sum_{k=a}^{R} \prod_{R} \prod_{m=1}^{R} \binom{f_{1,m-1} + f_{0,m}}{k_m} \left(\frac{m}{R+1}\right)^{k_m} \left(\frac{R+1-m}{R+1}\right)^{f_{1,m-1}+f_{0,m}-k_m}$$

$$+ \sum_{k=a+1}^{M_1} \prod_{R} \prod_{m=1}^{R} \binom{f_{1,m-1} + f_{0,m}}{k_m} \left(\frac{m}{R+1}\right)^{k_m} \left(\frac{R+1-m}{R+1}\right)^{f_{1,m-1}+f_{0,m}-k_m} \qquad [13\text{-}17]$$

where the notation is identical to that of formulas 13-13 and 13-14. Although formulas 13-16 and 13-17 are similar to formulas 13-13 and 13-14, their application is considerably more difficult because the number of possible outcomes corresponding to each value of k can be high. In Example 13-2, there is one binomial for R = 1 and two binomials for R = 2 to consider in the calculations; the total number of possible outcomes for the three binomials is 11 × 38 × 26 = 10,868. Of these, 3522 are in the upper-tail summation for formulas 13-16 and 13-17. There are 279 combinations of the three binomials that yield exactly 47 exposed cases, the observed number. Taking the sum of 3522 terms, each of which is the product of three binomial probabilities, is a task for a computer. An evaluation of expression 13-16 for the data in Example 13-2 gives 0.0038 for the upper-tail Fisher P-value and 0.0028 for the upper mid-P value.

The approximate test statistic in formula 13-15 can also be easily extended to accommodate a varying number of controls by taking the sums in the numerator and denominator over the values of R:

$$\chi = \frac{\displaystyle\sum_{R}\sum_{m=1}^{R}\left[f_{1,m-1} - \frac{m}{R+1}(f_{1,m-1}+f_{0,m})\right]}{\sqrt{\displaystyle\sum_{R}\sum_{m=1}^{R}(f_{1,m-1}+f_{0,m})\frac{m(R+1-m)}{(R+1)^2}}} \qquad [13\text{-}18]$$

For example 13-2, the approximate formula above gives

$$\chi = \frac{8 - \left(\frac{1}{2}\right)(11) + 16 - \left(\frac{1}{3}\right)(38) + 23 - \left(\frac{2}{3}\right)(26)}{\sqrt{11\left(\frac{1}{4}\right) + 38\left(\frac{2}{9}\right) + 26\left(\frac{2}{9}\right)}} = 2.79$$

which corresponds to a one-tail P-value of 0.0026, in close agreement with the upper mid-P value.

Interval Estimation of the Odds Ratio with Matched Case-Control Data
INTERVAL ESTIMATION FOR MATCHED CASE-CONTROL PAIRS

Exact confidence limits for the odds ratio from matched case-control pairs can be calculated based on the probability distribution of the possible discordant pairs, conditional on the total number of discordant pairs, by expressing the probability as a function of the odds ratio (see formula 13-1):

$$\alpha/2 = \sum_{k=f_{10}}^{f_{10}+f_{01}} \binom{f_{10}+f_{01}}{k} \left(\frac{OR}{OR+1}\right)^k \left(\frac{1}{OR+1}\right)^{f_{10}+f_{01}-k} \qquad [13\text{-}19]$$

$$1 - \alpha/2 = \sum_{k=f_{10}+1}^{f_{10}+f_{01}} \binom{f_{10}+f_{01}}{k} \left(\frac{\overline{OR}}{\overline{OR}+1}\right)^k \left(\frac{1}{\overline{OR}+1}\right)^{f_{10}+f_{01}-k} \qquad [13\text{-}20]$$

The above formulas, when solved for $\underline{OR}$ and $\overline{OR}$, give the exact Fisher confidence limits. To obtain the mid-P exact confidence limits, only half the probability that $k = f_{10}$ is added to the tail:

$$\alpha/2 = \frac{1}{2} \binom{f_{10}+f_{01}}{f_{10}} \left(\frac{OR}{OR+1}\right)^{f_{10}} \left(\frac{1}{OR+1}\right)^{f_{01}}$$
$$+ \sum_{k=f_{10}+1}^{f_{10}+f_{01}} \binom{f_{10}+f_{01}}{k} \left(\frac{OR}{OR+1}\right)^k \left(\frac{1}{OR+1}\right)^{f_{10}+f_{01}-k} \qquad [13\text{-}21]$$

and

$$1 - \alpha/2 = \frac{1}{2} \binom{f_{10}+f_{01}}{f_{10}} \left(\frac{\overline{OR}}{\overline{OR}+1}\right)^{f_{10}} \left(\frac{1}{\overline{OR}+1}\right)^{f_{01}}$$
$$+ \sum_{k=f_{10}+1}^{f_{10}+f_{01}} \binom{f_{10}+f_{01}}{k} \left(\frac{\overline{OR}}{\overline{OR}+1}\right)^k \left(\frac{1}{\overline{OR}+1}\right)^{f_{10}+f_{01}-k} \qquad [13\text{-}22]$$

The solution of equations 13-19 and 13-20 or 13-21 and 13-22 amounts to finding the exact confidence limits for a binomial parameter, p, which is a function of the odds ratio: $p = OR/(OR + 1)$. Consider the data in Example 13-2 relating to matched pairs. With 11 discordant pairs, 8 of which have an exposed case, the calculation of exact confidence limits for the odds ratio corresponds to setting exact confidence limits for the binomial parameter estimated by eight successes in 11 trials. The Fisher exact 90 percent confidence limits are, from formulas 13-19 and 13-20, 0.4356 and 0.9212 for the binomial parameter, which correspond to a 90 percent exact Fisher confidence interval of 0.77 and 11.7 for the odds ratio. If formulas 13-21 and 13-22 are used to get the mid-P exact limits, the results are 0.4702 and 0.9030 for the binomial parameter, corresponding to 0.89 and 9.31 for the 90 percent exact limits for the odds ratio. The wide limits reflect the small number of discordant pairs.

Approximate confidence limits for matched case-control pairs can be determined in several ways. One approach is to determine the confidence limits for the probability that a discordant pair has an exposed case, based on the large sample characteristics of the binomial distribution, and then convert these confidence limits to the corresponding limits for the odds ratio. Other approaches include the large sample characteristics of maximum likelihood estimators, the formula by Robins et al. [1986] for the variance of the logarithm of the Mantel-Haenszel estimate (formula 12-58), and the test-based procedure.

First let us consider basing the approximation on the sampling distribution of the binomial distribution, which has a variance of pq/n for large n, where n is the number of binomial trials, p is the probability of a "success," and $q = 1 - p$. For matched case-control pairs, $\hat{p} = f_{10}/(f_{10} + f_{01})$, and confidence limits for $\hat{p}$ can be approximated by

$$\frac{f_{10}}{f_{10} + f_{01}} \pm Z \sqrt{\frac{f_{10}f_{01}}{(f_{10} + f_{01})^3}} \qquad [13\text{-}23]$$

where Z is the value of the standard normal distribution corresponding to the desired level of confidence, the plus sign gives the upper confidence limit, and the minus sign gives the lower confidence limit. The corresponding limits for the odds ratio are given by $\underline{OR} = p/(1 - p)$ and $\overline{OR} = \bar{p}/(1 - \bar{p})$, or

$$\underline{OR} = \frac{\dfrac{f_{10}}{f_{10} + f_{01}} - Z \sqrt{\dfrac{f_{10}f_{01}}{(f_{10} + f_{01})^3}}}{1 - \dfrac{f_{10}}{f_{10} + f_{01}} + Z \sqrt{\dfrac{f_{10}f_{01}}{(f_{10} + f_{01})^3}}} \qquad [13\text{-}24]$$

$$\overline{OR} = \frac{\dfrac{f_{10}}{f_{10} + f_{01}} + Z \sqrt{\dfrac{f_{10}f_{01}}{(f_{10} + f_{01})^3}}}{1 - \dfrac{f_{10}}{f_{10} + f_{01}} - Z \sqrt{\dfrac{f_{10}f_{01}}{(f_{10} + f_{01})^3}}} \qquad [13\text{-}25]$$

The above approximate confidence limits are simple to calculate, but they are inaccurate unless the number of discordant pairs is reasonably large. For values of the odds ratio that are far from the null value, the number of discordant pairs must be very large for the approximation to be adequate. The difficulty is that the binomial distribution does not approximate a normal distribution very well if the number of trials is modest, especially if the probability of a success is far from 0.5. Formula 13-23 always produces confidence limits for p that are symmetric about $\hat{p}$ despite the fact that the sampling distribution can be strikingly asymmetric for values of p that depart from 0.5, the center of the range of the distribution. It is possible to calculate a confidence interval from formula 13-23 with a boundary outside the admissible range of 0 to 1 for p. For example, if two successes were observed in 10 trials, formula 13-23 gives a 90 percent confidence interval for $\hat{p}$ with a lower bound of -0.008; eight successes in 10 trials would give, from the same formula, an upper bound of 1.008. These limits outside the admissible range for p correspond to negative values of the odds ratio as determined from formulas 13-24 and 13-25.

A more accurate method for obtaining approximate confidence limits for the binomial parameter was proposed by Wilson [1927]. This approach takes into account the asymmetry of the distribution and consequently never gives results outside the admissible range. Wilson's formula is

$$\frac{T}{T + Z^2} \left[\frac{f_{10}}{T} + \frac{Z^2}{2T} \pm Z \sqrt{\frac{f_{10}f_{01}}{T^3} + \frac{Z^2}{4T^2}} \right] \qquad [13\text{-}26]$$

where T is $f_{10} + f_{01}$, Z is $Z_{1-\alpha/2}$, the plus sign gives the upper confidence limit for p, and the minus sign gives the lower confidence limit for p. Confidence limits for the odds ratio are taken, as before, as $p/(1 - p)$ and $\bar{p}/(1 - \bar{p})$. If $f_{10} = 8$ and $f_{01} = 2$, the 90 percent confidence limits for p from formula 13-26 are 0.541 and 0.931, well within the admissible range and reflective of the asymmetry of the sampling distribution.

For the 11 discordant matched pairs in the data of Example 13-2, formula 13-23 gives the 90 percent confidence limits of the binomial parameter of 0.506 and 0.948, corresponding to 1.03 and 18.3 for the odds ratio. These limits, especially the upper one, agree poorly with the exact limits calculated earlier. Formula 13-26, on the other hand, gives a 90 percent confidence interval for the binomial parameter of 0.479 and 0.885, corresponding to a confidence interval for the odds ratio of 0.92 to 7.72, which agrees much more closely with the mid-P exact 90 percent interval.

The ratio of discordant matched pairs is simultaneously the maximum likelihood estimate and the Mantel-Haenszel estimate of the odds ratio. For matched case-control data the variance of the maximum likelihood estimate of the odds ratio has been described by Miettinen [1970]. As is usual for ratio estimators, the confidence limits are set for the logarithmic transformation of the estimate, and then the transformation is reversed. For matched pairs, the large sample formula for the variance of the logarithm of the odds ratio is

$$\mathrm{Var}[\ln(\hat{\mathrm{OR}})] \doteq \frac{f_{10} + f_{01}}{f_{10}f_{01}} \qquad [13\text{-}27]$$

which gives approximate confidence limits for the odds ratio of

$$\underline{\mathrm{OR}} = \exp\left[\ln\left(\frac{f_{10}}{f_{01}}\right) - Z\sqrt{\frac{f_{10} + f_{01}}{f_{10}f_{01}}}\right] \qquad [13\text{-}28]$$

and

$$\overline{\mathrm{OR}} = \exp\left[\ln\left(\frac{f_{10}}{f_{01}}\right) + Z\sqrt{\frac{f_{10} + f_{01}}{f_{10}f_{01}}}\right] \qquad [13\text{-}29]$$

For the matched pair data in Example 13-2, the variance is estimated from formula 13-27 to be $11/24 = 0.458$, and the 90 percent confidence limits from formulas 13-28 and 13-29 are 0.88 and 8.12. Considering the few pairs involved, this approximation gives excellent results for these data; the lower bound is nearly equal to the mid-P exact lower limit, and the upper bound is reasonably close to the corresponding exact upper limit.

Since the maximum likelihood and Mantel-Haenszel estimators are the same for matched case-control pairs, it is not surprising to find that formula 12-58 for the variance of the logarithm of the Mantel-Haenszel estimator is identical to formula 13-27 when applied to matched pairs.

One other approach to approximate confidence limits for the odds ratio estimated from matched case-control pairs is the test-based approach. For matched pairs, the test-based limits are

$$\left(\frac{f_{10}}{f_{01}}\right)^{(1 \pm Z/\chi)} \qquad [13\text{-}30]$$

where the χ is the value from equation 13-12. Since equations 13-28 and 13-29 represent a straightforward and theoretically optimal approach to obtaining approximate confidence limits for matched case-control pairs, it is generally preferable to use them rather than the test-based approach, the binomial formulations in equations 13-24 through 13-26, or other alternatives. For comparison, the 90 percent test-based confidence limits for the matched pair data in Example 13-2 are 0.91 and 7.78, which are similar to the results obtained from formula 13-26 and slightly worse, compared with the mid-P exact limits, than the results obtained from equations 13-28 and 13-29.

INTERVAL ESTIMATION FOR R CONTROLS MATCHED TO EACH CASE

Exact interval estimation of the odds ratio with R matched controls for each case proceeds from the probability expression for the data written as a function of the odds ratio:

$$\Pr(\text{data}) = \prod_{m=1}^{R} \binom{f_{1,m-1} + f_{0,m}}{f_{1,m-1}} \left(\frac{OR}{OR + C_m}\right)^{f_{1,m-1}} \left(\frac{C_m}{OR + C_m}\right)^{f_{0,m}} \qquad [13\text{-}31]$$

where $C_m = (R + 1 - m)/m$ and the remaining notation follows Table 13-6. Expression 13-31 represents the product of R binomial probabilities, in which the binomial parameter corresponding to the probability of a "success" (i.e., a matched set with an exposed case, given that the set has m exposed subjects) is

$$\Pr(\text{exposed case given m exposed subjects}) = \frac{OR}{OR + (R + 1 - m)/m}$$

which can be derived from the noncentral hypergeometric distribution. The exact confidence limits are determined iteratively by summing the value of expression 13-31 for every possible outcome of the data that departs equally or more extremely from the null hypothesis, starting with the observed data; the sum is calculated for trial values of the odds ratio until the tail area equals the desired value. Thus, the Fisher exact limits are the solutions to the following equations:

$$\alpha/2 = \sum_{k=a}^{M_1} \prod_{m=1}^{R} \binom{f_{1,m-1} + f_{0,m}}{k_m} \left(\frac{OR}{OR + C_m}\right)^{k_m} \left(\frac{C_m}{OR + C_m}\right)^{f_{1,m-1} + f_{0,m} - k_m} \qquad [13\text{-}32]$$

and

$$1 - \alpha/2$$
$$= \sum_{k=a+1}^{M_1} \prod_{m=1}^{R} \binom{f_{1,m-1} + f_{0,m}}{k_m} \left(\frac{\overline{OR}}{\overline{OR} + C_m}\right)^{k_m} \left(\frac{C_m}{\overline{OR} + C_m}\right)^{f_{1,m-1} + f_{0,m} - k_m} \qquad [13\text{-}33]$$

where a is the total number of exposed cases in sets with at least one unexposed control,

$$a = \sum_{m=1}^{R} f_{1,m-1} \qquad\qquad M_1 = \sum_{m=1}^{R} f_{1,m-1} + f_{0,m}$$

M_1 is the total number of sets that are not completely concordant, the values $\{k_m\}$ represent the permutations of possible values for the number of matched case-control sets with an exposed case when there are m exposed subjects in a set,

$$k = \sum_{m=1}^{R} k_m$$

and

$$C_m = \frac{R + 1 - m}{m}$$

For mid-P exact confidence limits, only half the probability is included in the tail for

$$k = \sum_{m=1}^{R} f_{1,m-1}$$

These limits are the solution to the equations

$$\alpha/2 = \frac{1}{2} \sum_{k=a}^{R} \prod_{m=1}^{R} \binom{f_{1,m-1} + f_{0,m}}{k_m} \left(\frac{OR}{OR + C_m}\right)^{k_m} \left(\frac{C_m}{OR + C_m}\right)^{f_{1,m-1} + f_{0,m} - k_m}$$

$$+ \sum_{k=a+1}^{M_1} \prod_{m=1}^{R} \binom{f_{1,m-1} + f_{0,m}}{k_m} \left(\frac{OR}{OR + C_m}\right)^{k_m} \left(\frac{C_m}{OR + C_m}\right)^{f_{1,m-1} + f_{0,m} - k_m}$$

[13-34]

and

$$1 - \alpha/2$$
$$= \frac{1}{2} \sum_{k=a}^{R} \prod_{m=1}^{R} \binom{f_{1,m-1} + f_{0,m}}{k_m} \left(\frac{\overline{OR}}{\overline{OR} + C_m}\right)^{k_m} \left(\frac{C_m}{\overline{OR} + C_m}\right)^{f_{1,m-1} + f_{0,m} - k_m}$$

$$+ \sum_{k=a+1}^{M_1} \prod_{m=1}^{R} \binom{f_{1,m-1} + f_{0,m}}{k_m} \left(\frac{\overline{OR}}{\overline{OR} + C_m}\right)^{k_m} \left(\frac{C_m}{\overline{OR} + C_m}\right)^{f_{1,m-1} + f_{0,m} - k_m}$$

[13-35]

In considering exact hypothesis testing, we saw that for the data in Example 13-1 (Table 13-7) there were three outcomes, including the observed data, that give k = 11, and only one more extreme outcome, for which k = 12. Therefore, a = 11 and M_1 = 12. The four terms in the summation of the upper-tail probability are

$$P_1 = \binom{4}{3}\left(\frac{OR}{OR+4}\right)^3 \binom{4}{4}\left(\frac{4}{OR+4}\right)^1 \binom{5}{5}\left(\frac{OR}{OR+3/2}\right)^5 \binom{3}{3}\left(\frac{OR}{OR+2/3}\right)^3$$

(the probability of the observed data),

$$P_2 = \binom{4}{4}\left(\frac{OR}{OR+4}\right)^4 \binom{5}{4}\left(\frac{OR}{OR+3/2}\right)^4 \left(\frac{3/2}{OR+3/2}\right)^1 \binom{3}{3}\left(\frac{OR}{OR+2/3}\right)^3$$

$$P_3 = \binom{4}{4}\left(\frac{OR}{OR+4}\right)^4 \binom{5}{5}\left(\frac{OR}{OR+3/2}\right)^5 \binom{3}{2}\left(\frac{OR}{OR+2/3}\right)^2 \left(\frac{2/3}{OR+2/3}\right)^1$$

and

$$P_4 = \binom{4}{4}\left(\frac{OR}{OR+4}\right)^4 \binom{5}{5}\left(\frac{OR}{OR+3/2}\right)^5 \binom{3}{3}\left(\frac{OR}{OR+2/3}\right)^3$$

(the probability of the most extreme outcome).

For the exact Fisher lower confidence limit, trial values of the odds ratio should be substituted in these expressions until the sum of all four terms equals $\alpha/2$. The exact Fisher upper limit is obtained by finding the value of the odds ratio for which P_4 alone is $1 - \alpha/2$. (The remaining terms, P_1, P_2, and P_3 are included in the other tail for the Fisher upper limit.) If α is chosen to be 10 percent, the exact Fisher 90 percent confidence limits are found to be 3.78 for the lower limit and 496 for the upper limit.

To get the exact mid-P confidence limits, the same procedure is used except that only half the probabilities calculated for P_1, P_2, and P_3 are included in the summation: the lower limit is the value of the odds ratio for which $\frac{1}{2}(P_1 + P_2 + P_3) + P_4 = \alpha/2$, and the upper limit is the value for which $\frac{1}{2}(P_1 + P_2 + P_3) + P_4 = 1 - \alpha/2$. By trial and error, solutions for the 90 percent exact mid-P limits can thus be calculated to be 4.59 and 252. The large discrepancy between the two upper exact limits, the Fisher and the mid-P, results from the fact that there is only one possible outcome more extreme than that actually observed; the difference between an upper boundary of 252 and 496 for the confidence interval will hardly affect the epidemiologic interpretation.

Approximate confidence limits for the maximum likelihood estimate of the odds ratio with R matched controls can be obtained from formulas 13-28 and 13-29, extended to R controls. The variance formula [Miettinen, 1970] that represents the extension of expression 13-27 to R controls is

$$\text{Var}[\ln(\hat{OR})] \doteq \frac{1}{\hat{OR} \sum_{m-1}^{R} \frac{(f_{1,m-1} + f_{0,m})C_m}{(\hat{OR} + C_m)^2}} \qquad [13\text{-}36]$$

where $\hat{OR}$ is the conditional maximum likelihood estimate of the odds ratio, C_m is $(R + 1 - m)/m$, and the other notation follows Table 13-6. Approximate confidence limits are calculated as

$$\underline{OR} = \exp\left[\ln(\hat{OR}) - Z \cdot SE[\ln(\hat{OR})]\right] \qquad [13\text{-}37]$$

and

$$\overline{OR} = \exp\left[\ln(\hat{OR}) + Z \cdot SE[\ln(\hat{OR})]\right] \qquad [13\text{-}38]$$

where the standard error is the square root of the variance expression 13-36.

For the data in Example 13-1, the maximum likelihood estimate of the odds ratio is 22.6, and the variance of the logarithm of the odds ratio is

$$Var[\ln(\hat{OR})] \doteq \cfrac{1}{22.6\left[\dfrac{4\cdot4}{(22.6 + 4)^2} + \dfrac{5\cdot(3/2)}{(22.6 + 3/2)^2} + \dfrac{3\cdot(2/3)}{(22.6 + 2/3)^2}\right]} = \frac{1}{0.8864}$$

$$= 1.1282$$

which gives an approximate 90 percent confidence interval, from equations 13-37 and 13-38, of

$$\underline{OR} = \exp[\ln(22.6) - 1.645 \sqrt{1.1282}] = 3.94$$

and

$$\overline{OR} = \exp[\ln(22.6) + 1.645 \sqrt{1.1282}] = 130$$

The lower limit is a reasonably good approximation to the mid-P exact lower limit, but the upper limit is notably off. Nevertheless, there is no material difference in interpretability for upper limits of 130 and 252, so there is no practical problem despite the apparent inaccuracy. Discrepancies of this magnitude from different approaches to interval estimation are not unusual when the upper limit of the odds ratio is extremely high; it is important to remember that for these data the point estimate of the odds ratio is 22.6, itself an extremely high value.

For the Mantel-Haenszel estimator of the odds ratio, the variance formula is given by expression 12-58 [Robins et al., 1986]. The components of formula 12-58, when applied to matched data with a fixed R-to-1 matching ratio, are

$$\sum_i P_i R_i = \sum_{m=1}^{R} f_{1,m-1} \frac{(R + 2 - m)(R + 1 - m)}{(R + 1)^2} \qquad [13\text{-}39]$$

$$\sum_i Q_i R_i = \sum_{m=1}^{R} f_{1,m-1} \frac{(m - 1)(R + 1 - m)}{(R + 1)^2} \qquad [13\text{-}40]$$

$$\sum_i P_i S_i = \sum_{m=1}^{R} f_{0,m} \frac{m(R - m)}{(R + 1)^2} \qquad [13\text{-}41]$$

$$\sum_i Q_i S_i = \sum_{m=1}^{R} f_{0,m} \frac{m(m + 1)}{(R + 1)^2} \qquad [13\text{-}42]$$

$$\sum_i R_i = \sum_{m=1}^{R} f_{1,m-1} \frac{R + 1 - m}{R + 1} \qquad [13\text{-}43]$$

$$\sum_i S_i = \sum_{m=1}^{R} f_{0,m} \frac{m}{(R + 1)} \qquad [13\text{-}44]$$

Applying this formula to the data of Example 13-1, for which $\hat{O}R_{MH} = 33$, the variance is calculated to be 1.5179, for a 90 percent confidence interval of

$$\exp[\ln(33) \pm 1.645 \sqrt{1.5179}] = 4.35,\ 250$$

The variance estimate of 1.5179 is larger than the corresponding variance estimate for the maximum likelihood estimator, which might be expected in view of the extreme departure from the null state. It is only in the vicinity of the null condition that the Mantel-Haenszel estimator is as efficient as the conditional maximum likelihood estimator.

Another approach to approximate interval estimation of the odds ratio for R controls matched to each case is the test-based procedure. As usual, these limits are

$$\hat{O}R^{(1 \pm Z/\chi)}$$

where the χ is the result from expression 13-15. In principle, the test-based limits could be used with either the maximum likelihood estimate or the Mantel-Haenszel estimate as the anchor point. For the data in Example 13-1, the χ is 4.0, which gives a 90 percent confidence interval of 6.3 to 81 when the maximum likelihood estimate of 22.6 is used as the anchor point, and 7.8 to 139 when the Mantel-Haenszel estimate of 33 is used as the anchor point. In either case the test-based limits are evidently much too narrow and would not serve as an adequate approximation to the exact confidence limits. The test-based limits are usually adequate in the vicinity of the null value of the odds ratio, but for these data, which depart strongly from the null condition, the test-based limits are a poor approximation.

INTERVAL ESTIMATION FOR A VARYING NUMBER OF CONTROLS MATCHED TO EACH CASE

With a varying number of matched controls, the probability expression for the data as a function of the odds ratio is an extension of formula 13-31, taking the product of the probabilities over each value of R:

$$\Pr(\text{data}) = \prod_R \prod_{m=1}^{R} \left(\frac{f_{1,m-1} + f_{0,m}}{f_{1,m-1}} \right) \left(\frac{OR}{OR + C_m} \right)^{f_{1,m-1}} \left(\frac{C_m}{OR + C_m} \right)^{f_{0,m}} \quad [13\text{-}45]$$

where the notation is that used for equation 13-31. The tail probabilities for the calculation of exact confidence limits are calculated as they are for a fixed matching ratio (formulas 13-32 through 13-35) with expression 13-45 representing the probability for each realization of the data in the tail summation.

The data in Example 13-2, for which there are 3522 terms in the tail summation, would not ordinarily warrant an exact calculation of confidence limits because the large numbers ensure that most approximate formulas for the determination of confidence intervals would be satisfactory. The exact confidence limits must be determined iteratively, so that the tail summation involving 3522 terms must be calculated repeatedly until the solution is reached. This tedious task is not difficult, however, using a computer. The 90 percent exact Fisher confidence limits for the data in Example 13-2 are 1.28 and 3.10; the 90 percent exact mid-*P* limits are 1.32 and 3.01.

Approximate confidence limits for the conditional maximum likelihood estimate of the odds ratio with a varying number of matched controls can be based on formulas 13-37 and 13-38 after extending the variance formula (13-36) to accommodate more than one value for R, by extending the summation in the denominator of formula 13-36 to the various values for R:

$$\text{Var}[\ln(\hat{OR})] \doteq \frac{1}{\hat{OR} \sum_R \sum_{m-1}^{R} \dfrac{(f_{1,m-1} + f_{0,m})C_m}{(\hat{OR} + C_m)^2}} \quad [13\text{-}46]$$

where the notation follows that in formula 13-36.

For the data in Example 13-2, the maximum likelihood estimate of the odds ratio is, from equation 13-8, 1.9835. Substituting this value for $\hat{OR}$ in equation 13-46 along with the observed frequencies gives, for the variance of the logarithm of the odds ratio and approximate 90 percent confidence interval,

$$\text{Var}[\ln(\hat{OR})] \doteq \cfrac{1}{1.9835\left[\cfrac{11}{(1.9835+1)^2} + \cfrac{38(2)}{(1.9835+2)^2} + \cfrac{26\,(\frac{1}{2})}{(1.9835+\frac{1}{2})^2}\right]} = 0.0620$$

and

$$\underline{OR} = \exp[\ln(1.9835) - 1.645\ \sqrt{0.062}] = 1.32$$

$$\overline{OR} = \exp[\ln(1.9835) + 1.645\ \sqrt{0.062}] = 2.99$$

As one would expect with these moderately large numbers, these approximate confidence limits are extremely close to the mid-P exact limits of 1.32 and 3.01.

The Mantel-Haenszel estimator for the data of Example 13-2 is 2.062. The variance of the Mantel-Haenszel estimator for a varying ratio R of controls to cases can be obtained from formula 12-58 by extending the components of 12-58 given in formulas 13-39 through 13-44 for all values of R. Thus, each of the six summations should be summed for all values of R. For the data of Example 13-2, the variance of the Mantel-Haenszel estimator can be calculated in this way as 0.0659, which is slightly greater than the maximum likelihood variance estimator of 0.0620. The approximate 90 percent confidence limits for the Mantel-Haenszel estimator for the data of Example 13-2 are

$$\underline{OR}_{\text{MH}} = \exp[\ln(2.062) - 1.645\ \sqrt{0.0659}] = 1.35$$

$$\overline{OR}_{\text{MH}} = \exp[\ln(2.062) + 1.645\ \sqrt{0.0659}] = 3.14$$

Test-based approximate confidence limits can also be applied when the matching ratio varies, subject to the usual caution that their accuracy suffers according to how much the data depart from the null condition. Whereas test-based limits were a poor approximation for the data of Example 13-1, which indicated a strong effect, one might reasonably expect a better performance for the data of Example 13-2, which depart only modestly from the null state. For these data, the χ from formula 13-18 is 2.79. Using the maximum likelihood point estimate of 1.98, the test-based 90 percent confidence limits are 1.32 and 2.96, which are nearly identical to the interval obtained using the variance expression for the logarithm of the maximum likelihood estimator and nearly identical to the mid-P exact limits. Using the Mantel-Haenszel point estimate of 2.06, the test-based 90 percent confidence limits are 1.35 and 3.16, which are close to the results using the variance formula of Robins et al. [1986].

MATCHED FOLLOW-UP STUDIES

Matching can achieve in follow-up studies what it cannot achieve in case-control studies: It can prevent confounding. The crude risk comparisons from a matched follow-up study are unbiased with respect to the matching factors because of the absence of an association between exposure and the matching factors among the study subjects at the start of follow-up.

Despite this efficacy, matched follow-up studies are rare. The main reason is the great expense of matching large cohorts; follow-up studies ordinarily have many more subjects than case-control studies, and matching is usually a time-consuming process. Walker [1982] has suggested a method to improve this poor cost efficiency in matched follow-up studies by limiting data collection on unmatched confounders to those sets in which an event occurs. Another reason that matched follow-up studies are rare is that matching can reasonably be accomplished only for subjects themselves, whereas in any long-term follow-up study the optimal measure to use for follow-up experience is person-time. If matching were employed in a long-term follow-up study at the time of subject selection, the identical distributions of the compared series for the matched factors could change as the follow-up experience of the compared groups began to differ.

For matched follow-up studies in which the period of follow-up is short enough to warrant the use of cumulative incidence data rather than incidence rate data, a crude analysis of the data will give results that are unconfounded by the matching factors (although the crude analysis will yield a variance estimate that is too large [Greenland and Robins, 1985a]). In addition to preventing confounding, matching also contributes to study efficiency by reducing the variation of the effect estimate; the reduced variation stems from the correlation in the disease outcome for the matched subjects introduced by the matching.

Consider a matched follow-up study with T matched pairs of exposed and unexposed subjects. Suppose that the frequency distribution of matched pairs according to the outcome in exposed and unexposed subjects is f_{11} for pairs in which both the exposed and unexposed subjects develop the disease, f_{10} for pairs in which only the exposed subject develops the disease, f_{01} for pairs in which only the unexposed subject develops the disease, and f_{00} for pairs in which neither subject develops the disease. The risk difference can be estimated by

$$\hat{RD} = \hat{R}_1 - \hat{R}_0 = \frac{f_{11} + f_{10}}{T} - \frac{f_{11} + f_{01}}{T} = \frac{f_{10} - f_{01}}{T} \qquad [13\text{-}47]$$

and the risk ratio can be estimated as

$$\hat{RR} = \frac{(f_{11} + f_{10})/T}{(f_{11} + f_{01})/T} = \frac{f_{11} + f_{10}}{f_{11} + f_{01}} \qquad [13\text{-}48]$$

Statistical hypothesis testing for these data is identical to the procedures used for case-control data; both the exact and approximate methods apply equally well for follow-up data in which all of the observations are frequencies. Exact confidence limits for the above measures are difficult to obtain, but excellent approximate methods exist that take into account the reduced variation introduced by the matching.

The most direct approach involves variance formulas corresponding to the estimators given in formulas 13-47 and 13-48. For the rate difference estimate, the variance is

$$\text{Var}(\hat{RD}) \doteq \frac{T(f_{10} + f_{01}) - (f_{10} - f_{01})^2}{T^3} \qquad [13\text{-}49]$$

The variance estimate for the logarithmically transformed rate ratio measure is

$$\text{Var}[\ln(\hat{RR})] \doteq \frac{f_{10} + f_{01}}{(f_{11} + f_{10})(f_{11} + f_{01})} \qquad [13\text{-}50]$$

The estimates of effect derived from formulas 13-47 and 13-48 are those obtained from the crude data, but the corresponding variances in formulas 13-49 and 13-50 are generally smaller than those obtained from a crude analysis. Another possible approach to confidence interval estimation is the use of test-based confidence limits, using the χ from formula 13-12.

Example 13-3 illustrates data from a follow-up study of 458 pregnant women who had previously used oral contraceptives; the comparison

Example 13-3. Distribution of matched pairs of
pregnant women exposed and unexposed to oral contraceptives
according to selected abnormalities in the offspring [Robinson, 1971]

	Unexposed mother		
	Abnormality present	Abnormality absent	Total
Exposed mother			
Abnormality present	28	85	113
Abnormality absent	61	284	345
Totals	89	369	458

Table 13-8. Crude data for example 13-3

	Oral contraceptive exposure		
	Yes	No	Total
Abnormal baby			
Yes	113	89	202
No	345	369	714
Total	458	458	916

group consists of an equal number of women who had never used oral contraceptives and who were individually matched to the exposed women for age and parity [Robinson, 1971]. The pairs are classified according to whether or not each mother delivered a baby with one of a group of abnormalities potentially related to the exposure. (The reader should note that these data, although they resemble cumulative incidence data, are actually prevalence data, since miscarriages are excluded.)

The estimate of risk difference from these data, from formula 13-47, is $(85 - 61)/458 = 0.052$. A 90 percent confidence interval may be calculated from the variance as determined by formula 13-49,

$$\text{Var}(\hat{\text{RD}}) \doteq \frac{458(85 + 61) - (85 - 61)^2}{458^3} = 0.000690$$

giving for the confidence limits

$$0.0524 \pm 1.645 \sqrt{0.000690} = 0.009, 0.096$$

It is also possible to use the test-based approach, based on the χ obtained from formula 13-12 applied to the data in Example 13-3. The χ value for this example is $(85 - 61)/\sqrt{146} = 1.986$, giving a 90 percent confidence interval for the rate difference of

$$0.0524(1 \pm 1.645/1.986) = 0.009, 0.096$$

which is essentially identical to the result obtained using formula 13-49.

It is interesting to compare these results with the confidence limits obtained from the crude data, ignoring the matching. The 2×2 table for the crude data is shown in Table 13-8; the cell entries for this table are the marginal totals for the pairs in Example 13-3. Using the square of formula 11-17, the variance for the risk difference is

$$\text{Var}(\hat{\text{RD}}) \doteq \frac{(113)(345)}{458^2} + \frac{(89)(369)}{458^2} = 0.000748$$

which is somewhat larger than the variance estimate that takes the matching ratio into account. From this value a 90 percent confidence interval can be calculated as

$$0.0524 \pm 1.645 \sqrt{0.000748} = 0.007, 0.097$$

The risk ratio can be estimated from the data in Example 13-3 as 113/89 = 1.27 using formula 13-48. The variance of the logarithmic transformation, taking the matching into account, is, from formula 13-50,

$$\text{Var}[\ln(\hat{\text{RR}})] \doteq \frac{85 + 61}{(113)\ (89)} = 0.0145$$

which gives a 90 percent confidence interval of

$$\exp[\ln(1.27) \pm 1.645 \sqrt{0.0145}] = 1.04, 1.55$$

Test-based 90 percent confidence limits for the risk ratio are

$$1.27^{(1 \pm 1.645/1.986)} = 1.04, 1.55$$

which is essentially the same result. From the crude data in Table 13-8, using formula 11-18, we have

$$\text{Var}\ [\ln(\hat{\text{RR}})] \doteq \frac{345}{(113)\ (458)} + \frac{369}{(89)\ (458)} = 0.0157$$

which corresponds to a 90 percent confidence interval of

$$\exp[\ln(1.27) \pm 1.645 \sqrt{0.0157}] = 1.03, 1.56$$

just slightly larger than the confidence intervals that take matching into account.

The analysis of matched follow-up studies with several unexposed subjects matched to each exposed subject is analogous to the analysis for paired data. The crude data provide an unbiased estimate of effect as long as the matching ratio is constant. If it varies, the methods of Chapter 12 for follow-up data should be applied, grouping the subjects into strata according to categories of the matching factor(s) to ensure control of confounding.

One of the differences between follow-up and case-control studies with respect to matching is the amount of information provided by the data about the effect of a matching factor on the disease occurrence. In a case-control study, there is no way to evaluate directly the effect of a factor that has been matched. An identical distribution in both cases and controls of any matched factor is ensured by the selection process. In a follow-up study, however, the identity of distribution is achieved for exposed and unexposed subjects before disease develops. The outcome among subjects classified at different levels of a matching factor is yet to be determined and can thus be evaluated by a straightforward comparison that is unconfounded by the exposure.

EVALUATION OF EFFECT MODIFICATION WITH MATCHED DATA

All of the estimation approaches described in this chapter involve the assumption that the effect is constant for all strata. Since the numbers within strata are usually extremely small for matched analyses, because the strata correspond to the matched sets, the usual statistical approaches to the evaluation of effect modification do not apply. It is still possible to evaluate whether the effect is constant over levels of a matching factor, however, if, for example, only a few categories of the matching factor are involved. We shall not consider this issue in detail but will discuss a simple case to demonstrate the idea.

Suppose a matched-pair case-control study were conducted with 200 pairs. Of the 200 pairs, suppose that 60 are discordant, 40 with the case exposed and 20 with the case unexposed, so that the overall estimate of the odds ratio is 2.0. The overall estimate is calculated on the assumption that the odds ratio is constant for all strata, but suppose that we want to evaluate statistically whether that is the case with respect to sex, which was one of the matching factors. To evaluate effect modification in these matched data by sex, it is necessary only to separate the discordant pairs into male and female subgroups and contrast the estimates of effect obtained from these subgroups. Of the 40 discordant pairs with an exposed case, suppose that 31 are male pairs and 9 are female, whereas 15 of the 20 discordant pairs in which the control is exposed are male pairs and 5 are female. Among males, the ratio of discordant pairs is $31/15 = 2.1$, compared with $9/5 = 1.8$ among females. The similarity of these ratios indicates that the data are reasonably comparable with a uniform rate ratio. A statistical test of the hypothesis that there is a uniform odds ratio for males and females amounts to a test of association of the 2×2 table shown in Table 13-9.

Table 13-9. Distribution of discordant pairs by exposure and gender for hypothetical matched data

	Male	Female	Totals
Case exposed	31	9	40
Control exposed	15	5	20
Totals	46	14	60

A χ test statistic for these data, from formula 11-6, gives $\chi = 0.21$, which corresponds to a *P*-value of 0.8 and is reasonably consistent with the hypothesis of a uniform effect.

More general tests of effect modification for matched data can be constructed by extending the procedure described above. Estimates of effect from several subcategories can be compared in a single test by using formula 12-60 coupled with formula 13-36 (or one of the simpler counterparts) to estimate the appropriate variances for each of the compared estimates.

EVALUATION OF THE EFFECT OF MATCHING WITH CASE-CONTROL DATA

We have seen that the process of matching itself can introduce confounding into a case-control study whenever the matching factor is a correlate of the exposure. The confounding that is introduced becomes a substitute for whatever confounding might have been observed for the factor in the absence of matching; there would be confounding as long as the factor in question, in addition to being correlated with the exposure, is also related to disease status. If the matching factor is not related to disease status and therefore is not inherently confounding, matching for it represents overmatching because the effort of matching and the loss of efficiency in the required matched analysis do not improve the validity of the study. The matched analysis is still required even if the factor matched for would not have been a confounding factor, since matching for any correlate of exposure introduces confounding that necessitates a stratified analysis to remove it.

The penalty for matching for a factor or a set of factors that jointly are not correlated with the exposure is not as severe. If the matching factors do not introduce a correlation in the exposure histories between cases and controls, the matching has not introduced any confounding into the data, and the matched analysis need not be retained. Avoiding the matched analysis may be useful to bolster study efficiency by avoiding the loss of information from the matched case-control sets with fully concordant exposure histories, or to permit stratification by factors that have not been matched. Matching factors that are uncorrelated with the exposure in the data probably represent factors that would not have been confounding even without matching, so the matching cannot be viewed as productive, but the ability to abandon the unnecessary matched analysis in this situation mitigates the problem.

Evaluation of the relation between the matched factors and the exposure is essentially an evaluation of the confounding introduced by the matching, and it proceeds in the same way as evaluation of confounding generally. The effect estimate is calculated in two ways, by preserving the matching and ignoring it. If the effect estimate from the matched analysis differs materially from the crude estimate, that difference can usually be ascribed to the confounding that results from the correlation between the matching factors and the exposure. The difference, if any exists, will usually be such that the crude estimate of the effect is closer to the null value than the confounded estimate, provided that the matching ratio of controls to cases is constant across sets. If no material difference exists between the crude estimate and the result of the matched analysis, then the investigator can conclude that the matching did not introduce or control any confounding, and the matching can be ignored in the analysis. It should be emphasized that the evaluation of matching, like the evaluation of confounding in general, should not be based on statistical tests but on the magnitude of the apparent bias reflected in the compared point estimates.

Consider as an example the data in Table 13-7. The maximum likelihood estimate of the relative risk from the stratified (matched) analysis is 23. The crude estimate, calculated from the crude exposure proportions of 12/18 for the cases and 16/72 for the controls, is 7.0. The discrepancy indicates that the matching factors were correlated with the exposure and therefore that the matched analysis must be retained.

If the matching ratio is constant across matched sets, the crude association between exposure and disease is usually closer to the null value than the association conditional on control of the matching factors. In unusual circumstances, however, the crude association between exposure and disease is farther from the null value than the association after stratification by the matching factors [Koepsell, 1984]. This anomaly occurs only if there is a negative correlation in exposure histories between cases and their matched controls. Ordinarily, the correlation is positive, but it may occasionally be negative either from sampling variability or from extreme effect modification. If stratification by the matching factors does lead to an effect estimate that is closer to the null value than the crude effect estimate, this result should be interpreted as a warning that the data are anomalous in some way. Koepsell has recommended an examination for effect modification in such situations; this step is generally a good idea even without the paradoxical effect of matching. It is also worthwhile verifying that no data processing or labeling errors have been overlooked.

MULTIVARIATE ANALYSIS OF MATCHED DATA

The conditional likelihood methods described in this chapter for estimating the odds ratio with individually matched data can be expressed mathematically in the form of a conditional logistic regression equation [Prentice and Breslow, 1978]. The two analytic approaches are equivalent as long as the exposure variable is dichotomous and no other factors, aside from the matching variables, are considered. The conditional logistic regression analysis does offer some advantages, however. A fundamental advantage is the ability to control conveniently for other factors that were measured but not matched for. Using the conventional stratified analysis, there is often no way to control effectively for the matching factors and for factors not included in the matching algorithm. It is possible that, on evaluating the effect of matching and determining that it has introduced little or no confounding by the matching factors, the matched sets can be disrupted and the data stratified by factors not matched on. If, on the other hand, the matching has introduced a material correlation in the exposure histories between cases and controls, conditional logistic regression analysis (or other conditional models) allows both the removal of the confounding introduced by the matching and the control of additional unmatched confounding factors. It is also possible, although unusual, that the matching factors are confounding only conditionally on the control of unmatched confounding factors [Fisher and Patil, 1974; Miettinen, 1974], a situation that conditional logistic analysis can diagnose and deal with effectively. The latter method also allows the evaluation of exposure at several levels simultaneously, a process that is otherwise especially difficult with matched data (see Chap. 16). The drawback of the multivariate approach is the requirement for a computer and the necessary software for the analysis; the conventional stratified approach requires only a pencil and paper and perhaps a pocket calculator.

The construction of the multivariate model for logistic regression analysis is discussed in the next chapter, along with the theory behind the approach.

REFERENCES

Breslow, N. Odds ratio estimators when the data are sparse. *Biometrika* 1981;68:73–84.

Fisher, L., and Patil, K. Matching and unrelatedness. *Am. J. Epidemiol.* 1974;100:347–349.

Gordis, L. Should dead cases be matched to dead controls? *Am. J. Epidemiol.* 1982;115:1–5.

Greenland, S. The effect of misclassification in matched pair case-control studies. *Am. J. Epidemiol.* 1982;116:402–406.

Greenland, S., and Robins, J. M. Estimation of a common effect parameter from sparse follow-up data. *Biometrics* 1985a;41:55–68.

Greenland, S., and Robins, J. M. Confounding and misclassification. *Am. J. Epidemiol.* 1985b;122:495–506.

Jick, H., Miettinen, O. S., Neff, R. K., et al. Coffee and myocardial infarction. *N. Engl. J. Med.* 1973;289:63–77.

Koepsell, T. Unmatched analysis of matched data: Is the bias always conservative? *Am. J. Epidemiol.* 1984;120:463–464.

Lubin, J. H. An empirical evaluation of the use of conditional and unconditional likelihoods for case-control data. *Biometrika* 1981;68:567–571.

McNemar, Q. Note on the sampling of the difference between corrected proportions or percentages. *Psychometrika* 1947;12:153–157.

Miettinen, O. S. Individual matching with multiple controls in the case of all-or-none responses. *Biometrics* 1969;25:339–355.

Miettinen, O. S. Estimation of relative risk from individually matched series. *Biometrics* 1970;26:75–86.

Miettinen, O. S. Confounding and effect modification. *Am. J. Epidemiol.* 1974;100:350–353.

Miettinen, O. S. Stratification by a multivariate confounder score. *Am. J. Epidemiol.* 1976;104:609–620.

Poole, C. Exposure opportunity in case-control studies. *Am. J. Epidemiol.* 1986;123:352–358.

Prentice, R. L., and Breslow, N. E. Retrospective studies and failure time models. *Biometrika* 1978;65:153–158.

Robins, J. M., Breslow, N., and Greenland, S. Estimators of the Mantel-Haenszel variance consistent in both sparse data and large strata limiting models. *Biometrics* 1986;42:in press.

Robinson, S. C. Pregnancy outcome following oral contraceptives. *Am. J. Obstet. Gynecol.* 1971;109:354–358.

Walker, A. M. Efficient assessment of confounder effects in matched follow-up studies. *Appl. Stat.* 1982;31:293–297.

Wilson, E. B. Probable inference. The law of succession and statistical inference. *J. Am. Stat. Assoc.* 1927;22:209–211.

The first experience with multivariate analysis is apt to leave the impression that a miracle in the technology of data analysis has been revealed; the method permits control for confounding and evaluation of interactions for a host of variables with great statistical efficiency. Even better, a computer does all the arithmetic and neatly prints out the results. The heady experience of commanding a computer to accomplish all these analytic goals and then simply gathering and publishing the sophisticated "output" with barely a pause for retyping is undeniably alluring. Indeed, it may even be a disappointment that the analysis culminating the work of weeks, months, or years of data collection is over in such a short time and the results compressed into such a compact form.

However useful it may be, multivariate analysis is not a statistical panacea. Its biggest drawback is the barrier it inserts between the investigator and the data. Other analytic methods facilitate an intimate understanding of the data, making the investigator aware of irregularities or deficiencies—a few critical cell entries with small frequencies, for example. Multivariate methods hinder this intimacy with the data. A related drawback is the lack of cogency in communicating the message in the results to others. Some readers are unfamiliar and uneasy with the mathematical models involved, and all readers, like the investigator, obtain a clearer understanding of the data when tabular frequencies are presented.

Increasing availability of computer hardware and software has triggered an avalanche of data crunching, much of it characterized by unstructured, poorly conceptualized analyses that carry the investigator toward the research goal by accident, if at all. One frequently encounters in the scientific literature situations in which the analytic methods described in earlier chapters of this book could have been applied but were overlooked in favor of multivariate analysis, and others in which many multivariate models are fitted to the data when one or two would suffice. The epidemiologist is better off to rely primarily on the more straightforward procedures of stratified analysis whenever possible, since these procedures engender greater familiarity with the data for both the investigator and the reader.

Multivariate analysis is undeniably useful as an analytic approach when stratified analysis becomes impractical. The feasibility of a stratified analysis depends on the number of subcategories over which the data must be dispersed; if these are too numerous, the data will be stratified too thinly over the subcategories, and the analysis will be inefficient, which is to say that the resulting estimates will be imprecise. Multivariate analysis provides a way to preserve precision while controlling many variables, by postulating a mathematical model that allows the data to be used more efficiently to estimate many effects simultaneously. The extent to which this analytic process represents improved efficiency rather than just bias depends on the adequacy of the assumptions built into the mathematical model. A stratified analysis, perhaps limited to some key variables, is often a sensible antecedent to a multivariate analysis, since it can shed light on the degree to which the data conform to the assumptions of a particular multivariate model. Although it is more time-consuming, a combination of analytic strategies should prove more fruitful of insights into the data than any single approach.

When multivariate analysis is undertaken, time spent planning the construction of one or few multivariate models rather than casually commanding the generation of many different models will lead to less work and clearer results. In the best circumstances, the end product will be an elegant summary of the data describing the complicated interrelation between many variables.

In the broadest sense, a multivariate analysis is any analysis of data that takes into account many variables. A unifying concept underlying different types of multivariate analyses is the use of a mathematical model to account for the interrelation among the variables in the analysis. The likelihood equations presented in Chapter 12 for estimating epidemiologic effect measures while controlling for confounding are examples of mathematical models that constitute a multivariate analysis. Many other multivariate methods have been developed, usually for specialized purposes. Factor analysis, for example, is a methodology intended to collapse a large number of predictor variables into a smaller number of "factors" that represent correlated subgroups of the original set of variables. Time-series analysis is a method directed at evaluating the association between variables while allowing for time-dependent variation and correlation between selected variables. The approach that has had the widest application in epidemiology is multiple regression analysis, which has numerous variants; in its most general forms it subsumes many other multivariate approaches, such as log-linear analysis, the likelihood approaches described in Chapter 12, analysis of covariance, and even time-series analysis.

Multivariate analysis is an advanced topic that has been the subject of many books. A full discussion of its applications is impossible here. Instead, the goal of this chapter is to describe in simple terms the basic mathematical models used and to discuss the strategy to be adopted by the epidemiologist in constructing and interpreting multivariate models.

BASIC MATHEMATICAL MODELS
The Linear Model

The most fundamental model describing the relation between two variables is the straight line. The linear model for two variables serves as a springboard for more complicated models between two or more variables. The equation for a straight line relating two variables has two parameters, usually formulated as the intercept, or constant, and the slope, or coefficient:

$$Y = a_0 + a_1 X_1 + \varepsilon \tag{14-1}$$

In equation 14-1, a_0 is the intercept, or constant; that is, a_0 is the average value of the variable Y when the variable X_1 is equal to zero. The other parameter, a_1, is the slope of the line relating X_1 and Y, representing the number of units change in Y for every unit change in X_1. The term ε is the error term, representing a random departure from the expected value of the dependent variable. The average error is generally assumed to be zero. The theoretical range for both a_0 and a_1 is from minus infinity to plus infinity. Figure 14-1 illustrates the two-variable linear model graphically.

It is seldom that the actual relation between two variables is linear; the assumption inherent in any analysis that is dependent on a mathematical model is that the model is a simplifying description that does not necessarily conform to the actual relation between the variables but does represent it closely enough so that inferences drawn on the basis of the model are reasonable. Departure of the data from the model may reflect the discrepancy between the model and nature as well as sources of inaccuracy in obtaining information. A sensible goal is to choose a model that fits the data closely enough so that the major source of departure of the data from

Fig. 14-1. Graphic representation of a straight line equation.

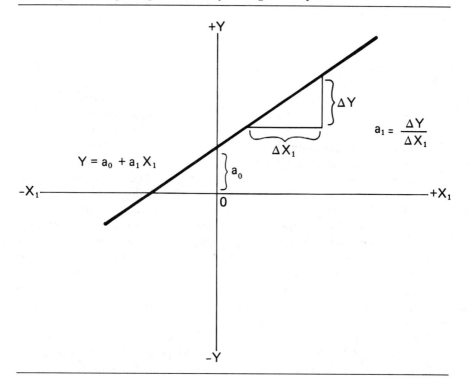

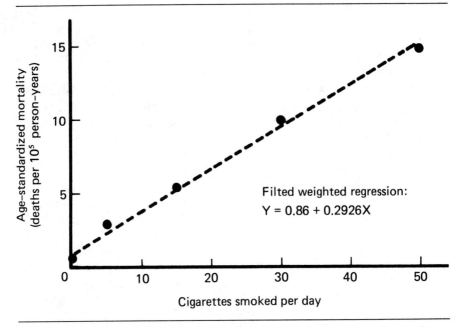

Fig. 14-2. Age-standardized mortality from laryngeal cancer according to the number of cigarettes smoked daily, derived from the data of Kahn [Rothman et al., 1980].

the model derives from inaccuracies inherent in the data rather than from the inappropriateness of the model.

Figure 14-2 illustrates a nearly linear relation between number of cigarettes smoked per day and age-standardized mortality from laryngeal cancer [Rothman et al., 1980]. Rarely do epidemiologic data follow a linear pattern as closely as these. When the observations do not fall exactly on a line but still demonstrate a basically linear pattern despite some scatter, the investigator must rely on statistical fitting methods to obtain the equation of the fitted line. The equation of the "best fitting" line can be determined through a variety of techniques. The best methods are those that take into account the amount of information reflected in each observation; a common method used is that of weighted least squares, which minimizes the sum of the squared vertical deviations of each observation from the line, weighting each squared deviation according to a value that reflects the amount of information for that observation. The equation of the fitted line for Figure 14-2 is $Y = 0.86 + 0.2926X$, where Y is the estimated mortality rate measured in deaths per 10^5 person-years and X is the number of cigarettes smoked daily. For nonsmokers, the mortality rate predicted from this linear model is 0.86 per 10^5 person-years; for smokers of 40 cigarettes a day, it is $0.86 + 40 \times (0.2926) = 11.70$ per 10^5 person-years.

In statistical parlance, equation 14-1 is referred to as a "regression" equation, which indicates that one set of variables, in this case just X_1, is used to predict or describe another variable, Y. The variable X_1 is referred to as the independent variable, and Y is referred to as the dependent variable. Equation 14-1 is the equation for a simple linear regression because the equation has only one independent variable. The equation could be expanded, however, by adding additional independent variables; with multiple independent variables, the equation is called a multiple linear regression:

$$Y = a_0 + a_1X_1 + a_2X_2 + a_3X_3 + \ldots \qquad [14\text{-}2]$$

Equation 14-2 is still linear, but the straight line crosses a space with more than two dimensions, there being one dimension for every variable in the equation, including the dependent variable.

The key feature of multivariate analysis that makes it such a useful technique in epidemiologic analysis is the fact that inference based on the coefficient for any independent variable in the model is conditional on the remaining independent variables in the model. This conditional interpretation means that confounding for a large number of factors can be controlled simultaneously in a single model, and the effect of each factor unconfounded by the other factors in the model can be determined from the fitted coefficients, provided that the mathematical assumptions of the model are reasonable.

Transformations of the Linear Model: Logistic Analysis

Equation 14-1 or its extension 14-2 represents the basic form for statistical modeling in virtually all epidemiologic applications. More complicated models can usually be written in a form that corresponds to one of these equations, the complexity deriving from transformations of one or more of the variables in the model. The transformations enable a linear model to describe inherently nonlinear relations. For example, suppose Y represents incidence rate and the independent variable is age, and the data follow the pattern demonstrated in Figure 14-3. A straight line relating incidence rate and age will be a poor fit, but consider defining the independent variable as the square of age: $X_1 = (\text{age})^2$. The relation between Y and the transformed age variable would now be perfectly linear. The inventive use of transformations enables a linear model to accommodate nearly any nonlinear relation.

Such flexibility does come at a price if the number of terms in the model is increased. Adding terms reduces the residual "degrees of freedom" in the model, thereby decreasing the efficiency of estimation. The loss of efficiency is usually small unless the model already has a relatively large number of constraints for the amount of data.

It is common for a variable in an epidemiologic analysis to have only

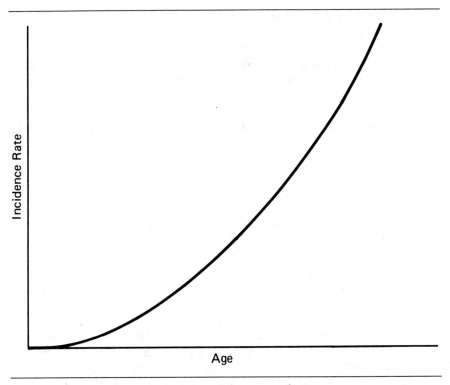

Fig. 14-3. Incidence rate increases as the square of age.

two values, corresponding to presence or absence of disease or presence or absence of exposure. Regression models based on dichotomous dependent variables are referred to as "binary regressions." Suppose a follow-up were conducted to evaluate disease outcome in an exposed and an unexposed group. In simplest form, the data would consist of two binary observations for each subject: whether exposed or not and whether diseased or not at the end of the follow-up period. The data in Example 11-4 illustrate such a situation: If both the independent and dependent variables are binary, then the data are summarized by a 2 × 2 table. A binary regression can be applied to such data; it is convenient to code each variable with the values 0 or 1 denoting the absence and presence, respectively, of exposure or disease. Using this coding scheme, the constant term a_0 corresponds to cumulative incidence among the unexposed group. Therefore a_1, the coefficient for the independent variable in the model, corresponds to the cumulative incidence difference (or risk difference) between those exposed and those unexposed. Of course, the risk difference can be easily estimated directly from the 2 × 2 table describing the data, so that the linear regression for simple binary data is unnecessary. The regression model, however, can be easily extended to accommodate many additional variables, wherein lies its advantage. If ten additional observations were made for each subject, representing ten confounding factors, these could be controlled simply by adding as few as ten additional terms to the linear model corresponding to the ten confounding factors. Simultaneous control of ten confounding factors using stratification, on the other hand, would be difficult, since it would call for a minimum of 2^{10} or 1024 strata.

Epidemiologic interpretation of the coefficient in the regression model is dependent on the type of data. If, for example, a simple binary regression model were applied to case-control data in a 2×2 table format, a_0 would correspond to the proportion of controls exposed and a_1 would correspond to the difference in proportion of cases and controls exposed. These values have little inherent epidemiologic interpretation; the measure of interest, the odds ratio, is not directly obtainable from the model, and hence the model is not appropriate for case-control data.

Even when a simple binary regression is applied to the appropriate type of data, there is a theoretical objection to its use. Cumulative incidence has a theoretical range of zero to one. A regression line, however, is theoretically unbounded. Consequently, it is possible that a regression model could give estimates of cumulative incidence outside its theoretical range. In practice, estimates of cumulative incidence would seldom be much below zero or above 1, and then only for extreme combinations of values of the independent variables. In place of such inadmissible estimates it is reasonable to substitute the theoretical minimum or maximum value, as appropriate, for the inadmissible value.

Although the theoretical objection is not a serious deterrent to the use of binary regression for follow-up data, it has motivated the use of other models that lack this problem. What is needed is a transformation of a variable measured as a proportion such that the transformed variable has a theoretical range of minus infinity to plus infinity rather than zero to one. This transformation can be accomplished in two stages: If Y is a proportion with a range of zero to one, then $Y/(1 - Y)$, referred to as the "odds" of Y, has a range from zero to infinity; the second step is to take the logarithm of the odds, $\ln[Y/(1 - Y)]$, which will have a range from minus infinity to plus infinity. The logarithm of the odds of Y is referred to as the "logit." A linear model with the logit as the dependent variable is a simple variant of equation 14-1:

$$\ln\left[\frac{Y}{1 - Y}\right] = a_0 + a_1 X_1 \qquad [14\text{-}3]$$

This is a regression model for the dependence of an expected proportion or probability Y on X_1. Equation 14-3 can be easily extended with additional independent variables. It can be rewritten in logistic form as

$$Y = \frac{e^{a_0 + a_1 X_1}}{1 + e^{a_0 + a_1 X_1}} = \frac{1}{1 + e^{-(a_0 + a_1 X_1)}} \qquad [14\text{-}4]$$

which is algebraically identical to equation 14-3. Equation 14-4 extended with additional independent variables is the *multiple logistic* regression model.

The definition of the logit ensures that the value of Y will always be in the range zero to one no matter what the value of the right hand side of equation 14-3. This constraint on the dependent variable may be construed as an advantage of the logistic model, although from the practical point of view it is a minor one.

The logistic model also has an important implication for the interpretation of the coefficients in the model. If the independent variable is binary, measured as 1 if exposed and 0 if unexposed, then a_0 corresponds to the logarithm of the odds for disease among the unexposed:

$$a_0 = \ln\left[\frac{CI_0}{1 - CI_0}\right] \qquad [14\text{-}5]$$

where CI_0 indicates disease risk among the unexposed. The logarithm of the odds for disease among the exposed is $a_0 + a_1$, so a_1 corresponds to the difference between the logarithms of the disease odds or, equivalently, the logarithm of the odds ratio,

$$a_1 = \ln\left[\frac{CI_1(1 - CI_0)}{CI_0(1 - CI_1)}\right] \qquad [14\text{-}6]$$

Therefore, the antilogarithm of the coefficient for a 0/1 binary independent variable in a logistic regression is an estimate of the odds ratio. If the data are cumulative incidence data, the interpretation of the odds ratio is subject to all the reservations that usually apply when using the odds ratio with cumulative incidence data (see Chap. 6 and Table 6-1).

Since the logistic model can provide estimates of the odds ratio, it can be applied to prevalence data or case-control data to obtain useful epidemiologic measures. Whereas the untransformed linear binary regression produced interpretable epidemiologic results only for cumulative incidence data and then provided an estimate of only the cumulative incidence difference, the logistic regression model is useful in a large number of applications, namely, those in which the odds ratio is of epidemiologic interest. This advantage of the logistic model is far more important than the theoretical advantage that motivated its development.

We have seen that the logistic transformation, in changing the range of the dependent variable, simultaneously changed the interpretation of the coefficients in the model, which also enhanced the utility of the model. The transformation has other concomitant aspects, however, that place limitations on its usefulness and should always be kept in mind by the thoughtful investigator. Suppose that rather than a binary independent variable a logistic model were fitted with an ordinal or a continuous independent variable. An example might be a variable indicating smoking behavior, with the variable taking on values of 0, 1, 2, 3, and so on, denoting the number of packs of cigarettes smoked daily. The coefficient for the smoking variable would represent the incremental amount in the logit that corresponds to a unit change in the independent variable—that is, the increase in the logit for every additional pack smoked per day. The antilogarithm of the coefficient is interpreted as the odds ratio describing the rate of disease at any given level of smoking relative to the rate corresponding to smoking one less pack per day. It is inherent in the model that each additional unit of increment in the independent variable or each additional pack smoked per day multiplies the odds ratio, or equivalently the rate of disease, by a constant factor. Therefore, each independent variable measured at more than two points inherently describes an exponential relation with disease frequency according to the model (see Fig. 14-4). This inherently multiplicative pattern is an important liability of the logistic model [Greenland, 1979]. Seldom will an investigator want to fit a model in which continuous or ordinal independent variables are automatically assumed to have an exponential relation to disease. Fortunately, the problem can be avoided by defining the independent variables as binary variables; this strategy is discussed in a later section, Designing Multivariate Models for Inference.

A related limitation of the multiple logistic model that cannot be easily avoided is the multiplicative relation of separate independent variables in the model with each other. Since each independent variable contributes toward a sum that is the logarithm of the odds for disease, the different variables in the model have a multiplicative relation with one another with regard to the rate of disease occurrence. A multiplicative relation is equivalent to an assumption that the ratio measure of effect for a given factor is constant over categories of the other factors. This assumption may not be a serious handicap—indeed, it is a frequently made assumption in stratified analysis—but unlike stratified analysis, the logistic model does not permit a direct evaluation of the adequacy of the assumption. It is possible to evaluate the multiplicative assumption by examining the magnitude of coefficients for terms that represent the product of two independent variables in the model. A more direct evaluation of the tenability of the mul-

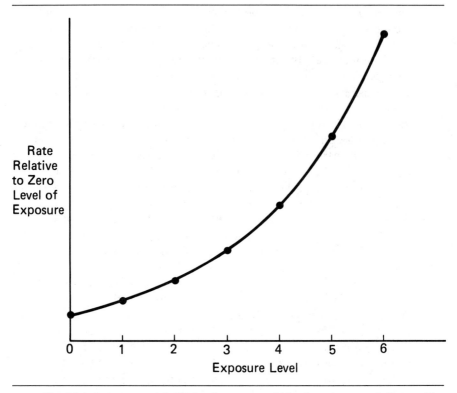

Fig. 14-4. An exponential relation between multi-level exposure and disease risk is implicit in the logistic model.

tiplicative assumption is possible using the generalized relative risk model of Thomas [1981], which embeds the logistic model in a more generalized multivariate model and enables the investigator to compare the adequacy of the mathematical assumptions for a broad range of specific models of which the logistic is but one.

Whether or not the multiplicative assumption inherent in the logistic model represents an adequate mathematical description of the data, the evaluation of biologic (as opposed to statistical) interaction between factors in a logistic model is complicated by the multiplicative nature of the model [Greenland, 1979]. This topic is discussed in Chapter 15.

It is worth noting that for case-control data in which the data on exposure and disease are dichotomous, a logistic regression can be formulated with either disease or exposure as the dependent variable. If disease is the dependent variable, the model is mathematically identical to the model used for follow-up studies [Prentice and Pyke, 1979]. If exposure is the dependent variable, the presence of disease must be included as an independent variable, and the odds ratio estimate is obtained as the antilogarithm of the coefficient for the disease term in the model [Prentice, 1976]. These two approaches are usually roughly, though not exactly, equivalent [Breslow and Powers, 1978]. It is generally easier to use disease as the dependent variable, since this approach allows the evaluation of the effect of several different exposure variables in the same model and can readily accommodate exposures measured with more than two categories.

The Proportional Hazards Model

The mathematical models described in the previous sections correspond to analyses in which the data can be summarized as frequencies in contingency tables. Indeed, the analyses for the odds ratio based on contingency table data that are presented in previous chapters can all be reformulated in logistic terms with identical results if the model is appropriately defined [Gart, 1971]. Logistic models can only be used, however, for frequency data; another approach is required to formulate mathematical models for incidence rate data, in which the denominators are person-time measures rather than frequencies.

One approach has been to use the amount of time until the event of interest for each subject, or some transformation of this amount of time, as the dependent variable in a linear regression model. The main difficulty with this straightforward approach is that in most studies the great majority of subjects are removed from observation before they develop the event of interest, either because the study ends, the individual becomes lost to follow-up, or the individual dies from another cause. The generalization of ordinary regression models for use with heavily censored data is problematic and poses computational difficulties [Breslow, 1979]. This approach might be appropriate if nearly every subject developed the event during the follow-up period.

A more flexible method has been developed by Cox [1972], who proposed a regression model that predicts as the dependent variable the ratio of incidence rates and in which the likelihood is evaluated conditionally on the set of subjects who remain under observation after each case occurrence. This model is known as the "proportional hazards" model because the incidence rate (hazard) ratio is assumed to be constant (i.e., hazards are proportional) over time. In the form originally proposed, this model is inherently multiplicative, as is the logistic model, to which it is closely related. The construction and interpretation of terms in the model are fundamentally the same as those for the logistic model. Indeed, when the event times are grouped into intervals, a logistic model can be adapted to the data and will often produce results that are nearly identical to those from the proportional hazards analysis [Abbott, 1985]. As with the logistic model, the proportional hazards model can be embedded within a generalized relative risk model [Thomas, 1981; McCullagh and Nelder, 1983] that allows evaluation of the multiplicative assumption.

Aside from the limitations mentioned earlier for the logistic model, a difficulty with the proportional hazards model is that relative to other multivariate models it is computationally onerous, since the likelihood evaluation is complicated and must be repeated for a large number of subsets of the data. For reasonably small sets of follow-up data such as those often encountered in clinical trials, the computations pose no serious difficulty for a high-speed computer. A recursive algorithm has been proposed by Howard [see discussion of Cox, 1972] and modified by Gail et al. [1981] that reduces the number of calculations considerably. Even with the recursive algorithm, however, the proportional hazards model may not be practical or feasible with today's computing equipment for the large data sets that are common for epidemiologic follow-up data relating to etiologic research. In such circumstances, a reasonable alternative is to group the data into time and/or age periods and consider a logistic model conditioning on the several time and/or age categories but not on the many subsets of individuals still under observation at each point in time [Breslow, 1979; Abbott, 1985]. With the expected continuation of progress in the technology of computer equipment, the time and cost of the calculations needed for fitting a proportional hazards model to a large set of data may soon prove to be inconsequential.

The proportional hazards model is one of a variety of methods for studying failure-time data. An excellent description of these methods is given by Kalbfleisch and Prentice [1980].

Log-Linear Models

Log-linear models are also closely related to logistic regression models. These are models for a contingency table that has one axis or dimension corresponding to each variable under study. The logarithm of the value expected for each cell in such a multidimensional contingency table is predicted as a linear function of terms. The terms correspond to each variable in the multidimensional table and various combinations of variables representing interaction terms. The marginal totals of the multidimensional table provide constraints for the fitted expected values of the cells.

With the appropriate model specified in the context of binary predictor and outcome variables, the maximum likelihood solution for a log-linear model will be identical to the maximum likelihood solution of the expected values for the common odds ratio estimation in a set of 2×2 tables as described in Chapter 12. The maximum likelihood estimate of the odds ratio can be obtained from the expected cell values of the fitted log-linear model just as it is from the fitted values stemming from equation 12-25. Furthermore, an appropriately specified logistic regression model will also give the same results. All these methods are mathematical reformulations of the same underlying model, that of an odds ratio that is constant across categories of one or more other factors; it is a multiplicative model because as the unexposed rate changes, the exposed rate must be multiplied by a constant factor for the incidence rate ratio, or odds ratio, to be constant.

Log-linear models have been popular with statisticians because they offer a kind of statistical flexibility: There is no specification of a dependent and a set of independent variables, nor of a disease and an exposure variable—all variables are treated equivalently as components of the model. Although this ecumenical treatment of variables offers an opportunity to explore the ways in which one confounder relates to another confounder as well as to the exposure, few epidemiologists will see this as an advantage. Epidemiologic analyses are usually focused on a specific interrelation of variables; if they are not, they probably should be. A disadvantage that has been cited for the log-linear model is that even continuous variables must be categorized to be put in contingency table format, whereas a logistic regression model can accommodate discrete or continuous predictor variables. This limitation is not serious, however, since, as argued in the later section, Designing Multivariate Models for Inference, the categorization of continuous variables is often desirable even in logistic regression models. The major drawback of the log-linear model is shared by the logistic regression model—namely, its inherent multiplicative assumption.

Multivariate Models for Matched Case-Control Studies

The analysis of matched case-control data usually requires that confounding by the matching factors introduced in the process of subject selection be controlled in the analysis. The specialized analyses discussed in the previous chapter are in fact just stratification techniques applied to matched data, with each matched set constituting a single stratum in the analysis. One important limitation to matched analysis by stratification is that it usually is not feasible to control for confounding by a factor that has not been matched in subject selection. This limitation can be overcome using multivariate models.

Since the odds ratio is the parameter of interest in case-control studies, the multivariate model that is pertinent is the logistic model and its generalizations [Thomas, 1981], from which the odds ratio can be easily estimated. If the only matching factors are variables with just a few categories, the multivariate model can be constructed with terms for these factors included as independent variables in the model, and the matching will be relevant to the analysis only to the extent that every variable matched in subject selection must be included in the model. Additional confounding variables that have not been matched in subject selection can also be added to the model.

A problem arises if the matching factors are variables with many categories, so that the model approaches the situation in which there is a term in the model for every matched set. This situation is analogous to a stratified analysis with a single stratum corresponding to every matched set.

Recall that maximum likelihood estimation of the odds ratio cannot be carried out in a stratified analysis with each matched set constituting a separate stratum using the unconditional approach of two independent binomials (formulas 12-22 and 12-24) because the estimation procedure gives rise to substantial bias when the marginal totals in each stratum are small. The bias is eliminated, however, by conditioning the estimation on both margins of each 2 × 2 table (formulas 12-22 and 12-23). Similarly, if the number of terms in a multivariate model becomes large relative to the number of subjects in the analysis, as occurs when a separate term is introduced for each matched set, unconditional maximum likelihood estimation becomes biased. The logistic model is usually fitted by a maximum likelihood procedure that is essentially the counterpart of the unconditional estimation procedure used in a stratified analysis. It is possible, however, to construct a logistic model in which the coefficients are estimated by a fitting procedure that is the counterpart of the conditional approach to the maximum likelihood estimation of the odds ratio [Prentice and Breslow, 1978]. This conditional structure is mathematically similar to, though not quite as complicated as, the proportional hazards model of Cox [1972], in which the survival experience of a group is modeled conditionally on those surviving at each point in time under observation. Like the proportional hazards model, the fitting of the conditional logistic regression can involve extensive computations, but the method allows matched case-control data to be analyzed with the necessary control of the matching factors as well as the control of additional confounding factors that were not matched. The recursive algorithm of Gail et al. [1981] reduces the computational burden considerably. Walker [1982] has noted that the conditional logistic model and the proportional hazards model are so similar that the computer programs for proportional hazards analysis can be used to fit a conditional logistic model.

General Relative Risk Models

Thomas [1981], noting the similarity in the statistical likelihood equations for matched case-control analysis, multiple logistic regression analysis, and the proportional hazards model proposed by Cox, has developed a more general model based on ratio measures of effect that subsumes these models and others. His general model allows for comparisons of, for example, additive versus multiplicative models of relative risk by creating mixtures of the two models within the format of the general model and evaluating the relative contribution of each component of the mixture. Walker and Rothman [1982] described a simple method for choosing between an additive and a multiplicative model for relative risk. With the general relative-risk model, however, a great variety of specific mathematical models of relative risk can be fitted, mixed, and compared. This methodology overcomes many of the limitations inherent in multiplicative models and is therefore an important expansion of the available options for epidemiologic multivariate analysis.

DESIGNING MULTIVARIATE MODELS FOR INFERENCE

The usual purpose for multivariate models in epidemiologic analysis is to permit the estimation of epidemiologic measures of effect while controlling efficiently for several confounding factors. Multivariate models may also be used to assess interaction; this application is discussed in Chapter 15. The dependent variable is usually an indicator term—that is, a binary variable with possible values of zero or one—that denotes the categorization with respect to disease for a given subject. The exposure variable and all confounding variables are included in the model as independent, or predictor, variables.

A variable in an epidemiologic analysis does not necessarily correspond to a single term in a multivariate model. At least one term will be required for each variable, but sometimes several will be required. The simplest type of variable is a nominal scale variable with only two categories, such as male and female. Such a variable would be included in a multivariate model as a single term; an indicator variable with values of one and zero corresponding to the two categories would be the numerical representation in a multivariate model for the variable "sex." Now consider a nominal scale variable with three categories such as white, black, and oriental, which, for the sake of example only, we shall assume are mutually exclusive and collectively exhaustive categories. It is inappropriate to assign different numerical values to these three categories and include them as a single term. Since the three categories do not represent quantitative aspects of a single measure, a single term will not allow a full description of the variable effect. For three categories, two terms are needed in the model: one of the three categories, for example, white, must be arbitrarily designated as a reference category; the two terms in the model are indicator terms that correspond to the presence of one of the two nonwhite categories. Suppose that the race terms are variables X_1 and X_2, and that X_1 indicates black and X_2 indicates oriental. If the subject is white, then both X_1 and X_2 take the value zero. If the subject is black, then $X_1 = 1$ and $X_2 = 0$, and if the subject is oriental then $X_1 = 0$ and $X_2 = 1$. The coefficients fitted for the terms X_1 and X_2 will represent measures of the effect of the characteristic black or oriental relative to the characteristic white. It makes little difference which category is selected as the reference category; it is usually a good idea, however, to select one that has a large proportion of the subjects, since the statistical stability of the coefficients in the model relative to the variable in question will depend on the choice of the reference category. If the variable has a "natural" reference category, then that group might take precedence even if it is not the largest. For example, in evaluating the risk of injury from participating in various school athletic activities, those who refrain from any activity form a natural reference group, even if some other groups in the classification are larger.

In general, if a nominal scale variable has n categories, then n − 1 terms are required in the model to describe the effect of each of n − 1 categories of the variable relative to a baseline category. If indicator terms are included for all n categories, the model will be redundant, and it will be impossible to solve the system of equations that give the estimates for the coefficients without some additional mathematical constraint. The different categories of a nominal scale variable may be thought of as a set of variables that must be evaluated separately in relation to an arbitrarily chosen reference category; what sets them apart as a collection is that they are mutually exclusive and therefore not independent. Theoretically, the lack of independence between terms in a multivariate model poses little problem unless there is a perfect correlation between two terms (or between any one term and any linear combination of other terms), in which case the model is redundant. In practice, very high correlations between two terms in the model, even if the correlation is not perfect, can lead to statistical instability in fitting the related coefficients, reflecting the difficult statistical problem of disentangling the effects of two highly correlated variables.

In constructing a model, the first step is to define the dependent variable. The investigator next proceeds to define the exposure term or terms. The exposure variable may be represented in the model as simply as with a single indicator variable, that is, a variable with a value of one if a subject is exposed and zero otherwise. If the exposure variable is nominal with more than two categories, it must be expressed in the model as several terms, as described in the previous paragraph. If the exposure variable is ordinal or interval, it is possible to express it in the model as a single term. To do so for an ordinal variable necessitates assigning scores to the categories, in effect translating the ordinal scale into an interval one. For either a scored ordinal variable or an interval one, the investigator must assess whether it is reasonable to allow the inherent shape of the curve that is built into the model relating the exposure and the effect measure to be used. With logistic regression, for example, a continuous exposure term will necessarily be related to the odds of disease risk exponentially, each added unit of exposure multiplying the baseline odds by a constant value that corresponds to the antilogarithm of the logistic regression coefficient. An exponential curve would rarely be appropriate since, as described earlier, it implies that a unit of exposure, for example, the twelfth cigarette smoked each day, adds more to the odds for disease than any of the units of exposure below it, such as the eighth or eleventh cigarette smoked each day. Consequently, the investigator should be wary of including continuous, interval, or scored ordinal terms in a multivariate model unless there is positive evidence that the curve implicit in the model is appropriate.

An alternative construction is to categorize an interval or continuous variable (an ordinal variable is already categorized) and treat it as if it were a nominal variable, including several exposure terms in the model. At first this approach may appear clumsy, since the ranked or continuous information in the data about exposure is lost, and several terms are now required in the model where only one term was required before. It is true that the statistical power of a trend test evaluating a dose-response relation, embodied in the P-value attached to a coefficient for a continuous variable, is lost with this approach. On the other hand, the inclusion of several exposure terms allows the information about each level of exposure to be used to generate effect estimates that are not constrained to follow any specific pattern. Simplicity of a multivariate model is often touted as being highly desirable, but the rationale is usually based on the adoption of models for predictive or descriptive purposes. When models are used, as they generally are in epidemiology, for inference about the role of specific factors, the simplicity of the model is not an important goal. Therefore, the inclusion of several terms rather than one presents no real drawback as far as the complexity of the model is concerned. The advantage of being able to estimate the effect separately, without an imposed pattern, at each level of exposure in relation to a baseline level outweighs the disadvantages of this approach in most situations. With sufficient data, complicated dose-response relations, such as U or inverted-U shapes, can be detected and estimated without fear that the model does not adequately describe the data.

After defining the exposure term or terms in the model, the investigator should focus on confounding factors. For these, the issues are much the same as for the exposure. Each variable must be translated into one or more terms in the model. Again, it is desirable to use a set of indicator terms to allow a less constrained relation between the confounder and the disease. The analytic goal is somewhat different for confounding variables: Rather than make inferences about the effect of the confounder, the goal is to allow for the effect of the confounder so that the effect of the exposure is not distorted. To achieve this goal, however, essentially the same treatment is needed in the model for a confounder as for the exposure. It is not nearly as important to pin down accurately the shape of the dose-response curve for a confounder, but on the other hand, there is usually little to gain, unless the data are sparse or poorly distributed, by reducing the number of terms in the model. Furthermore, in some analyses, a confounder of the exposure may hold some interest as an exposure in its own right. Inferences on exposure and several confounders can be made easily from a single model if the variables at issue are defined optimally in the model. On the other hand, if the confounder is known to have a monotonic relation with the disease outcome, it is possible to achieve better control of confounding by retaining the natural ordering of the categories in a single scored ordinal or continuous term. The trade-off between the ability to fit a better curve by using a set of indicator terms and the natural ordering and loss of fewer "degrees of freedom" that results from using a single term is not sufficiently well understood to make a general recommendation. It is clear, however, that uncertainty about the shape of the curve relating the confounder and the disease favors treating the confounder in the same way as the exposure, with a set of indicator terms.

A common method in the fitting of multivariate models is the stepwise approach, in which terms in the model are added or subtracted in successive stages according to a criterion of statistical "significance" that is related to the extent to which the fit of the model is affected by the loss or gain of the next term. An automatic selection process is alluring, especially for the model-builder who feels uncomfortable interpreting multivariate models. Nevertheless, this method is inappropriate for most epidemiologic applications and should be avoided. It posits as a goal that the model should be parsimonious with respect to the number of terms, but this goal is not pertinent to epidemiologic analysis that is focusing on the effect of specific factors. The method uses statistical "significance" to assess the adequacy of a model rather than judging the need to control confounding for specific factors on the basis of the extent of confounding involved. It is possible that ten different factors might each be confounding a moderate amount, but that none individually is related to the disease strongly enough to affect the fit of the model in a "statistically significant" way. A stepwise approach could lead to a model that excludes the terms relating to all ten factors. But what can be gained by censoring the model to exclude these terms? If most of the factors are confounding in the same direction, which is a possibility, then there might be a substantial amount of confounding for the excluded factors in the aggregate, even if none alone contributes in a "statistically significant" way to the model. Indeed, the primary advantage of employing a multivariate model in an epidemiologic analysis is the ability to control efficiently for a multitude of factors simultaneously. Using a stepwise approach is not merely wasteful but negates some of the advantage of the multivariate analysis. It simplifies and strengthens an analysis to avoid any stepwise option and instead attempt to construct a single comprehensive multivariate model that includes all important confounders along with the exposure term or terms.

Multivariate models can also be used to evaluate effect modification or interaction. The details will be discussed in Chapter 15, but it is important to note that if interaction terms involving the exposure are added to a model, it becomes difficult to assess the effect of the exposure. If the exposure or a given level of exposure is present in only a single term, the effect can be estimated from the coefficient for that term. If product terms between the exposure and other variables are included in the model, the effect of the exposure will be spread over the various terms that include it; a detailed examination of the terms may reveal information about the effect, but often a straightforward evaluation becomes impossible. For example, if an indicator term for exposure in a model is supplemented with an interaction term that involves the product of exposure and age, to allow for an age interaction, the investigator may find a negative coefficient for the exposure term and a positive coefficient for the exposure-age interaction term. Under such circumstances, it may not be easy to determine whether the overall effect of exposure is positive or negative. A sensible approach is to avoid interaction terms involving the exposure unless the evaluation of effect modification is a specific analytic goal, in which case the approach described in the next chapter should be adopted. In contrast, there is little problem posed by adding interaction terms that involve the product of two (or more) covariates; a model can usually be fitted with any level of complication desired for the confounders, including complicated interactions among them, usually without serious drawbacks. (The only concern is that sparseness in the data will lead to statistical instabilities in fitting the model with the added terms.) For example, age-sex interaction terms allow for different age effects for males and females to be fitted. The intricacy of a model that includes interaction terms between covariates does not inhibit a straightforward inference about the effect of the exposure, and it permits effective control of confounding by letting the model adapt to the pattern of the confounding factors that fits the data most closely.

One of the measures often associated with multivariate models is the correlation coefficient. The multiple correlation coefficient is the simple product-moment correlation between the dependent variable and the set of model-generated estimates of the dependent variable that correspond to the individual data points. The square of the multiple correlation corresponds to the proportion of the variance of the dependent variable explained by the model; however, it has no epidemiologic interpretation. Simple or partial correlations are measures of association between two variables; simple correlations are crude measures, whereas partial correlations are controlled for other factors. Correlation coefficients are generally inappropriate for epidemiologic inferences, since they do not offer any epidemiologic interpretability. The value of a correlation coefficient depends on the distribution and range of the component variables and consequently on design factors that should not bear on scientific inference. Within a narrow enough range of two variables, correlations will be small, whatever the degree of association over the wider range. Therefore, reliance on correlation coefficients for inference can be misleading and should be avoided. Inferences drawn from unstandardized regression coefficients are not subject to the same problem as those drawn from correlation coefficients, but the use of standardized regression coefficients for inference is problematic, since the standardized coefficient depends on overall frequency of the risk factor and the study outcome; path analysis, depending heavily on partial correlations, should be avoided as an analytic tool in epidemiology for the same reason [Greenland et al., 1986].

To summarize, the interpretation of a multivariate model used for epidemiologic analysis is facilitated by the use of indicator terms, even if it is necessary to break up ordinal or continuous variables to form them, to free the investigator to some extent of the mathematical constrictions of the multivariate model. This procedure complicates the model by adding more terms but allows for greater flexibility. A monotonic relation between a confounder and the disease, if known with assurance, could warrant the use of a single term to obtain optimum control but only if the slope of the curve corresponds well to what is imputed by the model. By avoiding stepwise algorithms, the overall complexity of the analysis can be reduced, since the investigator can focus on a single model with all the relevant terms. Interaction terms can be added to account for the interrelation among confounding factors, but it is desirable to avoid product terms involving the exposure because they hinder interpretation, unless the study of interaction is one of the analytic goals (see Chap. 15) or the investigator is confident about the accuracy of the model. Finally, correlation coefficients and standardized regression coefficients should not be used for epidemiologic analysis.

MULTIVARIATE MODELS IN ECOLOGIC ANALYSIS

Studies in which the unit of observation is a group of people rather than an individual are known as ecologic studies (see Chap. 6). The outcome measure in an ecologic study is usually a continuous variable, such as the mortality rate for a country, which distinguishes ecologic studies from other epidemiologic studies and necessitates an analytic approach different from studies that have a discrete outcome variable. Multivariate modeling is a convenient way to dissect the variability in the outcome variable and explain it as a function of several independent variables. Multivariate models applied to an ecologic analysis correspond well to a classic regression problem, since typically not only the outcome variable is measured on a continuous scale but also all the independent variables as well. Since the unit of observation is a population, information on predictor variables is measured as a population average, which is a continuous variable. Even discrete variables such as gender become continuous when averaged for a population: Gender is a binary variable, but the proportion of a population that is male is essentially continuous.

Although a classic regression model would seem to apply well to such data, some nuances in the analysis should be kept clearly in mind. First, since each unit of observation is a population and since populations differ in size, the amount of information in each observational unit will differ. To allow for this properly in the analysis, the regression should be a weighted regression. This procedure takes into account a weight assigned to each observation that reflects the relative amount of information embodied in the observation. The weights could be taken as the reciprocal of the estimated variance of the observation; for an incidence or mortality rate this would be the square of the denominator divided by the numerator. Another reasonable weighting scheme is to weight each observation simply by the size of the denominator of the rate.

A second point to bear in mind is that the coefficients in the model usually cannot be converted into the usual epidemiologic measures of effect. Although the outcome variable may be a measure such as incidence rate or mortality rate, the independent variables represent at best average values of exposure and cannot accurately reflect the effect of a change in exposure level on disease occurrence unless the linear assumption of the model is reasonably accurate. Most often the independent variables in the model are proxy variables anyway, so that epidemiologic interpretation of the coefficients is problematic, being at best subject to considerable bias. Effect estimates from epidemiologic studies may be greatly exaggerated by a phenomenon known as "cross-level" bias [Morgenstern, 1982]. Nevertheless, epidemiologic inferences are occasionally possible with ecologic data, and it may even be possible to assess the extent of bias [Stevens and Moolgavkar, 1984]. Examples of proxy variables include data on cigarette or alcohol tax in place of data on actual consumption of cigarettes or alcohol.

A third point is that the control of confounding is difficult in ecologic analyses, since the individual observations are average data or proxy data for populations, thereby leading to attenuated associations and intercorrelations between variables that limit the control of confounding [Greenland, 1980; Morgenstern, 1982]. Furthermore, it is usually more difficult in ecologic studies to obtain even proxy data for some factors that are known or suspected to be confounders. The lack of availability of relevant information is the most serious handicap in ecologic analysis.

In a linear regression model, the dependent variable can range from minus infinity to plus infinity, but the incidence rate ranges only from zero to plus infinity. The incomparability of ranges can be addressed by transforming the incidence rate with a logarithmic transformation. While this transformation is mathematically attractive because it prevents the model from providing negative estimates for incidence rate, the main consideration is whether the multiplicative model that results is a better description of the data than the additive model that applies without the logarithmic transformation. Continuous terms in the multiplicative model would have, as in a logistic model, an exponential relation to one another. It would be possible to use a set of indicator variables for each continuous variable in the model, but since the continuous variables are population averages, they become that much more difficult to interpret. Unless a specific reason demands it, it would appear preferable to conduct most multivariate ecologic analyses as untransformed linear regressions.

STRENGTHS AND LIMITATIONS OF MULTIVARIATE MODELS

Stratification has been presented as the first-line method for controlling confounding and evaluating effect modification in epidemiologic analysis. Cross-classification of data by many variables simultaneously may stretch the observations too thinly over the many subcategories required, thus making stratification infeasible when the investigator must account for a relatively large number of variables in the analysis. The specific point at which stratification becomes unmanageable depends on the amount of data, the number of variables and categories, the distribution of the data over these variables, and the judgment of the investigator about the price that is worth paying to conduct a stratified analysis. Certainly stratification offers some clear advantages: The analyses can usually be conducted with no more than a pocket calculator (although a computer is usually used and often necessary to generate the stratified data); the investigator develops a familiarity with the data and can observe the distribution of each variable over the strata; the pattern of effect estimates across strata is readily apparent; and the presentation of the analysis retains a cogency for readers, many of whom are more comfortable with stratified analysis than with multivariate analysis, especially when the stratified data are presented for the reader to scrutinize. The major limitation of stratified analysis is the inability to deal with more than a few variables at once, unless matching has provided similar distributions for the compared series across strata. Without matching, as the number of observations within strata decreases with an increasing number of strata, the ratio of controls to cases (or, in follow-up studies, the ratio of unexposed to exposed subjects) will fluctuate randomly in wild swings about the average value; these fluctuations inject too much random error into the estimation process, causing a loss in study efficiency that jeopardizes the interpretation of the results. In these circumstances, the only analytic alternative is some form of multivariate analysis.

The strengths and limitations of multivariate analysis are largely the mirror image of those of stratified analysis. Whereas stratified analysis becomes inefficient in the face of many covariates, multivariate analysis is usually highly efficient. On the other hand, the cogency of stratified analysis is missing from multivariate analysis. A computer must intrude between the raw observations and the epidemiologic measures that result from them, obscuring some of the most meaningful interrelations of the study variables from both the investigator and the reader. Only long experience with multivariate modeling will begin to simulate the feel for the data that is readily obtainable from a stratified analysis. The calculations are so intricate that the investigator must rely completely on the available computing equipment and software. Software errors may go undetected through many analyses, since there is no simple way to check the software thoroughly. In addition, the statistical efficiency of multivariate models comes at a price, which is the assumption that a given mathematical form describes the relation of study variables. Extrapolation beyond the limits of the observations, which many investigators are reluctant to do and which is easily avoided in stratified analysis, is difficult to avoid in multivariate models; indeed, extrapolation and interpolation are critical to the gain in efficiency in multivariate analysis. By assuming that the mathematical model will describe the conditional distribution of a variable over a range of values for which direct observations are lacking, the model can express the combined relation of many factors simultaneously with simplicity and elegance. If the model is incorrect, however, the improved efficiency may be negated by an intolerable degree of bias; furthermore, the bias will not be detected without special efforts, and the caution that such efforts characterize can easily be eroded by the seductive appeal of a neat, efficient-looking model.

These drawbacks of multivariate analysis make stratified analysis the more desirable alternative when the data permit it. In many situations stratified and multivariate analysis may be complementary in providing useful insights about the data. The great strength of multivariate analysis is its ability to control for a large number of variables simultaneously, a goal that stratified analysis cannot often attain. Similarly, a matched case-control analysis using stratification can efficiently control only those factors that have been matched; a conditional logistic regression analysis permits control of additional factors beyond those that were matched. For such applications multivariate analysis is a necessary component of the epidemiologist's analytic repertoire.

USE OF A CONFOUNDER SUMMARY SCORE

Since the advantages and disadvantages of stratification and multivariate modeling are complementary, it is reasonable to consider how the two approaches might be combined into a single methodology to gain the advantages of both. The primary disadvantage of stratification is the loss of efficiency that results from creating a large number of strata to control confounding by many variables simultaneously. In principle it should be possible to combine many of these strata without introducing any substantial confounding, but the difficulty is to identify which ones. If there were only one confounding variable, say age, and strata had been created for every single year of age, the large number of resulting strata would be unnecessary, since nearly all the confounding by age could be controlled with a handful of age categories [Cochran, 1968]. Collapsing redundant age strata presents no difficulty, because age is a continuous variable, and neighboring categories can be coalesced into a few broader age strata.

The idea behind confounder summarization is to define a single continuous variable that pulls together the relevant information on the confounding properties of all variables [Bunker et al., 1969; Miettinen, 1976; Rosenbaum and Rubin, 1983]. Consider a randomized experiment. A propensity for developing disease, if the randomization works well, should be distributed equally across the intervention groups. There is no direct way, however, to check these distributions, since propensity for disease cannot be measured directly except by measuring disease incidence, which is the outcome of the study and which could be influenced by the intervention itself. What is needed to evaluate the efficacy of the randomization is some indication of disease risk among the individuals in the different treatment groups apart from the effect of the intervention. The distribution of known risk factors serves as an indicator of this propensity for disease. A study may have little or no confounding, however, even if the distributions of known risk factors are not identical, since it is possible that imbalances for some risk factors are offset by imbalances for other risk factors. The overall confounding that exists could be easily controlled if the contribution of all the known risk factors to the propensity to develop disease could be summarized into a single measure.

A multivariate model can be used to combine the risk factor information into a single measure, a confounder summary score. The method can be applied to nonexperimental studies as well as to experiments. In follow-up studies, the score is a proxy for disease risk. In case-control studies, the score cannot be a proxy for disease risk; the analogous measure may be thought of as the probability of being classified as a case conditional on being in the study. Some of the disadvantages that accompany multivariate analysis do not apply in using multivariate models to generate confounder summary scores. If the multivariate model is used simply to generate scores that will be used for stratification rather than directly for inference, the problem of lack of cogency of the model is alleviated.

Construction of a multivariate model to generate summary confounder scores is straightforward. Not only will nearly any type of mathematical model do, but the definition of terms in the model can be as complex as desired, even for exposure terms, without clouding the interpretation, since there is no interpretation based directly on the model. Exposure variables can be represented by several terms in the model, including interaction terms and higher order polynomial terms if desired. It is desirable to omit from the model factors that are strong predictors of outcome but are not related to the exposure of interest and therefore not confounding; including such factors does not improve validity but can adversely affect efficiency by introducing less overlap of the case and noncase distributions. After fitting the model, scores must be estimated for each subject. Since it is the disease risk (or disease classification probability) score conditional on the absence of exposure that is desired, the scores should be calculated by setting the exposure to the nonexposed value, regardless of the actual exposure, for all subjects and then using the other data for each subject to calculate the summary score from the fitted multivariate model [Miettinen, 1976]. Alternatively, scores can be calculated from a model fitted to the data relating to unexposed subjects only.

Once the scores are calculated, they can be used as a confounder summary variable on which a stratified analysis can be based. The analysis proceeds as if there were a single continuous confounder such as age. The end product has many of the advantages of both stratified and multivariate analysis.

The method does have its drawbacks, however. One liability is the complexity of first fitting a multivariate model, calculating the scores, and then conducting a stratified analysis. Related to the complexity of the procedure is some added complexity of interpretation: From the strata, it is not always clear what variables have been controlled and how effectively they have been controlled. There are other problems: As with any multivariate modeling, the validity remains dependent on the adequacy of the model. The procedure is "circular" to the extent that the confounder scores used in stratification are estimated from a model fitted to the data to be stratified. Pike et al. [1979] have pointed out that the statistical hypothesis test based on the procedure is biased. Perhaps these drawbacks explain why the method has not become popular. Nevertheless, the principle is an appealing one that may prove useful as a way of gaining added insights in complicated analyses.

REFERENCES

Abbott, R. D. Logistic regression in survival analysis. *Am. J. Epidemiol.* 1985;121:465–471.

Breslow, N. Statistical methods for censored survival data. *Environ. Hlth. Perspect.* 1979;32:181–192.

Breslow, N. E., and Powers, W. E. Are there two logistic regressions for retrospective studies? *Biometrics* 1978;34:100–105.

Bunker, J. P., Forrest, W. H., Jr., Mosteller, F., et al. *The National Halothane Study — A Study of the Possible Association Between Halothane Anesthesia and Postoperative Hepatic Necrosis.* Bethesda: National Institutes of Health, National Institute of General Medical Sciences, 1969.

Cochran, W. G. The effectiveness of adjustment by subclassification in removing bias in observational studies. *Biometrics* 1968;24:295–313.

Cox, D. R. Regression models and life tables (with discussion). *J. R. Stat. Soc. B.* 1972;34:187–220.

Gail, M. H., Lubin, J. H., and Rubinstein, L. V. Likelihood calculations for matched case-control studies and survival studies with tied death times. *Biometrika* 1981;68:703–707.

Gart, J. J. The comparison of proportions: A review of significance tests, confidence intervals and adjustments for stratification. *Rev. Int. Stat. Inst.* 1971;39:148–169.

Greenland, S. Limitations of the logistic analysis of epidemiologic data. *Am. J. Epidemiol.* 1979;110:693–698.

Greenland, S. The effect of misclassification in the presence of covariates. *Am. J. Epidemiol.* 1980;112:564–569.

Greenland, S., Schlesselman, J. J., Criqui, M. H. The fallacy of employing standardized regression coefficients and correlations as measures of effect. *Am. J. Epidemiol.* 1986;123:203–208.

Kalbfleisch, J. D., and Prentice, R. L. *The Statistical Analysis of Failure-Time Data.* New York:Wiley, 1980.

McCullagh, P., and Nelder, J. A. *Generalized Linear Models.* New York: Chapman and Hall, 1983.

Miettinen, O. S. Stratification by a multivariate confounder score. *Am. J. Epidemiol.* 1976;104:609–620.

Morgenstern, H. Uses of ecologic analysis in epidemiologic research. *Am. J. Public Hlth.* 1982;72:1336–1344.

Pike, M. C., Anderson, J., and Day, N. Some insights into Miettinen's multivariate confounder score approach to case-control study analysis. *Epidemiol. Comm. Hlth.* 1979;33:104–106.

Prentice, R. Use of the logistic model in retrospective studies. *Biometrics* 1976;32:599–606.

Prentice, R. L., and Pyke, R. Logistic disease incidence models and case-control data. *Biometrika* 1979;66:408–412.

Prentice, R. L., and Breslow, N. E. Retrospective studies and failure time models. *Biometrika* 1978;65:153–158.

Rosenbaum, P. R., and Rubin, D. The central role of the propensity score in observational studies for causal effects. *Biometrika* 1983;70:41–45.

Rothman, K. J., Cann, C. I., Flanders, D., et al. Epidemiology of laryngeal cancer. *Epidemiol. Rev.* 1980;2:195–209.

Stevens, R. G., and Moolgavkar, S. H. A cohort analysis of lung cancer and smoking in British males. *Am. J. Epidemiol.* 1984;119:624–641.

Thomas, D. C. General relative risk models for survival time and matched case-control analysis. *Biometrics* 1981;37:673–676.

Walker, A. M. Efficient assessment of confounder effects in matched follow-up studies. *Appl. Stat.* 1982;31:293–297.

Walker, A. M., and Rothman, K. J. Models of varying parametric form. *Am. J. Epidemiol.* 1982;115:129–137.

15. INTERACTIONS BETWEEN CAUSES

The proper methodology for the evaluation of interactions has been hotly debated. On one side are those who would apply statistical or purely arbitrary criteria to the choice of a model for independence of effects; according to this view, interaction can be judged from a variety of vantage points, and the result of the evaluation can depend on the choice of vantage point. On the other side are epidemiologists who are increasingly convinced that there is a uniquely appropriate epidemiologic definition of independence that must be applied to obtain a meaningful evaluation of interaction.

The discussion has been conducted on two levels. On the first level is an examination of the principles that govern the definition of independence of effects for epidemiologic purposes, presuming that there is a nonarbitrary reference point. On the second level is a discussion of whether any meaningful interpretation can emerge from an evaluation of interaction that begins with an arbitrary definition of independence.

To illustrate the argument, suppose that incidence rates for lung cancer depended on exposure to cigarette smoke and asbestos according to the pattern of rates shown in Table 15-1. What interpretation can be drawn from these rates regarding the interaction between smoking and asbestos?

With respect to the absolute measure of effect, the rate difference, there is substantial effect modification in these data. Specifically, the effect of smoking is an increase in incidence of lung cancer of $9/100,000 \ yr^{-1}$ among those not exposed to asbestos, but $45/100,000 \ yr^{-1}$ among those exposed to asbestos. The absolute effect of smoking is five times greater among those exposed to asbestos than among those unexposed. Similarly, the asbestos effect is substantially greater for smokers than for nonsmokers.

On the other hand, if ratio measures of effect are calculated for either exposure within each category of the other, the ratio is found to be uniform. Thus, smokers experience a tenfold incidence of lung cancer relative to nonsmokers in the presence or in the absence of exposure to asbestos. Similarly, asbestos exposure is related to a fivefold increase in incidence of lung cancer for smokers and for nonsmokers. Using the ratio measure of effect as a guide, there is no indication of any effect modification of smoking by asbestos or vice versa. Equivalently, any mathematical model based on proportional effects—that is to say, a multiplicative relation between factors, will indicate no interaction between asbestos and smoking based on these data. For example, the coefficient of a product term between asbestos and smoking in a multiple logistic regression analysis based on data conforming to the rates in Table 15-1 would be zero; a log-linear analysis, which is also premised on a multiplicative model, would also indicate no interaction. Indeed, any statistical evaluation of heterogeneity of the rate ratio would find no discrepancy from the null hypothesis of a uniform rate ratio for data conforming to these rates.

Table 15-1. *Hypothetical incidence rates for lung cancer (expressed as cases per hundred thousand person-years) according to exposure to cigarette smoke and asbestos*

Smoke	Asbestos	
	+	−
+	50	10
−	5	1

For those who have proposed that the concept of interaction between factors is inherently arbitrary, since it is dependent on the choice of reference point [Walter and Holford, 1978; Kupper and Hogan, 1978; Darroch, 1974], comparison of rate ratios, rate differences, or possibly some other measure of effect could all be used equally well to evaluate interaction. These investigators hold that statistical convenience in conducting the analysis is an integral part of the decision process determining which measure should be used to evaluate interaction between variables. Darroch [1974] used several statistical criteria of convenience and concluded that "the multiplicative definition (of no interaction) is preferable by a small margin." Similarly, Walter and Holford [1978], who also expressed a preference for multiplicative models, argued that "the definition of interaction, in the absence of a specific physiologic model, is indeed arbitrary, and that the choice of the definition should depend to some extent on statistical convenience in the analysis of observed data." This concept of interaction, in which the reference point corresponding to the absence of interaction is not anchored to any specific theoretical underpinning, has been termed "statistical interaction" [Rothman, 1978]. Statistical interaction is simultaneously both present and absent for the rates in Table 15-1, according to whether the reference point for independence of effects corresponds to an additive or multiplicative model.

It is certainly true that for statistical purposes a variety of models can be used with equal efficacy to describe the pattern of rates in Table 15-1. If the goal of an analysis is simply description or the development of a model for predictive purposes, it may be defensible to place economy of description ahead of other criteria in choosing a model. This process may justify selecting a model for a particular analysis that exhibits no interaction and therefore offers a more parsimonious description than alternative models. Interaction between factors is completely model-dependent in such a process; its presence or absence is a statistical artifice that indicates how well the chosen model describes the data and has no implication for inference beyond the model itself. Interaction viewed in this arbitrary way is equivalent to the concept of effect modification, which was also seen to be an arbitrary concept that depended on whether the effect was measured in absolute or relative terms.

Epidemiologic analysis, however, usually attempts to go beyond statistical modeling. The concept of statistical interaction, linked as it is to arbitrariness in the choice of model, is devoid of epidemiologic interpretability because it does not rest on an explicit theoretical foundation. Without implication for inference beyond the model, a purely statistical concept of interaction cannot contribute meaningfully to epidemiologic analysis. This point is illustrated sufficiently well by the dual interpretation that emerges with respect to the presence of statistical interaction from the rates in Table 15-1. If the phenomenon of interaction were merely a statistical construct that permitted contrary interpretations from the same data, it could not contribute to scientific knowledge.

DEFINING INTERACTION

It is possible to develop an unambiguous definition of epidemiologic interaction using as a conceptual framework the general causal model presented in Chapter 2. In that model, sufficient causes of disease were seen to comprise a constellation of component causes that correspond to the individual factors that are the intended objects of inference in epidemiologic analysis. Different causal mechanisms correspond to different sufficient causes of disease. If two component causes act to produce disease in a common sufficient cause, some cases of disease will consequently arise for which the two component causes share in the causal responsibility; in the absence of either of the components, these cases would not occur. This coparticipation in a sufficient cause is the conceptual basis for interaction.

If the two component causes act only through different sufficient causes, their actions are conceptually independent. It is axiomatic to epidemiologic theory that the absolute effect of a single component cause is measured by the incidence rate that corresponds to the rate of occurrence of sufficient causes that involve the factor in question. This rate cannot be observed, but it can be inferred: Among those exposed to a component cause, the incidence rate of disease is the sum of the rate of occurrence of two different classes of sufficient causes. One part of the sum is the rate of occurrence of sufficient causes that contain the factor, which is the rate of interest. The other part is the rate of occurrence of sufficient causes that lack the factor. If there is no confounding, the latter rate also corresponds to the rate among unexposed. Therefore, the difference between rates of disease occurrence in exposed and unexposed corresponds to the absolute effect, that is, the incidence rate of completion of sufficient causes that contain the component cause of interest. If the factor is denoted by A, we can represent this relation as follows:

$$RD = R(A) - R(\overline{A})$$

or, in terms of the causal "pies" corresponding to the components of the epidemiologic measures,

where U represents unidentified component causes of disease or components that are simply unspecified in this particular analysis. Thus, measuring the effect of exposure A requires separating the rate of disease occurrence among people with exposure A into two components, the first representing instances of disease resulting from sufficient causes that include A, and the second representing instances of disease from mechanisms that do not include A and for whom exposure to A is incidental.

If we extend the same model to a second specified component cause, B, there are four classes of sufficient causes of disease to consider: those with both A and B, those with A but not B, those with B but not A, and those with neither:

People exposed to both A and B may develop disease from any of these classes of mechanisms. The rate of occurrence of completed mechanisms containing both A and B, corresponding to the absolute measure of the interactive effect of factors A and B, can be defined as

$$I(AB) = R(AB) - R(A\bar{B}) - R(\bar{A}B) + R(\bar{A}\bar{B}) \qquad [15\text{-}1]$$

which can be depicted in terms of causal "pies" as

This definition for interaction is implicit in the conceptualization of causes and epidemiologic measures presented earlier in this book. The definition is equivalent to defining as independence of effects (i.e., assuming that $I(AB) = 0$) the relation

$$R(AB) = R(A\overline{B}) + R(\overline{A}B) - R(\overline{AB}) \qquad [15\text{-}2]$$

or

$$R(AB) - R(\overline{AB}) = [R(A\overline{B}) - R(\overline{AB})] + [R(\overline{A}B) - R(\overline{AB})] \qquad [15\text{-}3]$$

which represents the additivity of absolute effects, or, what is the same thing, uniformity of rate differences for one factor across strata of the other. Expression 15-3 can be restated in terms of relative effect (see formula 4-1) by dividing by $R(\overline{AB})$:

$$RR(AB) - 1 = [RR(A\overline{B}) - 1] + [RR(\overline{A}B) - 1] \qquad [15\text{-}4]$$

The measure $RR - 1$ has been described by Cole and MacMahon [1971] as the "relative excess risk." Expressions 15-3 and 15-4 indicate that under independence the joint effect of two factors is equal to the sum of the effects of each factor acting without the other, whether the effects are measured in absolute or in relative terms. The reference group for the comparisons must be the group unexposed to either factor. The additivity of effects, absolute or relative, is the point from which meaningful departures from independence of action should be measured. Statistical models, such as logistic regression, that implicitly pose alternative definitions of independence are consequently inconsistent with the theoretical epidemiologic underpinnings from which the basic measures in epidemiology are derived. This is not to say that multiplicative models, for example, cannot be used to evaluate interactive effects; in fact, they can, but not in the usual manner of estimating the coefficient of a product term in the model. The interaction must be evaluated on an additive scale, as described later in this chapter.

The importance of adhering to the appropriate epidemiologic definition of interaction is illustrated by a study that was intended to evaluate the interaction between oral contraceptives and hypertension in the causation of stroke in young women [Collaborative Group for the Study of Stroke in Young Women, 1975]. The results for thrombotic stroke for this case-control study are summarized in Table 15-2. Note that each relative risk estimate uses the same reference category: women who did not use oral contraceptives and who had normal blood pressure. The two risk factors have a less-than-multiplicative relation, since the relative risk estimates for each factor in the absence of the other, when multiplied together, yield a product greater than the estimate of relative risk that was actually observed for

Table 15-2. Relative risk for thrombotic stroke
according to oral contraceptive use and severity of hypertension
[Collaborative Group for the Study of Stroke in Young Women, 1975]

	Oral Contraceptive Use	
	Yes	No
Severity of hypertension		
Severe	13.6	6.9
Normal	3.1	1.0*

*Reference category.

women with both risk factors. A multiplicative relation would be satisfied if women with both risk factors, severe hypertension and oral contraceptive use, had a relative risk of 3.1 × 6.9 = 21.4 rather than the value of 13.6 that was observed.

On the assumption built into multiplicative models for independent effects, these two risk factors manifest a negative interaction, or "antagonism." On the other hand, when independence is construed as additivity of effects, these two risk factors exhibit a positive interaction, or "synergy," since the excess relative risk for those with both exposures is greater than the sum of the excess relative risk for each factor considered in isolation. For oral contraceptive use alone, the excess relative risk is 3.1 − 1.0 = 2.1; for severe hypertension alone it is 6.9 − 1.0 = 5.9; for both factors, it is 13.6 − 1.0 = 12.6, which is greater than the sum of 5.9 and 2.1. (The relative risks in Table 15-2 can be compared in the same way as the rates in Table 15-1 because the relative risk estimates all have a common referent category.) If the study of interaction were only a matter of statistical convenience, the choice between two apparently contradictory interpretations, of antagonism on the one hand and synergy on the other, would be totally dependent on the mathematical model used to define what the relative risk would be for women with both risk factors if the two risk factors were independent. In their report, the authors chose to use the multiplicative definition for independent effects rather than the additive definition.

The use of an inappropriate definition for independence violates more than just a sterile set of epidemiologic axioms: The practical and biologic interpretation of interactive effects follows from the epidemiologic principles [Koopman, 1981]. Consider what the investigators in the stroke example were trying to learn: Is oral contraceptive use more hazardous for women with hypertension than it is for normotensive women with regard to risk of stroke? If the two risk factors are independent, that should imply that an informed woman facing a decision to use oral contraceptives and weighing the risk of stroke in that decision would not need to take into account her blood pressure. Independence means that the risk evaluation of oral contraceptives can be made without reference to blood pressure.

It follows that negative interaction should imply to a user of oral contraceptives that hypertension, beyond the effect it has alone on stroke incidence, mitigates the effect of oral contraceptives on stroke, whereas positive interaction should imply that hypertension, in addition to its own effect, exacerbates the effect of oral contraceptives. A system of interpreting interactive effects that simultaneously permits an interpretation of mitigation and exacerbation of a biologic risk from the same data cannot serve a useful scientific purpose. Here it is clear that the arbitrariness that is inherent in the concept of statistical interaction must be studiously avoided in epidemiologic contexts, whatever the statistical exigencies may be. Epidemiologists cannot accept a definition of interaction so loose that it allows the data in Table 15-2 to be interpreted as synergy for some investigators and antagonism for other investigators: At least one of these interpretations must be incorrect.

The authors' use of a multiplicative criterion for independence leads to the inappropriate conclusion that the effect of oral contraceptives on stroke is greater among normotensive women than it is among women with severe hypertension; that is, that oral contraceptives are more dangerous, with regard to stroke, for normotensive women than for hypertensive women. A warning based on this interpretation would logically be a warning for the women more susceptible to the effect of oral contraceptives, namely, the women with normal blood pressure. In the actual paper, the warning stated was "... we believe that oral contraceptives should not be used by women with any degree of high blood pressure." [Collaborative Group for the Study of Stroke in Young Women, 1975]. The authors offer no justification for the logical inconsistency between their data and their conclusion, but the conclusion signals that somehow the authors must have understood that their initial methodologic assumption about independence was faulty.

In steady-state conditions, the number of cases of a disease occurring in a dynamic population free of the disease is proportional to the incidence rate. If a given agent, exposure A, increases the incidence rate among a population subgroup with exposure B by a larger absolute amount than among the subgroup lacking exposure B, then exposure A will produce more cases of the disease among a population with exposure B than among the same size population unexposed to B. It follows that the public health costs of exposure A will be greater for the subpopulation exposed to B than for the unexposed subpopulation. On the other hand, if the sum of the incidence rate differences attributable separately to exposures A and B were equal to the difference in incidence rates between those exposed to both and those exposed to neither, then the public health costs of exposure to either agent would be unrelated to exposure to the other agent [Rothman et al., 1980]. Thus, the public health consequences of interaction between factors are the manifestation of the biologic definition of interaction between component causes of disease applied to a population.

The inappropriateness of a multiplicative model to describe independent effects is especially important in light of the fact that most epidemiologic analyses involve such an assumption. Some analyses make the assumption explicitly, as in the Collaborative Stroke Study. In others, the assumption is implicit, stemming from the use of a multiplicative model such as logistic regression or from a stratified analysis in which the rate ratio is assumed to be uniform over the strata. The assumption of a uniform rate ratio can be defended as a statistical convenience in situations in which there is no interest in inference about interaction between the exposure and the stratification variable. If interaction is of interest, however, an assumption of uniformity of the rate ratio is inappropriate because it poses an incorrect description for the relation between risk factors under independence, making it difficult to judge departures from independence. If the relation between factors is thought to be multiplicative based on a specific biologic model of interaction, then a uniform rate ratio or multiplicative multivariate model is applicable for descriptive modeling, but this descriptive objective differs from that of inferring the extent of departures from independence of action for two or more factors.

The conceptual simplicity of the idea that interaction and independence correspond respectively to the joint action of factors in one or more sufficient causes and separate action in different sufficient causes has been questioned by Koopman [1977]. He has argued that to the extent that the complementary causes of independent component causes share common elements, the effects of causes that act through separate mechanisms are not completely independent. For example, if two factors, A and B, produce disease through separate sufficient causes with a single complementary cause C, so that AC and BC were each sufficient causes, then I(AB) in equation 15-1 is negative, implying that factors A and B are antagonistic. In biologic terms, A and B are competing factors for a single pool of susceptible individuals, those who have C. If the set of complementary component causes for factors A and B share one or more common elements, there will be some degree of competition for susceptible persons between factors A and B, and in that sense some antagonism between the factors. Only if the sets of complementary causes are completely distinct with no common elements will A and B be completely independent.

Competition for susceptible individuals is presumably a common phenomenon. Does this phenomenon invalidate the postulate that component causes acting in different sufficient causes are independent? Suppose, for example, that there are two sufficient causes for a disease, as in Figure 15-1.

C is a necessary cause, being present in both sufficient causes. Does A interact with B? Since there is some overlap of complementary causes for

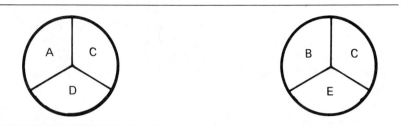

Fig. 15-1. Two sufficient causes of disease with a common component cause.

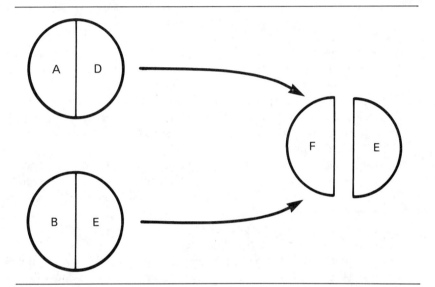

Fig. 15-2. Two sufficient causes of disease with a common component cause.

A and B, namely C, A and B must compete for the susceptible pool of people with C and are thus antagonistic. This is an indirect form of antagonism, since we could imagine more direct forms where an effect was somehow blocked when A and B were present together. A simple example of this direct form of antagonism might be a burn injury that could result from strongly alkaline or strongly acidic solutions coming into contact with skin; admixture of the two causes of burn might literally neutralize one another to have no effect. One way to diagram the indirect form of antagonism resulting from competition for susceptible individuals is shown in Figure 15-2.

F is a factor that is complementary to C and results from either the complex AD or BE. Since C is necessary for disease, we can consider what is required for a sufficient cause among those with factor C. In this restricted domain, factors A and B are independent, since there is no overlap of their complementary causes. The point is that the model of sufficient and component causes is a simple but completely general conceptualization that can be elaborated to accommodate more complicated causal models and various types of interaction. Thus, Koopman's argument does not force an abandonment of the sufficient-component causal model as a conceptualization of interaction.

Koopman [1977] has also pointed out that interactions can result because of causal connections between various component causes in different sufficient causes, but these too can be accommodated easily by elaborating the model. A causal mechanism presumably exists that leads to the action of each component cause in a sufficient cause as a result; the simple representation of causal pies is not intended to describe such intricacies, but neither does it deny them. Because the set of complementary component causes in a sufficient cause generally cannot be specified beyond a superficial level except in odd or contrived examples, and because the usually unknown distribution of these complementary component causes in a given population will influence the extent of departure from independence of effects for two component causes that act in different sufficient causes, the evaluation of causal interaction is not possible with much precision except in extreme cases. (Indeed, the same could be said about the evaluation of causal action itself, since the unknown distribution of complementary component causes will determine the magnitude and even the presence of an effect in specific circumstances.) For example, if two factors are observed never to have an effect, however defined, in the absence of one another but do have an effect when acting "together," it is logical to conclude that they both have a role in a common causal mechanism that leads to the outcome. Analogously, an agent for which the dose-response curve is a step function with a sharp threshold below which there is no effect and above which there is a clear effect demonstrates a self-interaction, that is, small "doses" of the agent interact with subsequent doses to cause the effect [Rothman, 1974]. Outside of such extreme examples, however, a wide variety of possible causal mechanisms can be hypothesized to explain a set of observations involving two risk factors.

MEASURING INTERACTION

Many methods have been proposed to evaluate interactions with statistical hypothesis tests. Few methods, however, focus on the estimation of parameters that offer some epidemiologic interpretation of interactive effects analogous to the estimation of single effects.

The measure of interaction defined in equation 15-1 is the analogue for interactive effects of the absolute measure of simple effects; as such, it should be viewed as the most fundamental epidemiologic measure of interaction [Koopman, 1981]. It may be rewritten as

$$I(AB) = [R(AB) - R(\overline{AB})] - \left\{[R(A\overline{B}) - R(\overline{AB})] + [R(\overline{A}B) - R(\overline{AB})]\right\} \quad [15\text{-}5]$$

in which the structure of the measure can be seen as the difference between the absolute effect of joint exposure to A and B and the sum of the absolute effects of A and B individually, with each of the effects being assessed with $R(\overline{AB})$ as the reference rate. Alternatively, the rate of disease among those jointly exposed can be expressed as

$$R(AB) = R(\overline{AB}) + [R(A\overline{B}) - R(\overline{AB})] + [R(\overline{A}B) - R(\overline{AB})] + I(AB) \quad [15\text{-}6]$$

which demonstrates the additive components of the rate among those with joint exposure to be the background rate, the rate attributable to factor A alone, the rate attributable to factor B alone, and the rate attributable to interaction [Environmental Protection Agency, 1980; Walker, 1981]. The proportion of disease among those with both exposures that is attributable to their interaction is

$$AP(AB) = \frac{I(AB)}{R(AB)} = \frac{R(AB) - R(A\overline{B}) - R(\overline{A}B) + R(\overline{AB})}{R(AB)} \quad [15\text{-}7]$$

This expression can be rewritten in terms of rate ratios (relative to the rate $R(\overline{AB})$) as

$$AP(AB) = \frac{RR(AB) - RR(A\overline{B}) - RR(\overline{A}B) + 1}{RR(AB)} \quad [15\text{-}8]$$

Another measure of potential epidemiologic interest is

$$AP^*(AB) = \frac{AP(AB)}{AP(A + B)} = \quad$$

$$[15\text{-}9]$$

where AP(A + B) is the proportion of disease attributable to factors A and B together or singly; AP*(AB) represents that part of the proportion of the disease attributable to factors A and B that is attributable to their interaction [Walker, 1981]. The denominator of expression 15-9 is calculated using expression 4-2 as

$$AP(A + B) = \frac{RR(AB) - 1}{RR(AB)} \qquad [15\text{-}10]$$

If standardization is needed, the corresponding SMR for those exposed to both A and B in relation to those exposed to neither should be used in place of RR(AB). AP*(AB) will be 100 percent if neither factor A nor B have an effect in isolation but together produce disease. However, AP(AB) and AP*(AB) will be zero when the factors have additive effects.

Another measure of interaction that has been proposed [Rothman, 1974; Rothman, 1976] is the synergy index S, defined as

$$S = \frac{R(AB) - R(\overline{AB})}{[R(A\overline{B}) - R(\overline{AB})] + [R(\overline{A}B) - R(\overline{AB})]} \qquad [15\text{-}11]$$

$$= \frac{\left(\begin{smallmatrix}A & B\\ & U\end{smallmatrix}\right) + \left(\begin{smallmatrix}A & U\end{smallmatrix}\right) + \left(\begin{smallmatrix}B & U\end{smallmatrix}\right)}{\left(\begin{smallmatrix}A & U\end{smallmatrix}\right) + \left(\begin{smallmatrix}B & U\end{smallmatrix}\right)}$$

The ratio S will be equal to unity under additivity, will exceed unity if the observed rate difference for joint exposure exceeds the magnitude predicted based on the sum of rate differences, and will be less than unity when additivity of the separate effects predicts a value greater than that observed. The presentation of formula 15-11 was initially framed for risk differences, but a formulation based on rate differences is simpler and conceptually equivalent. The ratio S is analogous to the rate ratio parameter to the extent that it provides a relative scale of measurement for the interaction of two risk factors, with unity representing the null point demarcating the domains of positive and negative effects. Dividing the numerator and denominator of expression 15-11 by R(\overline{AB}) gives

$$S = \frac{RR(AB) - 1}{RR(A\overline{B}) + RR(\overline{A}B) - 2} \qquad [15\text{-}12]$$

in which RR( ) denotes rate ratio relative to the rate $R(\overline{AB})$. The addition of "excess relative risks" to evaluate synergy [Cole and MacMahon, 1971] is logically equivalent to the use of the index S, as is evident from the structure of expression 15-4.

Other measures of interaction can easily be constructed using the above principles. For example, a measure such as

$$\mathrm{RERI} \ = \ \frac{I(AB)}{R(\overline{\overline{AB}})} \ = \ \frac{\text{⊘}}{\text{◯}}$$

$$= \ RR(AB) \ - \ RR(A\overline{B}) \ - \ RR(\overline{A}B) \ + \ 1 \quad [15\text{-}13]$$

where RERI signifies "*relative excess risk due to interaction*," might be useful as a relative measure of the strength of an interactive effect.

There is a connection that exists between the synergy index S and the measure AP*(AB) analogous to the relation between the rate ratio measure and the attributable proportion. From expression 15-12, we have that

$$\frac{S \ - \ 1}{S} \ = \ \frac{RR(AB) \ - \ RR(A\overline{B}) \ - \ RR(\overline{A}B) \ + \ 1}{RR(AB) \ - \ 1} \ = \ AP^*(AB) \quad [15\text{-}14]$$

analogous to expression 15-9. Thus a value of $S \ = \ 2$ would imply that $AP^*(AB) \ = \ 50$ percent, or that 50 percent of the disease burden caused by factors A and B is attributable to their interaction.

Point estimation of the above measures from crude data is straightforward, involving only the substitution of the appropriate rates or rate ratio estimates into the formulas. It is worth noting, however, that there is often an important practical problem in the estimation of interaction, namely, getting adequate numbers of subjects in the necessary categories. The calculation of confidence intervals is more complicated and will not be treated here. Walker [1981] has discussed interval estimation for AP(AB), and Rothman [1974; 1976] has discussed interval estimation for S.

Estimation of interaction in the presence of confounding is more difficult. A likelihood approach for estimation of S from stratified case-control data was presented by Flanders and Rothman [1982]. This approach is adequate for one or possibly two confounding factors, but if several factors must be controlled, it is necessary to consider multivariate methods because the number of subjects within categories quickly becomes exhausted as the number of stratification factors increase.

*Example 15-1. Smoking and alcohol in relation to
oral cancer among male veterans under age 60
(From Walker, [1981]; modified from Rothman and Keller, [1972])*

Alcohol use	Smoker	
	No	Yes
No		
Cases	3	8
Controls	20	18
Yes		
Cases	6	225
Controls	12	166

As explained in the previous chapter, the primary problem with the evaluation of interaction in multivariate models is that the interpretation of product-term coefficients depends on the mathematical structure underlying the model. Specifically, if the model is a multiplicative one, such as logistic regression, departures from additivity do not correspond to departures of a product-term coefficient from zero. Nevertheless, a multiple logistic model may be used to evaluate departures from additivity. The model should be constructed with indicator terms from each category of joint exposure. Defining the reference category to be those unexposed to both of two risk factors, we would need three indicator terms: one for the presence of each exposure in the absence of the other and one indicating the presence of joint exposure. The odds ratio estimating the effect of each exposure in the absence of the other is obtained as the antilogarithm of the coefficient for the corresponding term; the odds ratio estimating the effect of joint exposure is the antilogarithm of the sum of the coefficients for all three indicator terms. These three effect estimates can be inserted into equations 15-8 to estimate AP(AB), 15-12 to estimate S, 15-13 to estimate RERI, and 15-14 to estimate AP*(AB). Confounding factors can be controlled by including terms for those factors in the multiple logistic model, although this extension carries the usual caveat, namely, that the mathematical constraints imposed by the model are realistic. Appropriate confidence intervals could be obtained from the variance-covariance matrix of the fitted logistic model.

Example 15-1 presents case-control data for male veterans under age 60 with oral cancer and an independent control series. The rate ratio estimate for smoking in the absence of alcohol drinking is

$$\hat{RR}_s = \frac{(8)\,(20)}{(18)\,(3)} = 2.96$$

The rate ratio estimate for alcohol use in the absence of smoking is

$$\hat{RR}_a = \frac{(6)\,(20)}{(12)\,(3)} = 3.33$$

The rate ratio estimate for combined exposure, relative to exposure to neither factor, is

$$\hat{RR}_{as} = \frac{(225)\,(20)}{(166)\,(3)} = 9.04$$

Because these are case-control data, no rates are available from which $I(AB)$ can be estimated. It is possible, however, to estimate any relative measure of interaction.

The relative excess risk due to interaction, RERI, is estimated from formula 15-13 as

$$\hat{RERI} = 9.04 - 3.33 - 2.96 + 1 = 3.75$$

The proportion of oral cancer among these veterans that is attributable to the interaction of smoking and alcohol use is, from formula 15-8,

$$\hat{AP}(as) = \frac{9.04 - 3.33 - 2.96 + 1}{9.04} = \frac{\hat{RERI}}{\hat{RR}(AB)} = \frac{3.75}{9.04} = 0.41$$

Since $\hat{AP}(a + s) = (9.04 - 1)/9.04 = 0.89$ from formula 15-10, we can calculate $\hat{AP}^*(as)$ as

$$\hat{AP}^*(as) = \frac{\hat{AP}(AB)}{\hat{AP}(A + B)} = \frac{0.41}{0.89} = 0.47$$

Thus, the data provide an estimate that of all cases of oral cancer caused by smoking and alcohol use combined, the interaction of the two factors is responsible for nearly half of these cases.

Using the synergy index, S, from formula 15-12 to measure the interaction between smoking and alcohol use in oral cancer occurrence yields

$$\hat{S} = \frac{9.04 - 1}{2.96 + 3.33 - 2} = 1.87$$

which indicates a moderate amount of departure from an additive relation. Note that the rate due to interaction is greater than the rate due to either of the individual factors, since $\hat{RERI} = 3.75$, which is greater than 2.33 or 1.96.

$\widehat{AP}^*(as)$ can also be calculated from $\hat{S}$ as

$$\widehat{AP}^*(as) = \frac{\hat{S} - 1}{\hat{S}} = \frac{1.87 - 1}{1.87} = 0.47$$

REFERENCES

Cole, P., and MacMahon, B. Attributable risk percent in case-control studies. *Br. J. Prev. Soc. Med.* 1971;25:242–244.

Collaborative Group for the Study of Stroke in Young Women. Oral contraceptives and stroke in young women. *J.A.M.A.* 1975;231:718–722.

Darroch, J. N. Multiplicative and additive interaction in contingency tables. *Biometrika* 1974;61:207–214.

Environmental Protection Agency, Office of Pesticides and Toxic Substances. Support Document: Asbestos-containing materials in schools. Health effects and magnitude of exposure. EPA-560/12-80-003. Washington, D.C.: U.S. Government Printing Office, October, 1980.

Flanders, W. D., and Rothman, K. J. Interaction of alcohol and tobacco in laryngeal cancer. *Am. J. Epidemiol.* 1982;115:371–379.

Koopman, J. S. Causal models and sources of interaction. *Am. J. Epidemiol.* 1977;106:439–444.

Koopman, J. S. Interaction between discrete causes. *Am. J. Epidemiol.* 1981;113:716–724.

Kupper, L., and Hogan, M. D. Interaction in epidemiologic studies. *Am. J. Epidemiol.* 1978;108:447–453.

Rothman, K. J., and Keller, A. Z. The effect of joint exposure to alcohol and tobacco on risk of cancer of the mouth and pharynx. *J. Chron. Dis.* 1972;23:711–716.

Rothman, K. J. Synergy and antagonism in cause-effect relationships. *Am. J. Epidemiol.* 1974;99:385–388.

Rothman, K. J. The estimation of synergy or antagonism. *Am. J. Epidemiol.* 1976;103:506–511.

Rothman, K. J. Occam's razor pares the choice among statistical models. *Am. J. Epidemiol.* 1978;108:347–349.

Rothman, K. J., Greenland, S., and Walker, A. M. Concepts of interaction. *Am. J. Epidemiol.* 1980;112:467–470.

Walker, A. M. Proportion of disease attributable to the combined effect of two factors. *Int. J. Epidemiol.* 1981;10:81–85.

Walter, S. D., and Holford, T. R. Additive, multiplicative and other models for disease risks. *Am. J. Epidemiol.* 1978;108:341–346.

16. ANALYSIS WITH MULTIPLE LEVELS OF EXPOSURE

The discussion of data analysis thus far has presumed that exposure variables are measured on a dichotomous scale. Exposure variables that are measured on a nominal scale with more than two categories can be treated for analytic purposes as a set of dichotomous variables, comparing each category with a reference category; thus, a study relating the ethnic origin of residents of Hawaii to disease incidence could take Hawaiian ancestry as a reference category and consider Chinese, Japanese, and European ancestry as three different variables. Exposure variables that are ordinal or continuous can also be collapsed into dichotomies for analysis. The motivation is usually that the use of more than two categories would divide the data too finely to accommodate control of confounding and still maintain reasonable precision in estimation. Collapsing, however, does involve a degradation of the underlying scale of measurement and the loss of potentially important information. The extent to which the data indicate a trend in effect, or the absence of such a trend, over various levels of exposure can provide insight into the biology of the relation under study and guidance for any public health intervention.

Loss of information from collapsing a continuous variable into categories is mitigated by retaining more than two ranked categories for the variable. It is natural, however, to consider whether any collapsing into categories is necessary. Theoretically it should be possible to extract more information from the data by using in the analysis the actual values of the observations rather than the <u>frequency of observations in selected categories</u>. That is, rather than base an analysis on categories of people who, for example, smoke zero, 1 to 10, 11 to 20, 21 to 40, and 41 to 60 cigarettes a day, it should be more informative to use the actual number of cigarettes smoked per day for each individual subject. Many statistical techniques exist to extract from continuous measurements all the quantitative information present in the observations, and these techniques have often been applied in epidemiology. Applying these techniques, unfortunately, can open the door to serious problems that often outweigh the theoretical advantages.

A fundamental difficulty in follow-up studies is that disease occurrence is measured with incidence rates, which are not meaningful unless they are calculated for populations, that is, groups of individuals. If exposure is measured on a continuous scale without collapsing into groups, then no populations are defined for which incidence rates can be estimated directly. It is possible to conceptualize the incidence rate for an individual as a function of the individual's "waiting time" until disease onset (incidence rate is the reciprocal of waiting time if the rate is constant over time), but without a mathematical model to smooth the data it would be difficult in the absence of grouping to make sense of the distribution of waiting times for all subjects in a study. Thus, the need to calculate stable incidence rates motivates the aggregation of subjects with similar levels of exposure into categories. In case-control studies, a similar line of reasoning applies because the analysis focuses on the estimation of incidence rate ratios.

If the data analysis is (inappropriately) based on statistical hypothesis testing rather than on estimation the use of continuous rather than grouped data may seem indicated to improve statistical power. Statistical hypothesis testing for case-control data amounts to a comparison of the exposure distributions for the case and control series. Statistical tests such as the t-test can be used to evaluate whether samples from two continuous distributions differ; the tests may be based on the actual values observed rather than on a frequency distribution obtained by grouping. While some gain in power for statistical hypothesis testing is theoretically achievable in this way, statistical testing should not be a primary objective in epidemiologic analysis, so that the gain in statistical power adds very little information of interest. The format of the data for such testing does not readily lend itself to estimation of any meaningful epidemiologic effect measure, which is the central analytic objective. Thus the gain in statistical power serves to shift attention in the analysis away from estimation toward hypothesis testing, a shift that is inherently undesirable. A possible ramification of the focus on testing in such situations is that the qualitative inference that depends solely on the outcome of such a test can be extraordinarily misleading. Since a t-test is basically a test of differences in mean values, the test can be unduly influenced by a single observation or a few outliers (extreme data points).

Consider the following hypothetical example. Suppose that a case-control study of brain cancer were conducted in a population of nuclear energy workers. Let us imagine that the study groups comprise 12 cases and 12 controls, for whom the cumulative radiation exposures are those given in Example 16-1. Let us assume that exposures of less than 0.1 rem cannot be measured with precision and are, on average, equal to 0.05 rem. The mean exposure for cases is 4.4 rem compared with only 0.59 rem for controls. The difference in means is substantial. A t-test comparing these two distributions would give $t = 1.71$ with 22 degrees of freedom, which corresponds to a one-tail P-value of 0.05.

Of course, t-tests should never be applied unless there is some indication that one is dealing with approximately normal sampling distributions, which is not the case for these data. Indeed, 94 percent of the total radiation exposure for the cases comes from cases 1, 2, and 7. A few extreme values can thus unduly influence the mean and can be extremely misleading [Baron et al., 1984].

A nonparametric test such as the Mann-Whitney test could be applied instead of the t-test. The Mann-Whitney test, based on the ranks of the observations, does not require an assumption of normality. Nevertheless, the problem remains that such an analysis would not be directed at epidemiologically interpretable measures [Poole et al., 1984]. By categorizing

Example 16-1. Hypothetical data for brain cancer
cases and controls on cumulative radiation exposure

Cases (rem)		Controls (rem)	
1.	15.6	1.	0.05
2.	21.8	2.	0.2
3.	0.05	3.	0.3
4.	0.05	4.	1.4
5.	0.2	5.	0.05
6.	0.05	6.	0.05
7.	12.4	7.	1.2
8.	0.05	8.	0.05
9.	0.05	9.	0.4
10.	0.2	10.	0.05
11.	0.05	11.	0.05
12.	2.3	12.	3.3

exposure, the problem can be simply avoided. If 0.1 rem is used to delineate high versus low exposure for the data in Example 16-1, a rate ratio estimate of 1.0 is obtained. If 1.0 rem is used instead for the category boundary, a rate ratio estimate of 1.5 is obtained. The interpretation of the data is still open to some discussion, since the effect estimate is based on only a few observations and depends heavily on where the category boundary is drawn; this dependence reflects the fact that the upper tails of the two exposure distributions differ considerably, but the medians are identical. With more data, this dependence of the effect on the placement of the category boundary might diminish, and it might be feasible to use several finer categories of exposure to evaluate the trend in effect with increasing exposure, avoiding an open-ended dichotomous categorization. Nevertheless, the interpretation is still clearer with this crude categorization, even with only two open-ended categories, whereas a misleading inference might be drawn from the observation that the mean exposure of cases is 7.5 times that of controls. It would be easy to imagine situations in which only one subject with an extreme value of exposure was sufficient to distort an analysis based on mean values.

The undue influence of outlier observations is but one possible problem arising from an analysis that does not categorize the exposure variables. It is also possible that a comparison of two exposure distributions will reveal only minor discrepancies in a measure of central tendency such as the mean or median, whereas the tails of the distributions could differ substantially, reflecting a strong relation between exposure and disease. This problem was noted by MacMahon et al. [1970], who first reported the strong relation between age at first birth and risk of breast cancer (Fig. 16-

1). Commenting on why this strong relation had not previously been reported, they noted that

This is by no means the first study in which a difference between breast cancer cases and controls in age at first birth has been observed. In many previous comparisons of breast cancer cases and unaffected women the cases have been found to be, on average, older at marriage, at first pregnancy, or at both. ... However, previous workers seem not to have considered the differences to be sufficiently important to warrant detailed exploration. An apparent lack of interest in the relationship may have resulted from failure to realize the magnitude of the differences in relative risk that underlie it. This lack of recognition of the strength of the relationship can be attributed primarily to analyses utilizing summary statistics such as means and ridits. In countries where most epidemiological studies of this disease have been undertaken, the proportion of women who have their first birth at an early age is relatively small, and summary statistics fail to reveal the high risks experienced by small segments of the population. For example, in the present data from Boston, the mean age at first birth was 27.1 years in the cases and 25.5 years in the controls. While this difference is statistically highly significant it would hardly lead one to suspect the almost four-fold range of relative risks shown in Table 3 (Fig. 16-1).

The lesson from these examples coincides with the primary theme of this book: The main objective of an epidemiologic analysis is to estimate the magnitude of effect (i.e., the difference in incidence rates) as a function of exposure status. The major problem with continuous measures of exposure is that their use is often accompanied by summary procedures that focus either on statistical hypothesis testing or on the comparison of measures of central tendency of the exposure variable. Neither statistical hypothesis testing nor the comparison of measures of central tendency, however, can accomplish the desired measurement goal. Categorization of exposure facilitates the estimation of effect as a function of exposure using the categorical methods already discussed for dichotomous exposures. Of course, effect functions can also be estimated from continuous data using mathematical models, although the potentially detrimental influence of outliers needs to be considered in such analyses.

Indeed, categorization per se does not eliminate the problem of outliers. Categorization that lumps outlier observations with less extreme values will dilute the distorting effect of the outlier observation, but the broad or open-ended categories that are necessary to accomplish this dilution are undesirable because they are conducive to within-category distortion similar to that occurring with an overall reliance on mean values. Finer categorization will tend to isolate outliers in separate categories, where they may be automatically discarded if there are no comparison data available within the category. Nevertheless, an analysis based on scoring of categories is still susceptible in principle to distortion by groups of out-

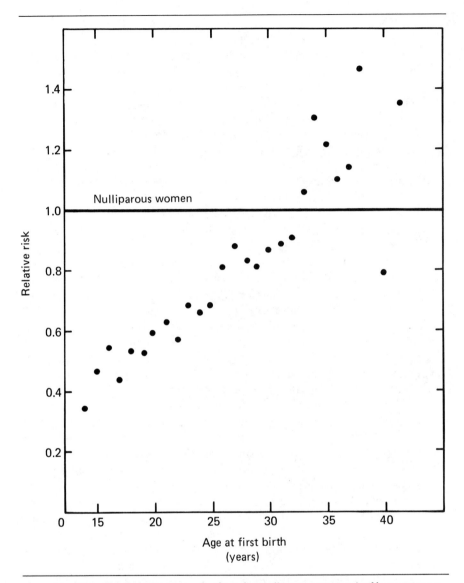

Fig. 16-1. Risk (relative to a risk of 1.0 for nulliparous women) of breast cancer according to age at first birth, from MacMahon et al. [1970].

liers in extreme categories. Consequently, it is often desirable to conduct an analysis with several levels of exposure using only a nominal scale categorization for the exposure (i.e., without scoring of categories) as an initial analysis or as a supplement to other approaches. This approach may reveal outliers that should be ignored or given less weight in further analyses based on category scores or continuous measurements.

ESTIMATION OF EFFECTS FOR MULTIPLE LEVELS OF EXPOSURE
Point Estimation Separately by Category

In an epidemiologic analysis dealing with exposure at more than two levels, a straightforward approach is to consider each level separately in comparison with a reference category of exposure, reducing the analysis to a series of analyses based on dichotomized exposure categories. For example, if the exposure variable is mean daily skin exposure to direct sunlight, the variable might be categorized as follows: *less than 0.5 hours, 0.5 to 1.9 hours, 2.0 to 3.9 hours, 4.0 to 6.9 hours,* and *7.0 to 8.9 hours.* The natural reference group would be the category *less than 0.5 hours.* Each of the remaining four categories could be contrasted with the reference category to obtain four separate estimates of effect, essentially conducting four analyses based on dichotomous comparisons. Point estimation would proceed as described in the earlier chapters dealing with dichotomous exposure variables.

If confounding is present, it can be dealt with in the same way as for dichotomous exposure variables, that is, by stratification. Since a major goal of the analysis is to examine the pattern of point estimates by exposure level, it is important to ensure that the point estimates are mutually comparable. Thus, if a standardization procedure is used to combine stratum-specific information across strata of a confounding factor or an effect modifier, it is imperative that a common standard be employed for each point estimate of effect that is obtained. Computing an SMR for each exposure category is invalid, since each SMR would involve a different standard, namely, the distribution of the exposure category at issue (see Chap. 5). It would be reasonable, however, to use any exposure category, including the reference category, as a common standard for weighting the stratum-specific data at each exposure level. Other reasonable choices for a standard include the distribution of all subjects with some exposure or some outside standard.

If pooling rather than standardization is used to obtain an overall point estimate of effect at each level of exposure, the weighting of each stratum will be a function of the number of observations in each stratum and will not necessarily be equivalent for each exposure level. If the assumption of a uniform parameter across strata of the confounding factor is valid, differences in weighting for different exposure categories are not crucial to validity. The assumption of uniformity can be difficult to defend, however: It is not sufficient to demonstrate lack of "statistical significance" for a test of a null hypothesis that the effect is uniform. Moreover, for ratio measures of effect, uniformity should be present only under the special circumstances in which there is interaction between the stratification variable and the exposure that happens to conform to a multiplicative model. Consequently, pooling under an assumption of uniformity should be used with caution if the analysis calls for a comparison of exposure level–spe-

Example 16-2. Number of patients with lung cancer and control patients by sex and by most recent amount of tobacco consumed regularly [Doll and Hill, 1954]

	Males			
	No. cigarettes smoked daily			
	0	1–4	5–14	15+
Cases	2	33	250	364
Controls	27	55	293	274
$\widehat{RR}$	1.0	8.1	11.5	17.9
	Females			
	No. cigarettes smoked daily			
	0	1–4	5–14	15+
Cases	19	7	19	15
Controls	32	12	10	6
$\widehat{RR}$	1.0	1.0	3.2	4.2

cific effect estimates. Standardization using a common standard should be used unless there is strong assurance that an assumption of uniformity at each level of exposure is reasonable.

The data in Example 16-2 are from a case-control study of lung cancer [Doll and Hill, 1954]. Maximum likelihood estimates of a uniform rate ratio over the two strata of gender, from the lowest level of cigarette smoking to the highest, are 1.0 (the reference category), 2.5, 5.3, and 8.3. These estimates are inappropriate, however, because the data exhibit striking differences in the effect estimates for males and females at each level of exposure. Instead, standardized estimates, with a common standard, should be obtained. For these case-control data, the general formula for standardized rate ratios (expression 12-66) becomes

$$\text{SRR} = \frac{\sum_i w_i \dfrac{a_i}{c_i}}{\sum_i w_i \dfrac{b_i}{d_i}} \qquad [16\text{-}1]$$

where w_i is the weight for standardization for stratum i of the stratification factor, and a_i, b_i, c_i, and d_i are the cell frequencies for stratum i following the notation of Table 11-2. The weights must be a function of the control frequencies [Miettinen, 1972] (see Chap. 12). Formula 16-1 reduces to formula 12-68 when the weight for standardization is taken as the reference category. The variance for the $\hat{SRR}$ computed from expression 16-1 is

$$\text{Var}(\hat{SRR}) \doteq (\hat{SRR})^2 \left[\frac{\sum_i w_i^2 \left[\frac{a_i}{c_i^2} + \frac{a_i^2}{c_i^3} \right]}{\left[\sum_i w_i \frac{a_i}{c_i} \right]^2} + \frac{\sum_i w_i^2 \left[\frac{b_i}{d_i^2} + \frac{b_i^2}{d_i^3} \right]}{\left[\sum_i w_i \frac{b_i}{d_i} \right]^2} \right] \quad [16\text{-}2]$$

If the reference group is chosen as the standard, formula 12-71 should be used instead of formula 16-2 for the variance. In this example, the use of the distribution of all control subjects as a standard would assign a weight of 649 to the male data and 60 to the female data. From formula 16-1, the standardized rate ratio estimates would be 1.0 (the reference category), 5.1, 8.0, and 12.1. Another reasonable choice of standard would be the distribution of all exposed controls, thereby assigning a weight of 622 to the male data and 28 to the female data; this standard yields effect estimates of 6.2, 9.3, and 14.3 for the three nonzero exposure categories.

With pooling, a problem that arises from treating each category separately in an independent analysis is that the set of effect estimates may not be mutually consistent. For example, the maximum likelihood estimates of rate ratio for the data in Example 16-1 for exposure levels 2 and 3 are 2.5 and 5.3, respectively; the ratio of these estimates is $5.3/2.5 = 2.1$. An analysis of the same data using level 2 as the reference category would give a maximum likelihood rate ratio estimate for level 3 relative to level 2 of 1.6, which is considerably different from the ratio of 2.1 implied by the effect estimates obtained when levels 2 and 3 are each compared with level 1. The difference arises from the fact that pooling uses ad hoc weights determined by the data, and the weighting differs in the two analyses. A standardized procedure using a common set of weights would lead to consistent results. Consistent pooled estimates can also be obtained using a likelihood approach [Pike et al., 1975; Hill et al., 1978], by multivariate analysis, or by a proposed modification of the Mantel-Haenszel estimators [Mickey, 1985].

Estimation of Overall Trend

The main difficulty with estimation of effects separately for each level of exposure is that information is lost in not considering the continuity of the underlying variable. An analysis based on separate consideration of each category proceeds identically if the categorized variable is measured on a nominal scale, ordinal scale, or continuous scale. Treating each category separately produces confidence intervals that do not take into account the overall pattern, if any, in the data. A large number of categories can lead to few data within each, resulting in imprecision in category-specific estimates of effect. When there is a regular trend in the data, how-

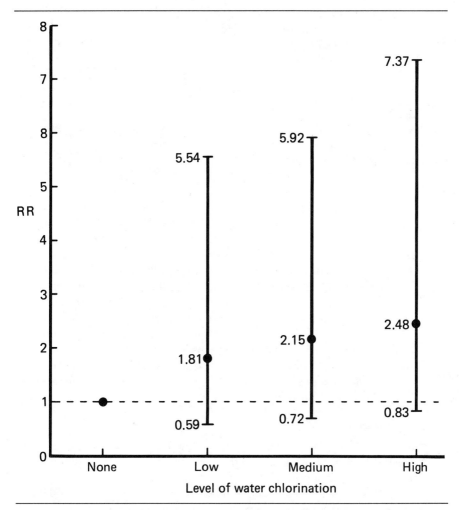

Fig. 16-2. Estimated rate ratios (RR) and 95 percent confidence intervals for brain cancer among Wisconsin white females according to level of water chlorination, from Young et al. [1981].

ever, the estimates of effect from bordering categories do provide information about the effect in a given category. Indeed, if the effect is estimated precisely in the categories below and above a category of interest, that may be enough to give an excellent indication of the effect for a category that has only few data.

An example of the ways in which information can be lost by considering each category separately appears in a study of female cancer mortality and water chlorination [Young et al., 1981]. The amount of chlorine in the water supply, inherently a continuous variable, was categorized into none, low, medium, and high. Figure 16-2 indicates the estimated effects for

Example 16-3. Cases of breast cancer and person-years at risk
for women of Hiroshima and Nagasaki age 10 or more at the time
of the atomic blast, according to dose of radiation in rad [McGregor et al., 1977]

	Dose (Rad)			
	Nonexposed	0–9	10–99	100+
Cases	38	105	48	34
Person-years	208,515	463,086	164,639	52,185
Incidence (× 10^6 yr)	182	227	292	652

brain cancer. A consistent trend is evident in the point estimates. Although each of the confidence intervals taken alone is wide, the consistent pattern provides added information. Since the confidence intervals do not reflect this additional information, they overstate the variability with which the overall effect of chlorine on brain cancer mortality might be estimated. In this example, the authors compounded the problem by relying on *P*-values for interpretation; since none was "significant," they inferred no relation between brain cancer and water chlorination.

There are two important lessons from this example: (1) It is a mistake to rely on statistical hypothesis testing for inference; and (2) it is desirable to estimate a single overall measure of trend in effect rather than a set of separate effect estimates. A reanalysis of these data using a single measure of trend is given later in this chapter.

FOLLOW-UP STUDIES

To take account of the pattern of effects over an ordered series of exposure categories, the investigator can fit a regression equation. A straight-line regression is the simplest expression of trend.

Let us consider fitting a simple linear regression to a set of crude incidence rate data. The incidence of breast cancer among women in Hiroshima and Nagasaki who were age 10 or more at the time of the atomic blast is given in Example 16-3 according to dose of radiation in rad [McGregor et al., 1977]. The data demonstrate a monotonic increase in incidence with increasing dose.

To estimate the linear component of trend, it is necessary to assign scores representing the magnitude of the exposure for each category. Score assignment is necessary simply to locate the points in a meaningful way on a graph, since the horizontal distance between points is not inherent in an ordered ranking. The distance between categories in Figure 16-2, for example, is arbitrarily set and may not characterize the actual increments in chlorine concentration. For the data in Example 16-3, let us assign scores of 0, 5, 55, and 150 to the four categories. These represent the midcategory points, except for the highest category, which requires an

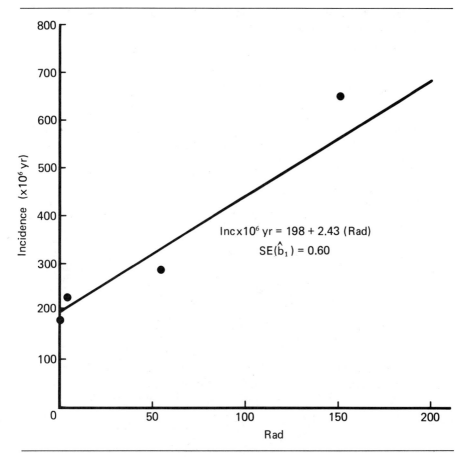

Fig. 16-3. Incidence (Inc) of breast cancer according to radiation dose in rad for the data of example 16-3, with estimated linear trend.

arbitrary score because it is open-ended. If the information is available, it would be preferable to assign scores that represent the mean value of exposure within the category. (Note that for these follow-up data the mean value would ideally not be the unweighted mean for all subjects within a category but rather a mean that is weighted according to the person-time contribution of each subject.) For ordinal data with no inherent exposure values, it is still necessary to assign scores to estimate trend, however arbitrarily. Uniformly incremented scores that correspond to the rank of each category are usually used in such instances.

With scores assigned, the data points can be plotted on a graph (Fig. 16-3). It is straightforward to fit a regression line through four data points, but the points each reflect a different amount of information and should therefore be assigned different weights. A least-squares approach to weighted regression gives the following formulas for the slope and intercept [Kleinbaum and Kupper, 1978]:

slope:

$$\hat{b}_1 = \frac{\sum_{j=1}^{n} w_j x_j y_j - \left(\sum_{j=1}^{n} w_j x_j\right)\left(\sum_{j=1}^{n} w_j y_j\right) \Big/ \sum_{j=1}^{n} w_j}{\sum_{j=1}^{n} w_j x_j^2 - \left(\sum_{j=1}^{n} w_j x_j\right)^2 \Big/ \sum_{j=1}^{n} w_j}$$ [16-3]

intercept:

$$\hat{b}_0 = \overline{Y} - \hat{b}_1 \overline{X}$$ [16-4]

where

$$\overline{Y} = \frac{\sum_{j=1}^{n} w_j y_j}{\sum_{j=1}^{n} w_j} \qquad \overline{X} = \frac{\sum_{j=1}^{n} w_j x_j}{\sum_{j=1}^{n} w_j}$$

n is the number of data points, j is an index for each point, w_j is the weight for each point, X is the exposure variable, and Y is the incidence rate. The standard error of the slope can be taken as [Grizzle et al., 1969]

$$SE(\hat{b}_1) \doteq \sqrt{\frac{\sum_{j=1}^{n} w_j}{\left(\sum_{j=1}^{n} w_j x_j^2\right)\left(\sum_{j=1}^{n} w_j\right) - \left(\sum_{j=1}^{n} w_j x_j\right)^2}}$$ [16-5]

In each of the preceding formulas, the weight for each data point should be calculated as the inverse of the variance for that point. For crude data, such as those of Example 16-3, the variance is given by

$$Var\left(\frac{a}{N}\right) \doteq \frac{a}{N^2}$$

where a is the number of cases and N is the number of person-years. Therefore, the weight would be

$$w_j = \frac{N_j^2}{a_j}$$

for each data point j. (Rates of zero magnitude can pose a problem, since the weight would be infinite. One solution is to add an arbitrary amount such as 0.5 to the numerator of each rate; another is to use a modified weighting scheme, such as $w_j = N_j$.)

For standardized incidence rates (SIR), the variance is

$$\text{Var(SIR)} \doteq \frac{\sum_i w_i^2 \frac{a_i}{N_i^2}}{\left(\sum_i w_i\right)^2}$$

where w_i refers to the standardization weight for stratum i. (The weights for standardization of each rate and for the regression of the trend in the standardized rates should not be confused.) The regression weight for each standardized rate in calculating the regression coefficients is the reciprocal of the above variance,

$$w_j = \frac{\left(\sum_i w_i\right)^2}{\sum_i w_i^2 \frac{a_i}{N_i^2}}$$

Some caution is advised in using regression methods with standardized rates, since the standardization process itself can, in certain circumstances, introduce a bias in the regression [Rosenbaum and Rubin, 1984].

The standard error of the intercept, $\hat{b}_0$, is given by

$$\text{SE}(\hat{b}_0) \doteq \sqrt{\frac{\sum_{j=1}^{n} w_j x_j^2}{\left(\sum_{j=1}^{n} w_j x_j^2\right)\left(\sum_{j=1}^{n} w_j\right) - \left(\sum_{j=1}^{n} w_j x_j\right)^2}}$$

and the covariance of $\hat{b}_0$ with $\hat{b}_1$ is

$$\text{Cov}(\hat{b}_0, \hat{b}_1) \doteq \frac{-\sum_{j=1}^{n} w_j x_j}{\left[\sum_{j=1}^{n} w_j x_j^2\right]\left[\sum_{j=1}^{n} w_j\right] - \left[\sum_{j=1}^{n} w_j x_j\right]^2}$$

The rate for any point x_k can be estimated as

$$\hat{Y}_k = \hat{b}_0 + \hat{b}_1 x_k$$

with

$$SE(\hat{Y}_k) \doteq \sqrt{\frac{\sum_{j=1}^{n} w_j x_j^2 - 2x_k \sum_{j=1}^{n} w_j x_j + x_k^2 \sum_{j=1}^{n} w_j}{\left[\sum_{j=1}^{n} w_j x_j^2\right]\left[\sum_{j=1}^{n} w_j\right] - \left[\sum_{j=1}^{n} w_j x_j\right]^2}}$$

The application of formulas 16-3 through 16-5 to determine the least-squares weighted regression line is usually simple, since typically only a few data points are involved. The resulting trend line offers a way to describe the effect mathematically as a function of exposure. The fitted line for the data of Example 16-3 is given in Figure 16-3. The slope, $2.43 \times 10^{-6}\text{yr}^{-1}\text{rad}^{-1}$, indicates the estimated amount that the incidence rate increases for each rad increase in dose. From the estimated standard error for the slope, we can calculate an approximate 90 percent confidence interval for the slope as

$$2.43 \times 10^{-6}\text{yr}^{-1}\text{rad}^{-1} \pm 1.645(0.60 \times 10^{-6}\text{yr}^{-1}\text{rad}^{-1})$$

$$= 1.45 \times 10^{-6}\text{yr}^{-1}\text{rad}^{-1}, 3.41 \times 10^{-6}\text{yr}^{-1}\text{rad}^{-1}$$

To estimate the incidence rate of breast cancer for women exposed to 100 rad using the regression equation, we assign $x = 100$ and get a predicted rate of

$$\frac{198 + 2.43(100)}{10^6 \text{ yr}} = 441 \times 10^{-6}\text{yr}^{-1}$$

with a standard error of $62 \times 10^{-6}\text{yr}^{-1}$. Thus, a 90 percent confidence interval for the rate at 100 rad, estimated from the linear regression, would be

$$\frac{441 \pm 1.645(62)}{10^6 \text{ yr}} = 339 \times 10^{-6}\text{yr}^{-1}, 543 \times 10^{-6}\text{yr}^{-1}$$

Nonlinear trends may be estimated using modifications of the above approach. One modification involves the assignment of scores for the exposure variable. Nonlinear trends can be "linearized" by score assignment that reflects the nonlinear pattern. For example, the exposure scores can be the square of the exposure value, reflecting a quadratic relation. It is even possible to reorder the categories by score assignment: Five categories with scores of 1, 2, 3, 2, 1 describe an inverted-V relation with exposure after a linear relation is fitted to the exposure scores. Another way to estimate nonlinear trends is to use scale transformations for the incidence rates and then fit a linear regression to the transformed rates. If using transformed rates, it is important to take the transformation into account when determining the weights.

CASE-CONTROL STUDIES

With case-control studies, only relative measures of effect can be estimated without recourse to external information. The effect at each level of exposure is estimated relative to the reference level, usually the lowest category of exposure. The value of the rate ratio is defined as 1.0 for the reference category. A linear trend in effect would thus follow the equation

$$RR = 1 + b'X \qquad [16\text{-}6]$$

where RR represents the rate ratio, X is the exposure, and b' is the slope for the RR.

To estimate b' in this equation, the same regression model described in the previous section for follow-up data can be applied, substituting the ratio of cases to controls at each level of exposure for the rate:

$$\text{Case-control odds} = b_0 + b_1 X$$

The slope b' in equation 16-6 can then be estimated by the quotient $\hat{b}_1/\hat{b}_0$, where $\hat{b}_1$ and $\hat{b}_0$ are determined from equations 16-3 and 16-4 (using the case-control odds instead of the rate for each y_j).

The weights assigned to each point in fitting the regression should reflect the variance of the case-control odds. For crude data, the regression weight w_j for each data point should be taken as

$$w_j = \cfrac{1}{\cfrac{a_j(a_j + b_j)}{b_j^3} - \left[\cfrac{a_j^2}{b_j^2}\right]\left[\cfrac{N_1 + N_0}{N_1 N_0}\right]}$$

where a_j and b_j are the frequencies for cases and controls, respectively, at exposure level j, N_1 is the total number of cases, and N_0 is the total number of controls. For stratified data, the odds at each exposure level should be standardized by taking

$$SO_j = \cfrac{\sum_i w_i \cfrac{a_{ij}}{b_{ij}}}{\sum_i w_i}$$

where SO_j is the standardized odds and w_i is the weight for standardization in stratum i. The regression weight should then be taken as

$$w_j = \frac{\left[\sum_i w_i\right]^2}{\sum_i w_i^2 \left[\frac{a_{ij}(a_{ij} + b_{ij})}{b_{ij}^3} - \left[\frac{a_{ij}^2}{b_{ij}^2}\right]\left[\frac{N_{i1} + N_{i0}}{N_{i1}N_{i0}}\right]\right]}$$

The standard error for $\hat{b}'$ is estimated as

$$SE(\hat{b}') \doteq \frac{\hat{b}_1}{\hat{b}_0}\sqrt{\frac{\frac{\Sigma w_j}{\hat{b}_1^2} + \frac{\Sigma w_j x_j^2}{\hat{b}_0^2} + \frac{2\Sigma w_j x_j}{\hat{b}_0 \hat{b}_1}}{\left[\Sigma w_j x_j^2\right]\left[\Sigma w_j\right] - \left[\Sigma w_j x_j\right]^2}}$$

and the standard error for a rate ratio estimate, $\hat{RR}_k$, predicted from equation 16-6 is

$$SE(\hat{RR}_k) \doteq x_k SE(\hat{b}')$$

Consider the stratified case-control data in Example 16-2. The standardized odds, the variances of each odds, the regression weights and the exposure scores are given in Table 16-1.

The application of formulas 16-3 and 16-4 give $\hat{b}_1 = 0.0654$ and $\hat{b}_0 = 0.1671$. Thus we can estimate $b' = \hat{b}_1/\hat{b}_0$ as $0.0654/0.1671 = 0.392$, with a standard error of 0.1305. For one pack a day smokers ($x = 20$), the estimated rate ratio from the regression model would be $1 + 0.392(20) = 8.83$, with a standard error of $20(0.1305) = 2.61$. To obtain confidence limits, it is desirable, as usual for ratio measures, to use a logarithmic transformation, with

$$SE[\ln(\hat{RR})] \doteq \frac{SE(\hat{RR})}{\hat{RR}}$$

A 90 percent confidence interval for the rate ratio for one pack a day smokers would therefore be

$$\exp[\ln(8.83) \pm 1.645(2.61/8.83)] = 5.42, 14.4$$

The above calculations can be done without much difficulty using a hand calculator. Ideally, a regression fitted to the case-control odds should take into account the covariances between the odds at the various exposure levels, which are not independent. To do this, however, a more com-

Table 16-1. Standardized case-control odds, variances,
regression weights and exposure scores for the data of example 16-2

	Number of cigarettes smoked daily			
	0	1–4	5–14	15+
SO	0.09646	0.59928	0.89833	1.37893
Var (SO)	0.00272	0.01509	0.00369	0.00768
Weight	368.204	66.273	271.251	130.257
Exposure score	0.0	2.5	10	20

plicated fitting procedure is required [Draper and Smith, 1966] that would not be possible without a computer and the appropriate software. The above approach, which fails to take these covariances into account, is consequently not optimally efficient, but it is unbiased [Silvey, 1970] and offers the advantage that it is feasible with minimal computing assistance.

Occasionally it may be desirable to fit a trend line to rate-ratio estimates when the raw data are unavailable. A reanalysis of the data in Figure 16-2 to evaluate trends is an example: These data derive from a logistic regression\analysis, and neither the raw frequencies nor the case-control odds are available. Nevertheless, it is still possible to estimate a linear trend line in the estimates, albeit less efficiently than with access to the raw data. The parameter b' in equation 16-6 can be estimated directly from the equation

$$\hat{b}' = \frac{\sum_{j=2}^{n} w_j x_j \hat{RR}_j - \sum_{j=2}^{n} w_j x_j}{\sum_{j=2}^{n} w_j x_j^2} \qquad [16\text{-}7]$$

where $\hat{RR}_j$ is the category-specific rate ratio estimate at level j, the reference category (j = 1) is ignored, and

$$w_j = \frac{1}{\hat{RR}_j^2 \left[\dfrac{1}{a} + \dfrac{1}{b} + \dfrac{1}{c} + \dfrac{1}{d} \right]}$$

For standardized rate ratios, the $\{w_j\}$ should be taken as the reciprocal of the variance given in formula 16-2 or, when applicable, formula 12-70. In the absence of the actual data, w_j can be estimated from a standard error, test statistic, or a confidence interval (see later).

This regression model, like the previous one, ignores the covariances between the point estimates, which can be substantial for this model if the frequencies for the reference category are small. The standard error for the slope can be estimated as

$$SE(\hat{b}') \doteq \sqrt{\dfrac{1}{\displaystyle\sum_{j=2}^{n} w_j x_j^2}}$$

For any exposure value x_k, the estimated value of the rate ratio, $\hat{RR}_k$, can be obtained from formula 16-6 using the slope estimate from expression 16-7. The standard error of the estimated rate ratio is simply

$$SE(\hat{RR}_k) \doteq x_k SE(\hat{b}')$$

The rate ratio estimates for the data of Figure 16-2 come from a multiple logistic regression model that includes terms for several confounding factors. The weights for fitting a trend line to the data points in Figure 16-2 can be determined from the confidence intervals. Since the 95 percent confidence interval spans a distance, on the logarithmic scale, that is equal to $2 \times 1.96 \cdot SE[\ln(\hat{RR})]$, the variance of $\ln(\hat{RR})$ can be taken as

$$Var[\ln(\hat{RR})] \doteq \left[\dfrac{\ln(\overline{RR}) - \ln(RR)}{2 \times 1.96}\right]^2 \doteq \dfrac{[\ln(\overline{RR}) - \ln(RR)]^2}{15.37} \qquad [16\text{-}8]$$

and the variance of the rate ratio can be estimated as

$$Var(\hat{RR}) \doteq \hat{RR}^2 Var[\ln(\hat{RR})] \qquad [16\text{-}9]$$

The regression weight can be taken as the reciprocal of $Var(\hat{RR})$. The preceding approach presumes that the confidence limits were set using a logarithmic transformation, which is usually true and is always the case if the estimate derives from a multiple logistic or Cox proportional hazards model. To verify the validity of this assumption, it is prudent to check that on the logarithmic scale the point estimate is the arithmetic mean of the upper and lower limits or that the untransformed upper bound multiplied by the untransformed lower bound equals the square of the point estimate. We note that for the data in Figure 16-2, this condition is met for the first and third data points but not for the middle point. Since all the estimates come from the same model, the explanation must be a reporting error. Based on the P-value that was reported in the original paper, it appears that the upper bound of the middle data point should have been approximately 6.4 rather than 5.92. Using formulas 16-8 and 16-9 and the value 6.4 for the upper bound for the middle data point gives weights for the three data points of 0.9370, 0.6944, and 0.5265 for low, medium, and high chlorine levels, respectively (Table 16-2). From formula 16-7, the

Table 16-2. Rate ratio estimates, variances, regression weights and exposure scores for the data of Figure 16-2

	Chlorine dose category			
	None	Low	Medium	High
$\widehat{RR}$	1.00	1.81	2.15	2.28
Var ($\widehat{RR}$)	—	1.0672	1.4401	1.8992
Weight	—	0.9370	0.6944	0.5265
Exposure score	—	1	2	3

slope is estimated to be 0.555 with an estimated standard error of 0.344. The slope estimate is interpreted as an increase of 0.56 in the rate ratio for brain cancer for each category of increase in level of water chlorination (e.g., low to medium).

Estimating the effect at the high level of chlorination ($x = 3$) in relation to none, using the regression equation, we have

$$\widehat{RR}_{high} = 1 + (0.555)3 = 2.66$$

$$SE(\widehat{RR}_{high}) \doteq 3(0.344) = 1.032$$

and, for comparison with the data of Figure 16-2, a 95 percent confidence interval of

$$\exp[\ln(2.66) \pm 1.96(1.032/2.66)] = 1.25, 5.69$$

The comparison of this result with the findings in Figure 16-2 suggests that the regression analysis uses the data in a considerably more efficient way.

The simplicity and directness of the least-squares model, which leads to formula 16-7, are attractive, but the method has its drawbacks. By forcing the regression line through the reference point, this regression model effectively places an extremely large weight on the location of that point in relation to the remaining array of points. The relative position of the reference point, however, is determined in part by the sampling variability of the observations at that level of exposure. If the reference category has small frequencies, then the relation of the remaining points to one another will reflect the trend better than their relation to the arbitrarily fixed reference point. Consequently, this model can be considerably less efficient than the model that fits a linear trend to the case-control odds, the degree of inefficiency depending on the numbers of subjects in the reference category. Even without specific knowledge of the frequencies that would allow assessment of the extent of inefficiency in this model, however, the rate ratio model may be useful. It is clear that some evaluation of trend, even using a statistically inefficient model, is better than no trend evaluation, as the water chlorination and brain cancer example illustrates.

STATISTICAL HYPOTHESIS TESTING FOR TREND

Throughout this book the emphasis has been placed firmly on estimation of meaningful epidemiologic measures in preference to hypothesis testing. Many investigators who agree with the objectives of estimation nevertheless resort to testing when they face evaluation of trends. Why should trend evaluation predispose to statistical testing? Perhaps these investigators understand that information can be lost when estimating effects separately by category, and they simply turn to the most widely used methods that extend the basic epidemiologic analyses of 2 × 2 tables. The main extensions are methods described by Mantel [1963] that include regression estimation but emphasize statistical testing. Although the regression methods of the previous section accomplish the epidemiologic objectives of estimating trends in terms of epidemiologically interpretable measures, it is worthwhile to examine Mantel's methodology because it is so widely used.

The Mantel-Haenszel test statistic (formula 12-38) addresses data summarized as a set of 2 × 2 tables. Mantel [1963] extended the test to accommodate data summarized as a set of contingency tables with any number of categories of exposure or disease. The extension also enabled the study variables to be treated as continuous measures. In most epidemiologic applications, the disease variable remains dichotomous but the exposure variable is categorized into several levels. Using the notation in Table 16-3, the Mantel extension test is

$$\chi = \frac{\sum_i \left[\sum_j a_j x_j - \frac{\sum_j a_j}{\sum_j N_j} \sum_j N_j x_j \right]}{\sqrt{\sum_i \frac{\sum_j a_j \sum_j b_j}{(\sum_j N_j)^2 (\sum_j N_j - 1)} \left[\sum_j N_j \sum_j N_j x_j^2 - (\sum_j N_j x_j)^2 \right]}}$$

where x_j represents the score assigned to level j of exposure, and i represents the index for the stratification factor, for which the data layout in Table 16-3 represents one stratum. The Mantel extension test in the form given here may be thought of as a generalization over strata of a test for linear trend in proportions. While it is an asymptotic test, like the Mantel-Haenszel test it does not require large numbers in any one stratum. In fact, the test works well when each stratum is simply a matched case-control pair, provided that there are enough such pairs for the asymptotic conditions to be met.

Table 16-3. Notation for epidemiologic data with several levels of exposure

	Exposure level					
	0	1	2	...	j	...
Cases	a_0	a_1	a_2	...	a_j	...
Noncases	b_0	b_1	b_2	...	b_j	...
Total	N_0	N_1	N_2	...	N_j	...

Example 16-4. Hypothetical case-control data demonstrating a linear trend in the proportion of subjects who are cases

	Exposure level				
	0	1	2	3	Total
Cases	20	40	60	80	200
Controls	80	60	40	20	200
Total	100	100	100	100	400
Rate ratio	1.0	2.7	6.0	16.0	

A test for linear trend does not have a built-in assumption about linearity; it amounts to a test of the linear *component* of trend, whatever the actual trend may be. Thus, the test is useful for detecting any monotonic relation between exposure and disease, even if the relation is not linear. Of course, there can be striking nonmonotonic associations with a linear component that is, on balance, zero. To the extent that such complex associations are suspected a priori, they can be evaluated by an assignment of exposure scores that reflect the a priori view.

Mantel [1963] also gave formulas for regression coefficients that measure the linear trend that is being tested, but these regression coefficients cannot be interpreted readily in epidemiologic terms for case-control data. The linear trend measured is a trend in the proportion of subjects who are cases. For follow-up data representing fixed cohorts, this is a trend in the cumulative incidence, but for case-control data, this trend is not equivalent to a linear increase in rate or rate ratio. Consider the hypothetical data in Example 16-4. The increase in the proportion of subjects who are cases is perfectly linear, but the rate ratio is increasing more than exponentially with uniform increments in exposure. In contrast, Example 16-5 shows a trend in rate ratio that increases linearly with exposure, but the proportion of subjects who are cases is increasing less than linearly. Thus, the regression coefficient from Mantel's procedure should not be applied to case-control data.

Although the regression coefficient proposed by Mantel has no application for case-control data, the Mantel extension test is nevertheless a

*Example 16-5. Hypothetical case-control data
demonstrating a linear trend in the rate ratio*

	Exposure level				
	0	1	2	3	Total
Cases	20	33	43	50	146
Controls	80	67	57	50	254
Total	100	100	100	100	400
Rate ratio	1.0	2.0	3.0	4.0	

valid test of the null hypothesis of no monotone relation between exposure and disease, even for case-control data. The interpretability of the test derives from the fact that an absence of trend is equivalent, whether expressed in terms of rate ratio or proportion of subjects who are cases at each level of exposure: There is a common null hypothesis, making the test valid; indeed, it is statistically powerful over a wide range of alternatives to the null hypothesis [Tarone and Gart, 1980]. Nevertheless, the test suffers the drawback that it is only a test, yielding only a *P*-value. To obtain a meaningful epidemiologic measure of trend, a method akin to that described in the previous section of this chapter is necessary.

MULTIVARIATE ANALYSIS OF TREND

The generalized relative risk models described by Thomas [1981] offer a means to evaluate trend in rate ratio with a multivariate model. In contrast, logistic regression analysis is much more restrictive, since it presumes an exponential relation between uniform increments of exposure and disease odds. The coefficient of a continuous exposure term in a logistic regression model implicitly describes an exponential relation. Transformations of the exposure scale can accommodate other exposure-disease relations, but more flexibility is attainable, as usual, by categorizing the exposure variable and using indicator terms in the logistic model for each nonzero level of exposure.

With indicator terms, the logistic regression model provides rate ratio estimates for each level of exposure. The model also provides estimates of variance, so that the output of the logistic regression could be employed in the weighted regression analyses for trend described above. The resulting trend evaluation will be unconfounded by all the factors taken into account in the logistic model. By obtaining separate estimates of effect at several levels of exposure from the logistic model, the investigator can maintain some "feel" for the data. The separate estimates also provide a clear picture of the actual trend without the built-in dose-response assumption of the logistic model using continuous independent variables. Furthermore, categorization into a nominal scale limits the problem of outliers influencing the data excessively.

The effect estimates in Figure 16-2 were derived from a logistic regression analysis; as we have seen, a linear regression analysis of these effect estimates is readily feasible by using only a few calculations based solely on these published results, without any access to the original data. The simplicity of the regression analysis of linear trend and its adaptability to anything ranging from crude data to the results of a logistic regression analysis make it an attractive approach for the initial epidemiologic evaluation of trend. The generalized relative risk model of Thomas [1981] is an efficient and flexible multivariate alternative, but logistic regression usually is not appropriate; to evaluate a trend in effect, logistic models should be considered only a preliminary step to the use of other methods.

REFERENCES

Baron, J. A., Vessey, M., McPherson, K., et al. Maternal age and breast cancer risk. *J. Nat. Cancer Inst.* 1984;72:1307–1309.

Doll, R., and Hill, A. B. Mortality of British doctors in relation to their smoking habits. A preliminary report. *Br. Med. J.* 1954;1:1451–1455.

Draper, N. R., and Smith, H. *Applied Regression Analysis.* New York: Wiley, 1966.

Grizzle, J. E., Starmer, C. F., and Koch, G. G. Analysis of categorical data by linear models. *Biometrics* 1969;25:489–503.

Hill, A. P., Pike, M. C., Smith, P. G., et al. Stratified analysis of case-control studies with the factor under study taking multiple values. *J. Chron. Dis.* 1978;31:547–555.

Kleinbaum, D. G., and Kupper, L. L. *Applied Regression Analysis and Other Multivariable Methods.* North Scituate, MA. Duxbury Press, 1978.

MacMahon, B., Cole, P., Lin, T. M., et al. Age at first birth and breast cancer risk. *Bull. WHO* 1970;43:209–221.

Mantel, N. Chi-square tests with one degree of freedom: Extensions of the Mantel-Haenszel procedure. *J. Am. Stat. Assoc.* 1963;58:690–700.

McGregor, D. H., Land, C. E., Choi, K., et al. Breast cancer incidence among atomic bomb survivors, Hiroshima and Nagasaki, 1950–69. *J. Nat. Cancer Inst.* 1977;59:799–811.

Mickey, R. M., and Elashoff, R. M. A generalization of the Mantel-Haenszel estimator of partial association for $2 \times J \times K$ tables. *Biometrics* 1985; 41:623–635.

Miettinen, O. S. Standardization of risk ratios. *Am. J. Epidemiol.* 1972;96:383–388.

Pike, M. C., Casagrande, J., and Smith, P. G. Statistical analysis of individually matched case-control studies in epidemiology: Factor under study a discrete variable taking multiple values. *Br. J. Prev. Soc. Med.* 1975;29:196–201.

Poole, C., Lanes, S., and Rothman, K. J. Analysis of ordered data (Letter). *N. Engl. J. Med.* 1984;311:1382.

Rosenbaum, P. R., and Rubin, D. B. Difficulties with regression analyses of age-adjusted rates. *Biometrics* 1984;40:437–443.

Silvey, S. D. *Statistical Inference*. Middlesex, England: Penguin Books, 1970.

Tarone, R. E., and Gart, J. J. On the robustness of combined tests for trends in proportions. *J. Am. Stat. Assoc.* 1980;75:110–116.

Thomas, D. C. General relative risk models for survival time and matched case-control analysis. *Biometrics* 1981;37:673–676.

Young, T. B., Kanarek, M. S., and Tsiatis, A. A. Epidemiologic study of drinking water chlorination and Wisconsin female cancer mortality. *J. Nat. Cancer Inst.* 1981;67:1191–1198.

INDEX